Immune System Regulation

Lobat Tayebi • Mohsen Abdolmaleki

Immune System Regulation

Inhibitory Checkpoint Receptors

Springer

Lobat Tayebi
School of Dentistry
Institute for Engineering in Medicine,
Health and Human Performance (EnMed),
Batten College of Engineering and
Technology, Old Dominion University,
Norfolk, VA, USA

Mohsen Abdolmaleki
Department of Medical Sciences
Al.C., Islamic Azad University
Aligudarz, Iran

ISBN 978-981-95-8025-5 ISBN 978-981-95-8026-2 (eBook)
https://doi.org/10.1007/978-981-95-8026-2

This Springer imprint is published by the registered company Springer Nature Singapore Pte Ltd.
The registered company address is: 152 Beach Road, #21-01/04 Gateway East, Singapore 189721, Singapore

Acknowledgement

Authors would like to sincerely thank Maryam Sadr for her active contributions to the development of this book. Her dedication, expertise, and continued support throughout the planning and preparation stages were invaluable, and they significantly strengthened the final outcome.

Contents

Chapter 1
Immune Response Activation and Regulation

1.1 Introduction

The immune system consists of different cells and soluble factors and has evolved to protect the body against invading pathogens. The immune system is divided into two main branches including innate immunity and adaptive immunity. Macrophages, neutrophils, and dendritic cells (DCs) are among the most important innate immune cells with phagocytosis activity. Innate immune cells are located in the skin, respiratory or intestinal tracts, and other parts of the body, and as the first line of defense, they recognize and ingest pathogens. Another important function of the innate immune system is to activate the adaptive immune response. DCs are specialized antigen-presenting cells (APCs). DCs capture antigens and migrate to the lymph nodes for interaction with T cells. Adaptive immune cells, including T and B lymphocytes, are resident in lymphoid organs and are activated upon recognizing the antigens. T cells are divided into two subsets: $CD4^+$ cells and $CD8^+$ cells. $CD4^+$ T cells become activated by recognizing antigens on MHC class II and differentiate into T-helper (Th) cells. $CD4^+$ Th cells regulate the function of immune cells by secreting different cytokines. $CD8^+$ T cells bind to MHC class I and differentiate into cytotoxic T cells after activation. $CD8^+$ cytotoxic T cells destroy virus and tumor-infected cells. Unlike T cells, B cells, which represent humoral immunity, directly recognize antigens (independent of MHC). After activation, B cells differentiate into antibody-producing plasma cells. Antibodies are the key arm of the immune system to neutralize microbes [1]. While the immune system combats microbes, it should not destroy self-tissues. Precise mechanisms control the immune system to prevent damage to organs known as self-tolerance. Failure in discrimination of self from non-self leads to autoimmune diseases. The thymus is the main site of T cell development and selection. In the thymus, self-reactive T cells are eliminated. In addition, the tolerance mechanisms in peripheral tissues also control the activation of lymphocytes. Immune checkpoints are among these mechanisms.

L. Tayebi, M. Abdolmaleki, *Immune System Regulation*,
https://doi.org/10.1007/978-981-95-8026-2_1

Uncontrolled activation of T cells after clearance of infection leads to self-tissue damage. Cytotoxic T lymphocyte antigen 4 (CTLA-4) and programmed cell death 1 (PD-1) are two critical immune checkpoints for regulating the function and homeostasis of T cells. Nevertheless, in chronic infections and tumors, inhibitory receptors are widely expressed on T cells following continuous antigenic stimulation, which leads to T cell exhaustion. Exhausted T cells have reduced effector function, secrete low levels of cytokines, and are hypo-proliferative, therefore they are not competent for eliminating pathogens or tumor cells [2, 3]. In this chapter, the mechanism of activation of T cells by DCs is discussed. In the following, T cell exhaustion state and different exhausted T cell subsets based on expression of immune checkpoints and transcription factors profile are covered.

1.2 Thymic Selection of T Cells

The thymus is a specialized central lymphatic organ for the development of T lymphocytes. After the successful rearrangement and expression of T cell receptor (TCR) on their surface, T cells express CD4 and CD8 co-receptors and become double-positive T cells that are localized in the thymus cortex. Recognition of MHC molecules of cortical thymic epithelial cells (cTECs) by TCR leads to the positive selection of double-positive T cells. Those thymocytes that do not recognize self-MHC are eliminated. During negative selection, T cells with strong binding affinity to self-peptide/MHC presented by medullary thymic epithelial cells (mTECs) and DCs are removed by clonal deletion. At this stage, potential autoreactive T cells undergo apoptosis. Those that weakly interact with self-peptide/MHC are selected and finally differentiate into $CD4^+$ single-positive T cells or $CD8^+$ single-positive T cells. These self-tolerant T cells are allowed to enter the peripheral tissues. The expression of tissue-specific self-antigens in the thymus is mediated by the autoimmune regulator (AIRE) gene, and defects in this gene lead to autoimmune polyendocrine syndromes. $CD8^+$ T cells bind to MHC I molecules expressed on various cell types, while $CD4^+$ T cells interact with MHC II molecules that are restricted to APCs (DC, macrophage, and B cell) [4–7].

1.3 Dendritic Cells

DCs are among the main components of the innate immune system that play an important role in promoting the adaptive immune response. DCs are present in both central (thymus and bone marrow) and peripheral (lymph nodes and spleen) lymphatic organs. Thymic DCs are involved in the negative selection of T cells [8]. In the peripheral lymphatic organs, they mediate the initiation of the adaptive immune response. In addition, DCs are found in the epithelial surfaces of the skin and mucosa and many other organs such as lung, heart, kidney, and brain. Langerhans cells are epidermal resident DCs and are specialized cells for recognition and phagocytosis of antigens [9]. In general, DCs are divided into conventional DCs (cDCs), plasmacytoid DCs (pDCs), migratory DCs (mDCs), and the type that originates from monocytes under inflammatory conditions (mo-DCs). pDCs are involved in antiviral immunity by producing type I interferons. cDCs are the major types of DCs and highly express MHC II molecules on their surface. DCs recognize pathogenic antigens with their pattern recognition receptors, including Toll-like receptors (TLRs), Nod-like receptors (NLRs), and RIG-I-like receptors (RLRs). Unlike macrophages, lysosomes are less acidic in DCs and they contain low levels of proteases. As a result, peptide antigens are less digested and peptides with suitable lengths for loading on MHC are produced after uptaking exogenous antigens in skin and mucosal tissues by phagocytosis and endocytosis; DCs upregulate MHC II, co-stimulatory ligands CD80/CD86, and chemokine receptor CCR7. CCL19 and CCL21 are the CCR7 ligands that are secreted in lymph nodes. Therefore, DCs migrate to the draining lymph nodes and present the antigen to naïve $CD4^+$ T cells. TCR interaction with cognate peptide–MHC causes T cell activation. Exogenous antigens are presented by MHC II to $CD4^+$ T cells and endogenous antigens are presented by MHC I to $CD8^+$ T cells. Although by cross-presentation, exogenous viral or tumor antigens can also be loaded on MHC I [8, 10–13].

1.4 T Cell Subsets

$CD4^+$ T as a regulator of the activity of other immune cells plays an important role in the clearance of infections. $CD4^+$ $\alpha\beta$ T cells constitute the major population of T cells. Various subgroups of $CD4^+$ T cells have been identified including T helper 1 (Th1), Th2, Th17, and T follicular helper (Tfh) cells. Th1 cells produce IFN-γ and are involved in clearing intracellular pathogens and activating macrophages. T-bet is the main transcription factor in Th1 development. Th2 cells are characterized by producing IL-4, IL-5, and IL-13 cytokines and play a prominent role in immune responses against parasites such as helminths and hypersensitivity reactions. GATA3 is the master regulator of Th2 response. The polarization of Th17 cells is under the control of RORγt. Th17 cells participate in the immune response against extracellular bacteria and fungi by secreting IL-17 and IL-22. In addition, the Th17 cells are involved in several autoimmune diseases. Tfh cells are important in germinal center formation and antibody responses [14, 15]. $CD8^+$ T cells are an important part of the adaptive immune system, which plays a pivotal role in antivirus and tumor immune response.

$CD8^+$ T cells bind to the peptide–MHC I complex presented on APCs and target cells. Like $CD4^+$ T cells, the interaction of $CD8^+$ T cells with DCs in the lymph node leads to their activation and finally, they differentiate into cytotoxic $CD8^+$ T cells. Cytotoxic $CD8^+$ T cells by producing perforin, granzyme B, and Fas-FasL signaling pathway destroy tumor and infected cells. They also secrete a large amount of IFN-γ

and TNF-α. STAT4, T-bet, and EOMES are important transcription factors expressed in this T cell subset [16–18].

$FoxP3^+$ $CD4^+$ regulatory T cells (Tregs) are another subset of T cells that are differentiated in the thymus. Tregs are critical for the maintenance of self-tolerance and immune homeostasis in peripheral tissues and prevention of autoimmune reactions. In addition to thymus-derived Tregs, there is another group of regulatory cells that develop in peripheral tissues. These cells are known as peripherally induced Treg (pTreg) [19]. Furthermore, Tregs are also involved in tissue maintenance and repair, fetal–maternal tolerance, and transplantation tolerance. Tregs can enhance the regeneration of injured muscle, lung, and brain tissues. Regulation of metabolic organ function and induction of epithelial barrier and hair follicle growth are other effects of Tregs [20, 21]. Tregs can suppress the T cell response by different mechanisms. Along with the FoxP3 transcription factor, the high level expression of CTLA-4 and CD25 (α chain of the IL-2 receptor) and the production of IL-10 and TGF-β are the main characteristics of Tregs. Activation of T cells is dependent on IL-2 and Treg deprives IL-2 through the expression of CD25. CTLA-4 also can suppress the function of T cells. Antigen-specific Tregs can remove peptide–MHC complexes from the surface of DCs and inhibit the activation of conventional $CD4^+$ T cells. Tregs, by producing the inhibitory cytokine IL-10, reduce the expression of co-stimulatory ligands on DCs and dampen the production of inflammatory cytokines. In addition, Tregs convert extracellular ATP into adenosine in the bone marrow through the CD73/CD39 axis. Adenosine has anti-inflammatory property and quiescent the hematopoietic stem cell (HSC) niche [21, 22].

1.5 T Cell Signaling

T cell requires two signals for full activation: the first signal is provided by TCR/pMHC interaction and the co-stimulatory signal is induced by the CD28 receptor. CD80/CD86 expressed on APCs act as ligands for CD28 and are upregulated upon activation of APCs. The majority of T cells express TCRαβ (αβ T cells), while the minor population expresses TCRγδ (γδ T cells). The TCR–CD3 complex consists of TCR heterodimer and CD3 dimers (εɣ, εδ, ζζ) (Fig. 1.1) [23, 24]. In addition, CD4 and CD8 act as co-receptors. CD4 is a monomeric protein that can bind to the β2 domain of the MHC II molecule. CD8 in the form of a heterodimer composed of α and β chains (the most common isoform expressed on αβ T cells) binds to the α3 domain of MHC I [25]. The TCR lacks intracellular signaling motifs; instead, CD3 chains contain immunoreceptor tyrosine-based activation motifs (ITAMs) that participate in the initiation of the signaling cascade (Fig. 1.2) [26].

Several protein tyrosine kinases (PTKs) such as Lck, Fyn, and ZAP-70 are involved in the activation of TCR signaling. After TCR ligation, ITAMs of CD3 are phosphorylated by src protein tyrosine kinases (mostly by Lck and to some degree by Fyn), and ZAP-70 is recruited. Lck can be membrane-anchored or attached to the

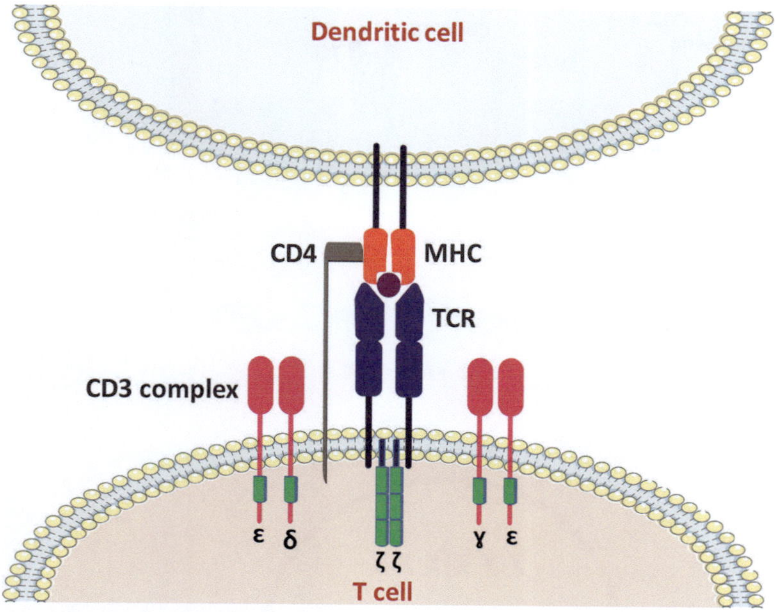

Fig. 1.1 T cell receptor complex structure. Created using elements from Servier Medical Art (https://smart.servier.com), licensed under CC BY 4.0 (https://creativecommons.org/licenses/by/4.0/)

cytoplasmic tail of CD4 and CD8. Lck also phosphorylates ZAP-70. ZAP-70 in turn phosphorylates and activates adapter proteins LAT and SLP-76. LAT is an important transmembrane protein for TCR signal transduction. Phospholipase Cγ1 (PLCγ1), p85 subunit of phosphoinositide 3-kinase (PI3K), the adapters growth factor receptor-bound protein 2 (GRB2), and GRB2-related adapter downstream of Shc (Gads) bind to phosphorylated LAT. SLP-76 is also an important cytoplasmic adapter protein in T cells. SLP-76 can bind to IL-2 inducible T cell kinase (Itk) as well as PLCγ1 and Gads. These associations lead to the formation of LAT–GADS–SLP76–PLCγ1 complex [27–30]. SLP-76 binds to Vav1, Nck, and Itk by its N-terminal domain. In addition, it can interact with Gads and PLCγ1 by its PRR and with ADAP and HPK1 through its C-terminal SH2 region. PLCγ1 can directly bind to SLP-76, LAT, Vav1, and Itk. Itk phosphorylates PLCγ1. Activated PLCγ1 hydrolyzes membrane-bound phosphatidylinositol-4,5-bisphosphate (PIP2) to inositol-3-phosphate (IP3) and diacylglycerol (DAG). Rlk is another kinase that can phosphorylate PLCγ1. DAG activates Ras and PKCθ pathways. Ras belongs to the family of guanine nucleotide-binding proteins and is active only when it is bound to GTP. The activation and deactivation of Ras is regulated by Guanine nucleotide exchange factors (GEFs) and GTPase activating proteins (GAPs), respectively. Two GEFs including Ras guanyl nucleotide-releasing protein (RasGRP) and son of sevenless (SOS) are present in T cells. PKCθ is responsible for phosphorylating RasGRP. Raf-1 is activated by Ras, which leads to the activation of Erk. Erk

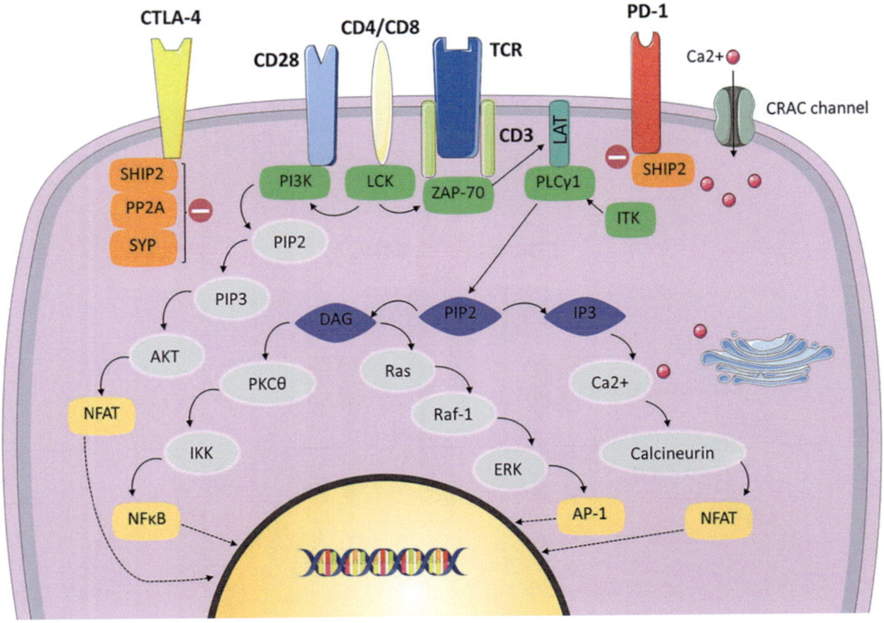

Fig. 1.2 T cell activation and related signaling molecules. *TCR*: T cell receptor, *LAT*: linker of activated T cells, *PLCγ1*: phospholipase C gamma 1, *ITK*: interleukin-2-inducible T cell kinase, *LCK:* lymphocyte-specific protein tyrosine kinase, *PI3K*: phosphoinositide 3-kinase, *PIP2*: phosphatidylinositol-4,5-bisphosphate, *PIP3*: phosphatidylinositol- [3, 4, 5]-trisphosphate, *IP3*: inositol-1,4,5-trisphosphate, *DAG:* diacylglycerol, *CRAC:* Ca^{2+} release-activated Ca^{2+}, *PKCθ*: protein kinase C-*theta*, *IKK*: inhibitor of κB (IκB) kinase, *ERK*: extracellular signal-regulated kinase, *NFAT*: nuclear factor of activated T cells. (The figure is adapted from Ref. (37), created using elements from Servier Medical Art (https://smart.servier.com), licensed under CC BY 4.0 (https://creativecommons.org/licenses/by/4.0/))

activates the transcription of Elk1 and STAT3. Ras also activates AP-1 (c-Jun/c-Fos) [31–33].

Another important pathway activated by DAG is PKCθ. PKCθ causes NFκB activation. Activated NFκB enters the nucleus. A trimolecular complex consisting of CARMA1 (caspase recruitment domain and membrane-associated guanylate kinase-containing scaffold protein), Bcl10, and MALT1 (mucosa-associated lymphoid tissue lymphoma translocation gene 1) is needed for the activation of NFκB. PKCθ mediates the formation of this complex through the phosphorylation of CARMA1. MALT1 breaks down the regulatory domain of IκB kinase (IKK) complex (gamma subunit). Subsequently, IKK catalytic subunits can phosphorylate IκB. After IκB is phosphorylated and degraded, NFκB is released, localizes in the nucleus, and activates gene transcription [29, 32].

Another part of TCR signaling is dependent on IP3 derived from PIP2. The binding of IP3 to IP3R (Ca^{2+}-permeable ion channel receptors) on the endoplasmic reticulum (ER) leads to the release of Ca^{2+} from the ER into the cytoplasm. The discharge of Ca^{2+} stored in the ER leads to the influx of extracellular Ca^{2+} into the cell through membrane CRAC (Ca^{2+} release activated Ca^{2+}) channels. As a second messenger, Ca^{2+} activates transcription factors MEF2, DREAM (downstream regulatory element antagonist modulator), and signaling proteins phosphatase calcineurin and CaMK (Ca^{2+}-calmodulin-dependent kinase). Calcineurin by dephosphorylating NFATs (nuclear factor of activated T cells) facilitates their entry into the nucleus. NFATs form transcriptional complexes with different transcription factors and regulate gene transcription. NFAT/AP-1 is one of the most important complexes that activate the IL-2 gene expression [32–34].

CD28-CD80/CD86 axis co-stimulatory signal is essential for T cell activation together with TCR. In the absence of CD28 signaling, T cells become anergic. CD28 is involved in the survival, proliferation, and metabolism of T cells. CD28 plays an important role in IL-2 gene expression through the activation of NFAT, AP-1, and NFκB. ligation of CD28 to CD80/CD86 on APCs results in the binding of the p85 subunit of PI3K to the phosphorylated YMNM motif of the CD28. Recruiting catalytic subunit of PI3K (p110) by p85 leads to phosphatidylinositol-[3, 4, 5]-trisphosphate (PIP3) production from PIP2. Membrane-localized PIP3 provides a docking site for PDK1 and Akt. Akt inactivates GSK-3 (glycogen-synthase kinase 3). GSK-3 restricts NFAT entry into the nucleus. Therefore, the inactivation of GSK-3 leads to NFAT localization in the nucleus. In addition, Akt increases the expression of the antiapoptotic protein Bcl-xl, which sustains cell survival. In addition, GRB2 and Gads can bind to the YMNM and PYAP motifs of CD28, which ultimately leads to the formation of the AP-1 complex. Upregulation of Glut1 (insulin transporter) and increase of glucose uptake are other effects of CD28 signaling. In addition to these activator proteins, some inhibitors inside T cells regulate TCR signaling. SHP1, Dok, HPK1, Sts family, and Cbla are proteins involved in reducing TCR-dependent signaling [32, 35, 36].

1.6 CTLA-4 Structure and Function

CTLA-4 is a CD28 homologous receptor expressed on T cells. In conventional T cells and Tregs, CTLA-4 is mainly localized in intracellular vesicles due to constitutive endocytosis. Internalized CTLA-4 can be recycled to the surface of plasma membrane or degraded by lysosome [38]. CTLA-4 by binding to its ligands (CD80 and CD86) on DC removes them from the plasma membrane through trans-endocytosis and therefore dampens the CD28-associated T cell activation [39]. CTLA-4 gene is located on chromosome 2 (Ch2q33) in humans and on chromosome 1 (Ch1C1) in mice. This gene contains four exons and three introns, which produces CTLA-4 protein with 223 amino acids. Exon 1 encodes the signal peptide, exon 2 the extracellular domain, exon 3 the transmembrane domain, and exon 4 the cytoplasmic tail. CTLA-4 is a member of the immunoglobulin (Ig) superfamily and has an Ig-V (variable)-like domain in its structure [40, 41]. CTLA-4 is found on activated T cells in the form of a homodimer. The conserved MYPPPY motif in the extracellular part of the CTLA-4 protein, which is shared with CD28, is responsible for binding to CD80 and CD86. CTLA-4 strongly binds to CD80/CD86. Therefore, it has an antagonistic effect on the CD28 signal. In addition to full-length CTLA-4, other isoforms are produced by alternative splicing. Resting lymphocytes produce soluble isoform CTLA-4 (sCTLA-4). sCTLA-4 lacks exon 3, which encodes the transmembrane domain. sCTLA-4 is able to bind to CD80 and CD86 and blocks the CD28-mediated T cell activation. Ligand-independent (liCTLA-4) is an isoform that is produced in mouse T cells and lacks the extracellular domain. liCTLA-4 also can exert an inhibitory effect. In addition, the super-short form of CTLA-4, consisting of the cytoplasmic tail, which is produced by exon 1, has been identified [41, 42]. Uncontrolled immune response during infections can lead to the expansion of autoreactive T cells. The expression of CTLA-4 on activated T cells is one of the main mechanisms of immune response regulation. Phosphorylation of CTLA-4 (by Fyn and Lck) causes the activation of SHIP2. As a result, CD3 and LAT are dephosphorylated and T cell activation signals are inhibited. CTLA-4 is also involved in the regulation of immune response through Treg cells. Tregs continuously express CTLA-4. The binding of CTLA-4 on Tregs with CD80/CD86 on DCs decreases the expression of these ligands on DCs. This interaction also promotes indoleamine-2,3-dioxygenase (IDO) expression in DCs. IDO suppresses T cell activation. CTLA-4 also increases the expression of FoxP3 in Treg. p52SHC is an adapter molecule that binds to CD3 following TCR signaling and is phosphorylated by Lck. Phosphorylated p52SHC participates in the formation of the p52SHC/GRB2/SOS/Ras complex, which enhances the Ras signaling. By binding the tyrosine phosphatase synaptophysin (SYP) to the cytoplasmic tail of CTLA-4, SYP is able to dephosphorylate p52SHC and disrupt the formation of the p52SHC/GRB2/SOS/Ras complex. In addition, CTLA-4 induces the dephosphorylation of CD3, PI3K, and AKT by recruiting SHIP2 and serine–threonine phosphatase PP2A. As a result, T cell activation is inhibited [43, 44].

1.7 PD-1 Structure and Function

PD-1 is one of the most important immune checkpoints that suppresses the T cell activation. PD-1 is a 288 amino acids long protein, which is expressed in a low amount on naïve T cells, but is overexpressed on activated T and B lymphocytes. PD-1 contains an IgV domain in the extracellular part, followed by a transmembrane domain and a cytoplasmic tail [45, 46]. PD-1 ligands (PD-L1 and PD-L2) are type 1 transmembrane glycoproteins and have IgC and IgV domains in their structures. PD-L1 is a protein of the B7 receptor family with a length of 290 amino acids, which is expressed on various immune and nonimmune cells, including lymphocytes and APCs, and its expression increases after stimulation. PD-L2 expression is more limited and is mainly found on DCs, macrophages, and B cells [47–49]. The binding of PD-1 to its ligands PD-L1 and PD-L2 leads to the phosphorylation of tyrosine residues of immunoreceptor tyrosine-based inhibitory motif (*ITIM*) and immunoreceptor tyrosine-based switch motif (*ITSM*) of the cytoplasmic tail of PD-1, then SHP-1 and SHP-2 are recruited. Binding of SHP-2 to phosphorylated ITSM tyrosine causes PD-1 dimerization [48, 50]. PD-1 signaling reduces the phosphorylation of CD3, ZAP70, and PKCθ. In addition, PD-1 can stop the cell cycle. p27kip1 is a member of Cdk inhibitors that hinder the Cdk2 function. PD-1 engagement increases p27kip1 levels and suppresses cell entry into the S phase [46].

1.8 T Cell Exhaustion

Studies of the T cells function in lymphocytic choriomeningitis virus (LCMV) infection of mice revealed that virus-specific $CD8^+$ T cells have decreased effector functions and cytokine production, and they are unable to eliminate the virus. In chronic infections, $CD4^+$ T cells also have a reduced response. This phenomenon, during which lymphocytes become nonfunctional due to persistent antigen, is called T cell exhaustion [51–53]. During acute viral infection, activated $CD8^+$ T cells destroy virus-infected cells. These cells strengthen the immune response by producing IL-2, TNF-α, and IFN-γ and inhibit virus replication. However, in long-term antigenic stimulation during chronic infection, the function of pathogen-specific $CD8^+$ T cells is progressively lost. Exhausted $CD8^+$ T cells have impaired cytolytic activity and their cytokine production and proliferation capacity are diminished. Exhausted $CD8^+$ T cells are unable to inhibit tumor growth or eliminate virus-infected cells. The hallmark of T cell exhaustion is the continuous expression of multiple inhibitory receptors. As noted above, CTLA-4 and PD-1 are important immune checkpoints in regulating the activation of T cells. CTLA-4 and PD-1 are widely expressed on exhausted T cells. In addition, several other inhibitory molecules, including TIGIT, LAG-3, TIM-3, are overexpressed on exhausted T cells (Chap. 2). Along with the increase in the expression of immune checkpoints, exhausted T cells show distinct transcriptional and epigenetic profiles (Chap. 3) [54, 55]. During acute infection, $CD8^+$ T cells undergo clonal expansion and differentiate into effector $CD8^+$ T cells to eliminate the pathogen. After the infection clearance, most of these cells die, but memory T cells can survive for a long time independently of the antigen and protect the body upon reexposure to the same pathogen. T cell exhaustion has been reported in many chronic infections such as hepatitis B virus (HBV), hepatitis C virus (HCV), human immunodeficiency virus (HIV), and many cancers. Tumor-specific $CD4^+$ T cells are also affected by exhaustion. These cells express various inhibitory molecules on their surface and have weakened effector functions. Overall, the characteristics of exhausted T cells include progressive functional and proliferative impairment, sustained upregulation of inhibitory receptors, skewed metabolism, epigenetic pattern, and transcription factors distinct from effector and memory T cells [56].

IL-2 is the first cytokine that is affected in exhausted $CD8^+$ T cells. As exhaustion progresses, TNF production reduces. At this stage, the cytotoxicity of T cells is suppressed. In more severe T cell exhaustion, the production of IFN-γ is impaired.

Terminally exhausted T cells may be physically removed. However, it should be noted that the pattern of changes in exhausted T cells may be different according to the type of disease and inflammatory environment. In infections, the type of pathogen, the severity of disease, and the microbial load are important factors [57].

Lymphocytes exhibit different metabolic profiles according to their activation state and the surrounding microenvironment. Naive T cells rely on oxidative phosphorylation for energy supply. The metabolism of activated effector T cells in acute infection switches from mitochondrial oxidative phosphorylation to glycolysis based on their bioenergetic demands for proliferation and effector functions. This metabolic shift is dependent on PI3K and mTOR pathways and CD28 positively regulates glycolysis. In the memory cells, in parallel with the clearance of the infection, the cellular metabolism returns to the oxidative phosphorylation state. CTLA-4 and PD-1 signaling change the metabolism of exhausted T cells by inhibiting the effect of CD28. Metabolic dysregulation in T cell exhaustion is associated with decreased cellular respiration and glucose uptake. In addition, in the tumor microenvironment, the consumption of glucose, fatty acids, and oxygen by tumor cells is involved in the development of exhaustion [57–59].

1.8.1 Effect of Cytokines and Other Factors

Soluble mediators secreted in inflammatory environments are important modulators of T cell exhaustion. The characteristics of tumor microenvironment (TME) affect the function of tumor-infiltrating T cells. Tregs are frequent in tumors and secrete large amounts of IL-10, IL-35, and TGF-β. IL-10 and IL-35 are anti-inflammatory cytokines and are involved in reducing T cell activation. $CD4^+$ T cells and APCs are the important sources of IL-10 production. In addition, the levels of these cytokines increase in chronic infections such as LCMV and HIV. IL-10 and IL-35 can increase the expression of immune checkpoints on tumor-specific T cells. TGF-β is a negative regulator of immune cell functions that increases in cancer and chronic infections and is associated with T cell exhaustion. IL-27 can also induce the expression of immune checkpoints such as TIM-3, TIGIT, LAG-3, and PD-L1 in T cells [54, 57, 59]. Type I interferons (IFN-α/β) inhibit virus replication. However, they also exert other effects in chronic inflammation conditions. They can induce the expression of PD-L1, IL-10, and IDO. Upregulation of PD-L1 in the TME by tumor cells, myeloid-derived suppressor cells (MDSCs), and immature DCs also escalates exhaustion. Extracellular ATP can be converted to adenosine by the CD73/CD39 axis. Adenosine suppresses the function of T cells by binding to adenosine A2A receptor (A2AR). Overexpression of CD39 and CD73 has been observed in the TME, including exhausted T cells. Prostaglandin E2 (PGE2) is another mediator produced during inflammation. Besides the proinflammatory effects, PGE2 can also inhibit the activity of effector T cells. Inhibition of PGE2 can enhance the effects of PD-1 blockers [57, 59]. Consumption of glucose by tumor cells and deprivation of tryptophan and arginine by IDO and arginase, which are secreted by DCs, MDSCs, and tumor-associated macrophages (TAMs), lead to suppression of the proliferation and function of lymphocytes [59].

1.8.2 *Transcriptional Regulation of T Cell Exhaustion*

Long survival and homeostatic self-renewing of memory T cells are dependent on IL-7 and IL-15 cytokines. However, in chronic infection, exhausted T cells are not able to properly respond to IL-7 and IL-15. Their survival depends on persisting antigen signals. A subset of exhausted T cells acts as a progenitor pool. They can proliferate and form a larger population of terminally exhausted T cells [57]. Naïve $CD8^+$ T cells express IL-7Rα on their surface but are negative for KLRG1 ($KLRG1^-$ IL-$7R\alpha^+$). Stimulation by APCs induces KLRG1 expression and decreases IL-7Rα on activated T cells. Terminally differentiated effector T $CD8^+$ cells have $KLRG1^{hi}$ IL-$7R\alpha^{lo}$ phenotype and are strong cytotoxic cells. These cells have a short lifespan and undergo activation-induced cell death (AICD) after clearance of the pathogen. Nevertheless, a subset of the effector $CD8^+$ T cells act as the precursors of long-lived memory $CD8^+$ T cells, which are characterized by downregulation of KLRG1 [60].

According to the findings of various studies, T cell exhaustion is a multistage process and exhausted T cells consist of a heterogeneous population that can be divided into different groups based on the expression of inhibitory receptors, especially PD-1, and their transcription factors [61].

T-bet and EOMES are two important transcription factors expressed in short-lived effector $CD8^+$ T cells (T-bet^{++} $EOMES^+$). Memory $CD8^+$ T cells are also positive for these two factors, but they express higher levels of EOMES (T-bet^+ $EOMES^{++}$). In chronic infection, the expression of T-bet in exhausted $CD8^+$ T cells is decreased while EOMES is upregulated (T-bet^+ $EOMES^{+++}$). Furthermore, PD-1 is increased on these cells, which indicates the relationship between EOMES and the expression of exhaustion markers [60].

The expression pattern of CXCR5 in $PD1^+$ $CD8^+$ T cells is helpful for the classification of exhausted T cells. CXCR5 is the receptor of CXCL13 chemokine, which is involved in the homing of B cells in lymphoid follicles. In addition, Tfh cells with CXCR5 expression reside in B cell follicles and are involved in promoting humoral immune response. Furthermore, some $CD8^+$ T cells also express CXCR5. The expression of inhibitory receptors and the intensity of exhaustion are lower in $CXCR5^+$ $CD8^+$ T cells. In chronic infection, the population of $PD1^+$ $CXCR5^+$ $CD8^+$ T cells is considered as the progenitor of fully exhausted $CD8^+$ cells. The differentiation to $PD1^+$ $CXCR5^+$ $CD8^+$ T cells is dependent on the expression of T cell factor 1 (TCF1) transcription factor. Deletion of TCF1 is associated with the absence of $PD1^+$ $CXCR5^+$ population [60].

In line with this, $KLRG1^+$ $PD1^-$ are negative for TCF1 but express T-bet, which is consistent with an effector-like phenotype. However, $KLRG1^-$ $PD1^+$ cells, which have reduced proliferation and are exhausted, express TCF1 and EOMES. These findings indicate the role of TCF1 in the process of T cell exhaustion [60].

It has been demonstrated that the population of PD-1$^+$ TCF1$^+$ TIM-3$^-$ CD8$^+$ T cells that are proliferative differentiate into PD-1$^+$ TCF1$^-$ TIM-3$^+$ CD8$^+$ T cells, which are terminally exhausted without proliferation ability. This progenitor population intermediately expresses PD-1, shows long survival and self-renewal properties, and is the source of more terminally exhausted T cells with high PD-1 expression [54, 58].

Exhausted T cells can be classified into four subsets based on the expression of Ly108 and CD69 (Fig. 1.3). Progenitor 1 exhausted T cells express Ly108 and CD69 (Ly108$^+$ CD69$^+$) and are a self-renewing population residing in secondary lymphoid organs. TCF1 and IL-7Rα are also expressed in these cells. Progenitor 2 exhausted T cells subset (Ly108$^+$ CD69$^-$) is highly proliferative and is found in lymphoid tissues and blood. Intermediate exhausted T cells are another subset that do not express Ly108 and CD69 (Ly108$^-$ CD69$^-$). Production of perforin and granzyme indicates that they have effector function. T-bet is highly expressed in these cells and they are present in blood. Progenitor 2 and intermediate exhausted cells severely expand in response to PD-1 pathway blockade. Terminal exhausted T cell (Ly108$^-$ CD69$^+$ Eomes^{hi}) express different inhibitory receptors such as PD-1, LAG-3, TIGIT, and CD244. They have minimal proliferative activity and effector function [61, 62].

Another study group has classified exhausted T cells based on the expression of CD101 and TIM-3. Accordingly, lymphoid organs resident stem cell-like CD8$^+$ T cells (TCF1$^+$CXCR5$^+$) produce CD101$^-$ TIM-3$^+$ subset. In the next step, this transitory population differentiates into CD101$^+$ TIM-3$^+$ CD8 T cells [63, 64].

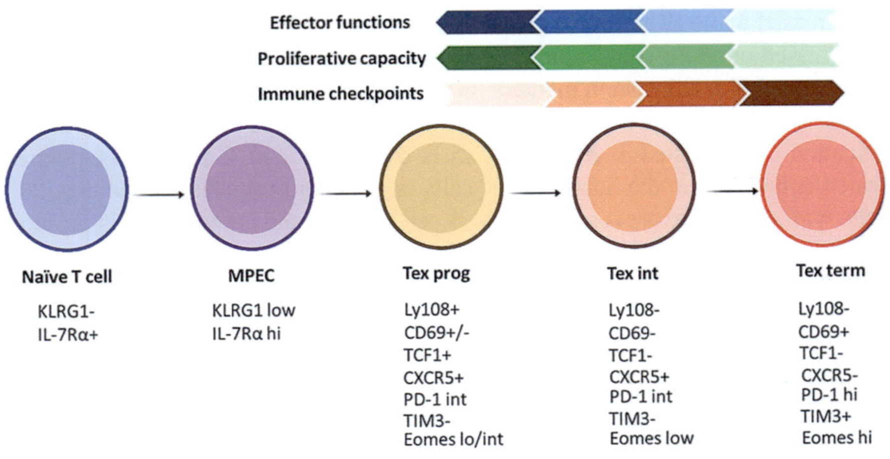

Fig. 1.3 Different subsets of exhausted T cells. *MPEC*: memory precursor effector cell, *Tex prog*: progenitor exhausted T cells, *Tex int*: intermediate exhausted T cells, *Tex term*: terminally exhausted T cells. Created using elements from NIAID NIH BioArt Source (bioart.niaid.nih.gov)

In summary, progenitor exhausted T cells express TCF1, Ly108, CXCR5, and low level of PD-1, without expression of TIM-3. They exhibit stem cell-like properties and have proliferation and self-renewing capacity and can produce more exhausted T cells.

1.8.3 CAR-T Cell Exhaustion

Chimeric antigen receptor T cell (CAR-T cell) therapy is one of the novel and effective methods in cancer treatment. CARs consist of an extracellular single-chain variable fragment (scFv) for binding to antigen, a hinge region, a transmembrane domain, and an intracellular signaling domain. CAR-T cells can recognize antigens directly and independently of MHC molecules [65, 66]. The efficacy of CAR-T cell therapy has been established in the treatment of hematological malignancies such as chronic lymphocytic leukemia (CLL), acute lymphoblastic leukemia (ALL), and diffuse large B-cell lymphoma (DLBCL). However, CAR-T cell therapy in solid tumors has not been very successful. One of the reasons for the low efficacy of CAR-T cell therapy is the exhaustion of CAR-T cells. Exhausted CAR-T cells have been reported in various cancers. In addition, CAR-T cells may be affected by exhaustion during in vitro expansion before injection. For example, adding IL-2 during CAR-T cell expansion can induce CAR-T cell exhaustion [67, 68]. Various strategies have been proposed to reverse CAR-T cell exhaustion. In chronic infections and cancers, the inhibitory receptors are upregulated on T cells. Overexpression of immune checkpoints such as PD-1, CTLA-4, and LAG-3 is also one of the main characteristics of exhausted CAR-T cells. Using PD-1 and CTLA-4 blockers or the development of engineered CAR-T cells lacking PD-1 can improve the function of CAR-T cells. Tumor cells express high levels of PD-L1 and the PD-1/PD-L1 axis is an important mechanism of tumor escape from the immune system. Manipulation of TME is also one of the potential approaches to enhance the function of CAR-T cells. Blockade of adenosine–A2AR interaction and inhibition of TGF-β signaling by biomolecules or generation of engineered CAR-T cells lacking TGF-β receptor or defective in TGF-β signaling can be effective in improving CAR-T cell exhaustion. Designing CAR-T cells with intracellular domains of co-stimulatory molecules such as 4-1BB and targeting transcription factors involved in CAR-T cell exhaustion such as NR4A and TOX are other potential strategies for reinvigoration of exhausted CAR-T cells [68–70].

1.9 Conclusion

The immune system's complicated balance between activation and regulation is important for maintaining health and combating pathogens. This chapter has explored the fundamental mechanisms of immune response activation, with a focus on T cell biology and the phenomenon of T cell exhaustion. T cells play a key role in adaptive immunity, with their activation carefully orchestrated through interactions with antigen-presenting cells, particularly dendritic cells. The complex signaling cascades initiated by T cell receptor engagement and co-stimulatory molecules lead to T cell proliferation, differentiation, and effector functions. However, the immune system has evolved regulatory mechanisms, such as immune checkpoints such as CTLA-4 and PD-1, to prevent excessive or prolonged immune responses that could lead to autoimmunity or tissue damage. In chronic infections and cancer, persistent antigen exposure can lead to T cell exhaustion, a state characterized by diminished effector functions, altered metabolism, and upregulation of multiple inhibitory receptors. This exhaustion process is now recognized as a major barrier to effective immune responses against tumors and chronic pathogens. Understanding the molecular mechanisms underlying T cell exhaustion, including the roles of transcription factors such as TCF1 and EOMES, has opened new avenues for therapeutic interventions. The development of strategies to reinvigorate exhausted T cells, such as checkpoint inhibitor therapies and engineered CAR-T cells, represents a significant advancement in immunotherapy. However, challenges remain in fully understanding the heterogeneity of exhausted T cell populations and in developing approaches to overcome exhaustion in diverse clinical contexts. As research in this field progresses, it is becoming increasingly clear that a good understanding of T cell biology, from activation to exhaustion, is essential for developing more effective immunotherapies. Future directions in this field may include refining our ability to manipulate T cell states, developing combination therapies that target multiple aspects of T cell function, and personalizing treatments based on individual patient immune profiles.

Acknowledgments The authors gratefully acknowledge the valuable assistance provided by Maryam Sadr.

References

1. Marshall JS, Warrington R, Watson W, Kim HL. An introduction to immunology and immunopathology. Allergy Asthma Clin Immunol. 2018;14(Suppl 2):49.
2. Chaplin DD. Overview of the immune response. J Allergy Clin Immunol. 2010;125(2 Suppl 2):S3–23.
3. Viganò S, Perreau M, Pantaleo G, Harari A. Positive and negative regulation of cellular immune responses in physiologic conditions and diseases. Clin Dev Immunol. 2012;2012:485781.
4. Hebbandi Nanjundappa R, Umeshappa C, Geuking M. The impact of the gut microbiota on T cell ontogeny in the thymus. Cell Mol Life Sci. 2022;79
5. Klein L, Kyewski B, Allen PM, Hogquist KA. Positive and negative selection of the T cell repertoire: what thymocytes see (and don't see). Nat Rev Immunol. 2014;14(6):377–91.
6. Bonilla FA, Oettgen HC. Adaptive immunity. J Allergy Clin Immunol. 2010;125(2 Suppl 2):S33–40.
7. Xing Y, Hogquist KA. T-cell tolerance: central and peripheral. Cold Spring Harb Perspect Biol. 2012;4(6)

8. Oh J, Shin JS. The role of dendritic cells in central tolerance. Immune Netw. 2015;15(3):111–20.
9. Chen K, Wang JM, Yuan R, Yi X, Li L, Gong W, et al. Tissue-resident dendritic cells and diseases involving dendritic cell malfunction. Int Immunopharmacol. 2016;34:1–15.
10. Merad M, Sathe P, Helft J, Miller J, Mortha A. The dendritic cell lineage: ontogeny and function of dendritic cells and their subsets in the steady state and the inflamed setting. Annu Rev Immunol. 2013;31:563–604.
11. Liu K. Dendritic cells: Encyclopedia of cell biology 2016:741–749. https://doi.org/10.1016/B978-0-12-394447-4.30111-0. Epub 2015 Aug 20.
12. Liu J, Zhang X, Cheng Y, Cao X. Dendritic cell migration in inflammation and immunity. Cell Mol Immunol. 2021;18(11):2461–71.
13. Cabeza-Cabrerizo M, Cardoso A, Minutti CM, Pereira da Costa M, Reis e Sousa C. Dendritic cells revisited. Ann Rev Immunol. 2021;39:131–66.
14. Zhu X, Zhu J. CD4 T helper cell subsets and related human immunological disorders. Int J Mol Sci. 2020;21(21)
15. Sun L, Su Y, Jiao A, Wang X, Zhang B. T cells in health and disease. Signal Transduct Target Ther. 2023;8(1):235.
16. Raskov H, Orhan A, Christensen JP, Gögenur I. Cytotoxic CD8(+) T cells in cancer and cancer immunotherapy. Br J Cancer. 2021;124(2):359–67.
17. Sigal LJ. Activation of CD8 T lymphocytes during viral infections: encyclopedia of Immunobiology. 2016:286–90. https://doi.org/10.1016/B978-0-12-374279-7.14009-3. Epub 2016 May 9
18. Koh CH, Lee S, Kwak M, Kim BS, Chung Y. CD8 T-cell subsets: heterogeneity, functions, and therapeutic potential. Exp Mol Med. 2023;55(11):2287–99.
19. Savage PA, Klawon DEJ, Miller CH. Regulatory T cell development. Annu Rev Immunol. 2020;38:421–53.
20. Okeke EB, Uzonna JE. The pivotal role of regulatory T cells in the regulation of innate immune cells. Front Immunol. 2019;10:680.
21. Dikiy S, Rudensky AY. Principles of regulatory T cell function. Immunity 2023;56(2):240–255.
22. Grover P, Goel PN, Greene MI. Regulatory T cells: regulation of identity and function. Front Immunol. 2021;12:750542.
23. Wang H, Kadlecek TA, Au-Yeung BB, Goodfellow HE, Hsu LY, Freedman TS, et al. ZAP-70: an essential kinase in T-cell signaling. Cold Spring Harb Perspect Biol. 2010;2(5):a002279.
24. Morath A, Schamel WW. αβ and γδ T cell receptors: similar but different. J Leukoc Biol. 2020;107(6):1045–55.
25. Li Y, Mariuzza R. Structural and biophysical insights into the role of CD4 and CD8 in T cell activation. Front Immunol. 2013;4
26. Mariuzza RA, Agnihotri P, Orban J. The structural basis of T-cell receptor (TCR) activation: an enduring enigma. J Biol Chem. 2020;295(4):914–25.
27. Shah K, Al-Haidari A, Sun J, Kazi JU. T cell receptor (TCR) signaling in health and disease. Signal Transduct Target Ther. 2021;6(1):412.
28. Courtney AH, Lo WL, Weiss A. TCR signaling: mechanisms of initiation and propagation. Trends Biochem Sci. 2018;43(2):108–23.
29. Liu Y, Chen S, Liu S, Wallace KL, Zille M, Zhang J, et al. T-cell receptor signaling modulated by the co-receptors: potential targets for stroke treatment. Pharmacol Res. 2023;192:106797.
30. Kane LP, Lin J, Weiss A. Signal transduction by the TCR for antigen. Curr Opin Immunol. 2000;12(3):242–9.
31. Hwang J-R, Byeon Y, Kim D, Park S-G. Recent insights of T cell receptor-mediated signaling pathways for T cell activation and development. Exp Mol Med. 2020;52(5):750–61.
32. Smith-Garvin JE, Koretzky GA, Jordan MS. T cell activation. Annu Rev Immunol. 2009;27:591–619.
33. Huse M. The T-cell-receptor signaling network. J Cell Sci. 2009;122(9):1269–73.
34. Huang Y, Wange RL. T cell receptor signaling: beyond complex complexes. J Biol Chem. 2004;279(28):28827–30.

35. Esensten JH, Helou YA, Chopra G, Weiss A, Bluestone JA. CD28 costimulation: from mechanism to therapy. Immunity. 2016;44(5):973–88.
36. Boomer JS, Green JM. An enigmatic tail of CD28 signaling. Cold Spring Harb Perspect Biol. 2010;2(8):a002436.
37. Servier Medical Art., https://smart.servier.com. Licensed under Creative Commons Attribution 4.0 (https://creativecommons.org/licenses/by/4.0/).
38. Rowshanravan B, Halliday N, Sansom DM. CTLA-4: a moving target in immunotherapy. Blood. 2018;131(1):58–67.
39. Qureshi OS, Zheng Y, Nakamura K, Attridge K, Manzotti C, Schmidt EM, et al. Trans-endocytosis of CD80 and CD86: a molecular basis for the cell-extrinsic function of CTLA-4. Science (New York, NY). 2011;332(6029):600–3.
40. Picardo SL, Doi J, Hansen AR. Structure and optimization of checkpoint inhibitors. Cancer. 2019;12(1)
41. Chikuma S. CTLA-4, an essential immune-checkpoint for T-cell activation. Curr Top Microbiol Immunol. 2017;410:99–126.
42. Kennedy PT, Saulters EL, Duckworth AD, Lim YJ, Woolley JF, Slupsky JR, et al. Soluble CTLA-4 attenuates T cell activation and modulates anti-tumor immunity. Mol Ther. 2024;32(2):457–68.
43. Hossen MM, Ma Y, Yin Z, Xia Y, Du J, Huang JY, et al. Current understanding of CTLA-4: from mechanism to autoimmune diseases. Front Immunol. 2023;14:1198365.
44. Lingel H, Brunner-Weinzierl MC. CTLA-4 (CD152): a versatile receptor for immune-based therapy. Semin Immunol. 2019;42:101298.
45. Patsoukis N, Wang Q, Strauss L, Boussiotis VA. Revisiting the PD-1 pathway. Sci Adv. 2020;6(38)
46. Ghosh C, Luong G, Sun Y. A snapshot of the PD-1/PD-L1 pathway. J Cancer. 2021;12(9):2735–46.
47. Pascolutti R, Sun X, Kao J, Maute RL, Ring AM, Bowman GR, et al. Structure and dynamics of PD-L1 and an ultra-high-affinity PD-1 receptor mutant. Structure (London: 1993). 2016;24(10):1719–28.
48. Schöniger S, Jasani B. The PD-1/PD-L1 pathway: a perspective on comparative immuno-oncology. Animals. 2022;12(19)
49. Zak KM, Grudnik P, Magiera K, Dömling A, Dubin G, Holak TA. Structural biology of the immune checkpoint receptor PD-1 and its ligands PD-L1/PD-L2. Structure (London: 1993). 2017;25(8):1163–74.
50. Freeman GJ. Structures of PD-1 with its ligands: sideways and dancing cheek to cheek. Proc Natl Acad Sci. 2008;105(30):10275–6.
51. Wherry EJ. T cell exhaustion. Nat Immunol. 2011;12(6):492–9.
52. Kim PS, Ahmed R. Features of responding T cells in cancer and chronic infection. Curr Opin Immunol. 2010;22(2):223–30.
53. Miggelbrink AM, Jackson JD, Lorrey SJ, Srinivasan ES, Waibl-Polania J, Wilkinson DS, et al. CD4 T-cell exhaustion: does it exist and what are its roles in cancer? Clin Cancer Res. 2021;27(21):5742–52.
54. Baessler A, Vignali DAA. T cell exhaustion. Annu Rev Immunol. 2024;42:179–206.
55. Yi JS, Cox MA, Zajac AJ. T-cell exhaustion: characteristics, causes and conversion. Immunology. 2010;129(4):474–81.
56. Zebley CC, Youngblood B. Mechanisms of T cell exhaustion guiding next-generation immunotherapy. Trend Cancer. 2022;8(9):726–34.
57. McLane LM, Abdel-Hakeem MS, Wherry EJ. CD8 T cell exhaustion during chronic viral infection and cancer. Annu Rev Immunol. 2019;37:457–95.
58. Brunell AE, Lahesmaa R, Autio A, Thotakura AK. Exhausted T cells hijacking the cancer-immunity cycle: assets and liabilities. Front Immunol. 2023;14
59. Franco F, Jaccard A, Romero P, Yu Y-R, Ho P-C. Metabolic and epigenetic regulation of T-cell exhaustion. Nat Metab. 2020;2(10):1001–12.

60. Seo W, Jerin C, Nishikawa H. Transcriptional regulatory network for the establishment of CD8(+) T cell exhaustion. Exp Mol Med. 2021;53(2):202–9.
61. Zhang J, Lei F, Tan H. The development of CD8 T-cell exhaustion heterogeneity and the therapeutic potentials in cancer. Front Immunol. 2023;14:1166128.
62. Beltra J-C, Manne S, Abdel-Hakeem MS, Kurachi M, Giles JR, Chen Z, et al. Developmental relationships of four exhausted CD8+ T cell subsets reveals underlying transcriptional and epigenetic landscape control mechanisms. Immunity. 2020;52(5):825–41.e8.
63. Hudson WH, Gensheimer J, Hashimoto M, Wieland A, Valanparambil RM, Li P, et al. Proliferating transitory T cells with an effector-like transcriptional signature emerge from PD-1(+) stem-like CD8(+) T cells during chronic infection. Immunity. 2019;51(6):1043–58.e4.
64. Im SJ, Ha SJ. Re-defining T-cell exhaustion: subset, function, and regulation. Immune Netw. 2020;20(1):e2.
65. Sun D, Shi X, Li S, Wang X, Yang X, Wan M. CAR-T cell therapy: a breakthrough in traditional cancer treatment strategies (review). Mol Med Rep. 2024;29(3)
66. Uscanga-Palomeque AC, Chávez-Escamilla AK, Alvizo-Báez CA, Saavedra-Alonso S, Terrazas-Armendáriz LD, Tamez-Guerra RS, et al. CAR-T cell therapy: from the shop to cancer therapy. Int J Mol Sci. 2023;24(21)
67. Yin X, He L, Guo Z. T-cell exhaustion in CAR-T-cell therapy and strategies to overcome it. Immunology. 2023;169(4):400–11.
68. Zhu X, Li Q, Zhu X. Mechanisms of CAR T cell exhaustion and current counteraction strategies. Front Cell Dev Biol. 2022;10:1034257.
69. Xiong D, Yu H, Sun ZJ. Unlocking T cell exhaustion: insights and implications for CAR-T cell therapy. Acta Pharm Sin B. 2024;14(8):3416–31.
70. Kouro T, Himuro H, Sasada T. Exhaustion of CAR T cells: potential causes and solutions. J Transl Med. 2022;20(1):239.

Chapter 2
Immune Checkpoint Molecules: Structure, Function, and Expression

2.1 Introduction

A competent immune system protects our body against infections and malignancies. Overactivation or dysfunction of the immune system can cause serious health problems. The function of immune cells is precisely regulated by several mechanisms including immune checkpoint receptors. Immune checkpoints are regulatory molecules that are expressed on immune cells. They can be divided into two categories: positive checkpoints that have a stimulatory role such as CD28 and CD40 and negative checkpoints that exert inhibitory effects [1]. Immune checkpoints play an important role in immune system homeostasis. Defects of cytotoxic T lymphocyte antigen 4 (CTLA-4) and programmed cell death 1 (PD-1) in mice can lead to severe autoimmune disorders. Therefore, signal induction through inhibitory molecules can maintain self-tolerance and prevent autoimmunity development. Various studies have shown the efficacy of the inhibitory molecule agonists in ameliorating autoimmune disease, for instance, the use of galectin 9 (TIM-3 ligand) and PD-1 or T cell immunoreceptor with Ig and ITIM domains (TIGIT) agonist antibodies in experimental autoimmune encephalomyelitis (EAE) and collagen-induced arthritis (CIA) mouse models [2]. Increased expression of inhibitory molecules leads to immune cells exhaustion. T cell exhaustion is a physiological phenomenon to modulate immune responses during the continuous presence of antigens but is considered as an immune escape mechanism in tumors and chronic infections. T cell exhaustion was first identified in lymphocytic choriomeningitis virus (LCMV) infection in which virus-specific cytotoxic T cells were dysfunctional. T cell exhaustion is characterized by the decrease in proliferative potential during the continuous presence of viral or tumor antigens, upregulation of several inhibitory molecules on the cell, and reduced production of cytokines including interferon-gamma (IFN-γ), interleukin-2 (IL-2), and tumor necrosis factor α (TNF-α) [3, 4]. Several inhibitory molecules have been identified in the immune system, which are summarized in Table 2.1

L. Tayebi, M. Abdolmaleki, *Immune System Regulation*,
https://doi.org/10.1007/978-981-95-8026-2_2

Table 2.1 List of immune checkpoint molecules

Molecule	Description	Ligand (or receptor)	Cellular expression
CTLA-4	CD28 family, discovered in 1991, negative regulator of T cell response, reducing T cell proliferation and cytokine production	CD80/CD86	$CD4^+$ T and $CD8^+$ T, Treg
PD-1	CD28 family, discovered in 1992, inhibition of immune cells function, contains ITIM and ITSM motifs	PD-L1, PD-L2	T cell, B cell, monocyte, NK cell, DC
TIM-3	TIM family, discovered in 2002, negative regulator of immune system, overexpression in cancer and viral infection	Galectin-9, CEACAM1, PtdSer, HMGB1	T cell, B cell, NK cell, monocyte, macrophage, DC
LAG-3	Ig superfamily, discovered in 1990, contains KIEELE, FXXL, and EP motifs for inhibitory signal transduction, reduces immune cells function in cancer	MHC-II, LSECtin, Galectin-3, FGL1, α-syn PFF, TCR–CD3	T cell, NK cell, B cell, NKT cell
CD244	SLAM family, discovered in 1993, initiates inhibitory signaling by ITSM motifs upon CD244–CD48 interaction, overexpression in cancer and chronic infection	CD48	T cell, NK cell, monocyte, basophil, DC, MDSC
CD160	Discovered in 1993, both activation and inhibitory functions, overexpression in cancer	MHC I, HVEM	T cell, NK cell, NKT cell
BTLA	CD28 family, discovered in 2003, contains ITIM and ITSM motifs in the cytoplasmic domain, induces inhibition of immune cells function	HVEM	T cell, NK cell, B cell, splenic macrophage, DC
TIGIT	PVR/nectin family, discovered in 2009, inhibitory immune checkpoint, contains ITIM and ITT-like motifs in the cytoplasmic tail, reduces cytotoxicity of tumor-specific T cells, overexpression in cancer and viral infection	PVR (CD155), PVRL2 (CD112), PVRL3 (CD113), PVRL4	T cell, NK cell
CD96	Immunoglobulin superfamily, discovered in 1992, reducing the CD226 activation signal by competing for CD155 binding	CD155, CD111	T cell, NK cell, B cell
PVRIG	Discovered in 2016, contains an ITIM-like motif in the intracellular domain, T cell suppression	CD112	T cell (predominantly $CD8^+$ T), NK cell
B7-H3	B7 family proteins, discovered in 2001, overexpression in cancer, both activation and inhibitory functions	TLT-2	T cell, DC, monocyte

(continued)

Table 2.1 (continued)

Molecule	Description	Ligand (or receptor)	Cellular expression
B7-H4	B7 family proteins, discovered in 2003, suppression of T cell function	Nrp1	Epithelial cell
VISTA	B7 family proteins, discovered in 2011, contains ITIM and ITSM motifs in its cytoplasmic domain for inhibitory signal transduction overexpression in cancer	VSIG-3, PSGL1	T cell, macrophage, DC, monocyte, neutrophils
B7-H7	B7 family proteins, both activation and inhibitory functions	TMIGD2, KIR3DL3	Macrophage, monocyte, activated lymphocyte
A2AR and A2BR	CD39 converts ATP to AMP and CD73 converts the AMP into adenosine Adenosine interacts with P1 receptors (mainly A2AR, A2BR) and causes T cell suppression	Adenosine	T cell, Treg
KLRG1	C-type lectin-like inhibitory receptor, senescence and differentiation marker, contains an ITIM motif	E-cadherin, N-cadherin, R-cadherin	$CD4^+$ T, $CD8^+$ T, NK
CD47	Discovered in 1988 as an unnamed cell-surface glycoprotein, SIRPα–CD47 signaling inhibits phagocytosis, overexpression in tumor	SIRPα	Myeloid cells
LILRB	Type I transmembrane glycoproteins including LILRB 1–7, contains ITIM motifs, inhibition of phagocytosis and lymphocytes function	MHC-I, nonclassical MHC-I, CD1d, ß-amyloid, APOE4	T cell, B cell, NK cell, monocyte, macrophage, neutrophil, DC
Siglecs	Sialic acid-binding Ig-like lectins, some of them have inhibitory functions including Siglec-5 to Siglec-11	Sialoglycans	Hematopoietic cells
CD200R	Ig super family, five types (CD200R1-R5), inhibitory function	CD200	T cell, NK cell, myeloid cells
LAIR-1	Ig superfamily, the leukocyte-associated inhibitory receptor family, contains two ITIMs in the cytoplasmic domain	Collagens	T cell, B cell, NK cell, monocyte, macrophage, eosinophils, basophil
CD300	Consists of seven members "a to g," CD300a and CD300f are inhibitory molecules, contains ITIMs in their intracellular domains	PtdSer, PE	T cell, B cell, NK cell, monocyte, DC, granulocyte
CD101	Type I integral membrane protein, inhibition of T cell function and cytokine production	Putative ligand	Activated T cell, monocyte, granulocyte

(continued)

Table 2.1 (continued)

Molecule	Description	Ligand (or receptor)	Cellular expression
Stabilin-1	Type I transmembrane protein, clearance of apoptotic cells, immune trafficking, T cell suppression in cancer	PtdSer	T cell, tissue macrophage, sinusoidal endothelial cell
CLEC12A	C-type lectin domain family, contains an ITIM in its intracellular region for inhibitory signal induction	MSU	Neutrophil, monocyte
DCIR	C-type lectin family, negative regulation of TLR response	Glycans	Myeloid cells
SIRL-1	Ig superfamily, contains two ITIMs for recruiting SHP-1 and SHP-2	S100 proteins, PSM, cathelicidin LL-37	Neutrophil, monocyte
Butyrophilins	Ig superfamily, activation of γδ T cells, inhibition of αβ T cells	Putative ligand	Lymphocyte, myeloid cell, epithelial cell

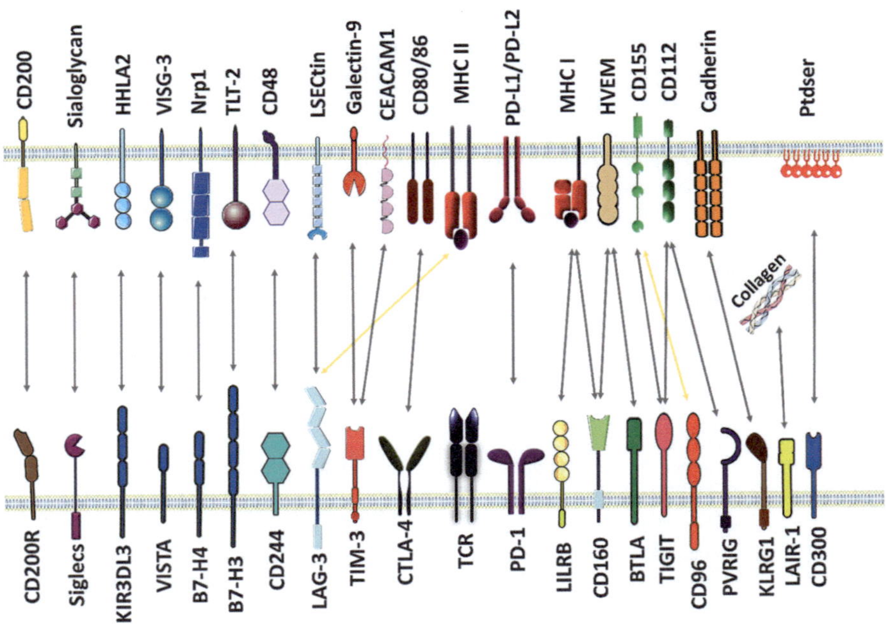

Fig. 2.1 Immune checkpoint molecules expressed on activated T cells with their relevant ligands. There are several receptor–ligand interactions that induce co-inhibitory signals in activated T cells and regulate their function. Signaling through the interaction of inhibitory receptors on T cells with their ligands on APCs or tumor cells suppresses T cell function. CTLA-4 and PD-1 are two classical immune checkpoints expressed on T cells. CTLA-4 binds to CD80/CD86 with high affinity and competes with CD28. PD-1 binds to PD-L1/PD-L2. Other inhibitory receptor-ligands include: TIM-3/Galectin-9 and TIM-3/CEACAM1, LAG-3/MHC-II and LAG- 3/LSECtin, CD244/CD48, CD160/MHC-I and CD160/ HVEM, BTLA/HVEM, TIGIT/CD155 and TIGIT/CD112, CD96/ CD155, PVRIG/CD112, B7-H3/TLT-2, B7-H4/Nrp1, VISTA/VSIG-3, KIR3DL3/HHLA2, KLRG1/Cadherin, LILRB/MHC-I, Siglecs/Sialoglycans, CD200R/CD200, CD300/PtdSer, and LAIR-1/collagens in extracellular matrix. Created using elements from Servier Medical Art (https://smart.servier.com), licensed under CC BY 4.0 (https://creativecommons.org/licenses/by/4.0/), and from NIAID NIH BioArt Source (bioart.niaid.nih.gov)

and Fig. 2.1. Here, the structure, mechanism of action, cellular expression, and clinical significance of inhibitory immune checkpoints are described.

2.2 CTLA-4

CTLA-4 or CD152 is an immune checkpoint that belongs to the immunoglobulin (Ig) superfamily [5]. CTLA-4 gene is located on chromosome two and consists of four exons [6]. It has an extracellular Ig variable-like (IgV) domain, a transmembrane part, and a cytoplasmic tail with a YVKM motif [7]. It continuously expresses on regulatory T cells (Tregs) while can be upregulated on conventional T cells after activation. CD28 is a co-stimulatory molecule that binds to CD80 and CD86 on antigen-presenting cells (APCs) to mediate T cell activation in conjunction with T cell receptor signals. CTLA-4 is a CD28 homolog that can bind to CD80 and CD86 with higher affinity than CD28 and compete for binding to these ligands. This competitive interaction prevents CD28 co-stimulatory signal [5, 8]. Furthermore, CTLA-4 also can directly generate inhibitory signals and act as a negative regulator of T cell function. Phosphorylation of the intracellular domain of CTLA-4 by Fyn and Lck tyrosine kinases leads to the recruitment of SH2 domain-containing inositol phosphate-2 (SHIP2) and protein phosphatase 2A (PP2A). SHIP2 disrupts T cell receptor (TCR)/CD3 signaling by dephosphorylating CD3 and inhibits phosphatidylinositol-3-kinase (PI3K)/protein kinase B (AKT) pathways in lymphocytes. PP2A also inhibits the T cell activation signaling by dephosphorylating AKT [6]. In naive T cells, CTLA-4 localized within the cells. Engagement of TCR and activation of T cell leads to an increase of CTLA-4 gene expression as well as translocation of CTLA-4 from endocytic vesicles to the cell surface [8, 9] and results in the reduction of IL-2 production, proliferation, and survival of T cells [7, 8]. In $CD8^+$ T cells, CTLA-4 can regulate IFN-γ and granzyme B production [7]. In Tregs, CTLA-4 regulates homeostasis and immunosuppressive properties [7]. Treg cells can induce an inhibitory signal through the binding of CTLA-4 to CD80/CD86 on dendritic cells (DCs) and turn them into tolerogenic APCs. CTLA-4 mutation leads to dysfunction of Treg cells, and uncontrolled proliferation and activation of lymphocytes [6]. CTLA-4 knock-out (KO) mice develop lymphoproliferative disorders and have auto-proliferating T cells in lymphoid and nonlymphoid tissues [10]. CTLA-4 is of particular importance in the pathogenesis of cancer and the overexpression of this molecule has been observed in many cancers. In this regard, several CTLA-4 inhibitors have been developed for the treatment of cancers [11].

2.3 PD-1

PD-1 (PDCD1, CD279) was discovered in 1992 as an apoptosis-related molecule [12]. PD-1 is a 288 amino acid protein encoded by the PDCD1 gene on chromosome 2 in humans and belongs to the CD28 family [12, 13]. It is expressed on activated T cells, B cells, monocytes, natural killer (NK) cells, and DCs [12]. PD-1 molecule contains an extracellular IgV domain, a transmembrane region, and a cytoplasmic tail comprising immunoreceptor tyrosine-based inhibitory motif (ITIM) and immunoreceptor tyrosine-based switch motif (ITSM) requiring for Src homology 2 domain-containing protein tyrosine phosphatase 1 (SHP-1) and SHP-2 recruitment and initiation of downstream inhibitory signal [12, 14]. Following the interaction of PD-1 with its ligands, SHP-2 stops PI3K/AKT and mitogen-activated protein kinase (MAPK)/extracellular signal-regulated kinase (ERK) and Janus kinase/signal transducers and activators of transcription (JAK-STAT) signaling pathways with its phosphatase activity and prevents lymphocytes activation [15]. Two types I transmembrane glycoproteins, programmed cell death ligand 1 (PD-L1, B7-H1, CD274) and PD-L2 (B7-DC, CD273), are ligands of PD-1. PD-L1 is a 33-kDa protein with 290 amino acid residues and its gene is located on chromosome 9. PD-L1 is expressed on a variety of immune and nonimmune cells including lymphocytes, myeloid cells, epithelial and vascular endothelial cells. The PD-1/PD-L1 interaction is an important tumor escape mechanism from the specific immune response. PD-L2 is a protein of 270 amino acid residues that binds to PD-1 with greater affinity than PD-L1, but its expression is mainly limited to macrophages and DCs, although it can be induced on other cells as well. PD-1 signaling inhibits cytokine production and proliferation of T cells. Increased expression of PD-1 and its ligands in autoimmune diseases such as inflammatory bowel disease (IBD) and systemic lupus erythematosus (SLE) indicates the essential role of PD-1 pathway in maintaining self-tolerance [15]. The regulatory effect of PD-1 has been observed in many diseases including infections and tumors. The overexpression of PD-1 has been reported in viral diseases such as hepatitis B virus (HBV), hepatitis C virus (HCV), and human immunodeficiency virus (HIV) and also in bacterial infections including *Helicobacter pylori*, *Mycobacterium tuberculosis*, and *Listeria monocytogenes* as well as parasitic infections including *Toxoplasma gondii*, *Leishmania*, and *Plasmodium falciparum*. PD-1 blocking can restore the activity of pathogen-specific $CD4^+$ T and $CD8^+$ T cells [16]. PD-1/PD-L1 signaling pathway is a critical immune escape mechanism in cancers. Like CTLA-4, PD-1 is one of the most important targets of cancer immunotherapy [17].

2.4 TIM-3

T cell immunoglobulin and mucin domain-containing protein 3 (TIM-3) or Hepatitis A virus cellular receptor 2 (HAVCR2) is an immune checkpoint that is first described as a specific marker for type I helper T cell (Th1) and cytotoxic T cells. TIM gene family is located on chromosome 5 and encodes three molecules with a similar structure including TIM-1, TIM-3, and TIM-4. TIM-3 is expressed on T cells, NK cells, monocytes, macrophages, and DCs. It is another marker of T cell exhaustion, which is overexpressed in chronic infections and cancers [18–20]. Structurally, TIM-3 is composed of an IgV domain in the N-terminal, a mucin domain with O-linked glycosylation sites, and a transmembrane section followed by a cytoplasmic domain. Typical inhibitory motifs are absent in the cytoplasmic tail; instead, there are conserved tyrosine residues and two of them (Tyr 265, 272 in human and Tyr 256, 263 in mouse) are critical for downstream inhibitory signaling of TIM-3 [18, 21, 22]. Following the binding of TIM-3 to its ligands, these tyrosine residues become phosphorylated and mediate intracellular signal transduction [18, 22]. Four ligands have been identified for TIM-3. Galectin-9 is a C-type lectin that binds to the IgV domain of TIM-3 and can induce cell death in TIM-3 expressing T cells [19, 23]. Carcinoembryonic antigen-related cell adhesion molecule 1 (CEACAM1) is another TIM-3 ligand that is expressed on activated T cells, DCs, monocytes, or tumor cells [24]. It seems that the *cis*-interaction of TIM-3 and CEACAM1 facilitates the TIM-3 inhibitory function. Trans-interaction also triggers inhibitory signaling [25]. Recent studies have shown that high-mobility group box 1 (HMGB1) acts as a ligand of TIM-3 [19]. HMGB1 plays an important role in transporting pathogens or tumor-derived nucleic acids into endosomal vesicles of DCs, which ultimately leads to an immune response against pathogens or tumors. HMGB1 can be released by dead/necrotic cells or actively be secreted by leukocytes or endothelial cells. In the tumor microenvironment (TME), TIM-3 is overexpressed on DCs; therefore, the interaction of TIM-3 and HMGB1 suppresses the DCs immune response via blocking the transfer of the nucleic acids into the endosomes [19, 26]. Furthermore, it has been shown that TIM-3 can bind to phosphatidylserine (PtdSer) [19]. PtdSer is a phospholipid component of the inner leaflet of the cell membrane and it appears on the cell surface during apoptosis [27]. Binding of the TIM-3 expressed on phagocyte cells to the PtdSer of apoptotic cells promotes inhibitory signaling in the cells [19, 28].

2.5 LAG-3

Lymphocyte activation gene-3 (LAG-3 or CD223), discovered in 1990, is another inhibitory molecule that belongs to the Ig superfamily. It is expressed by different immune cells such as $CD4^+$ and $CD8^+$ T cells, Tregs, NK cells, and B cells. Like the CD4 co-receptor, LAG-3 contains four extracellular Ig-like domains and a type I transmembrane domain. It can bind to major histocompatibility complex class II (MHC II) with an affinity higher than CD4. The cytoplasmic domain consists of four regions: a serine phosphorylation region, a KIEELE motif, a FXXL motif, and a glutamic acid-proline (EP) repeats motif [18, 22, 29, 30]. Other LAG-3 ligands include liver and lymph node sinusoidal endothelial cell C-type lectin (LSECtin), Galectin-3, fibrinogen-like protein 1 (FGL1), α-synuclein preformed fibrils (α-syn PFF), and TCR–CD3 complex [30]. LSECtin with a lectin structure is related to the DC-sign family and Galectin-3. Both of these ligands are expressed on tumor cells [18, 31]. FGL1 is a newly discovered ligand that binds to LAG-3 with high affinity and is overexpressed in cancers. FGL1 released by tumor cells interacts with the D1 domain of LAG-3 independently of MHC II [30, 32]. TCR–CD3 complex can also act as LAG-3 ligand. It has been found that in the absence of MHC II, TCR or CD3 can bind to LAG-3 by *cis*-interaction. LAG-3 can inhibit the intracellular signaling of CD4 and CD8 co-receptors by disrupting the function of Lck. This process is mediated by the EP motif. LAG-3 is also expressed in neural tissues and interacts with α-syn PFF, although the importance of this interaction is not clear; however, it seems to be essential in maintaining tolerance [30]. It has been shown that LAG-3 signaling can negatively affect the immune cells function in cancers and chronic infections [33, 34]. LAG-3 expressing T cells are defective in proliferation and cytokine production. The expression of LAG-3 along with PD-1 on T lymphocytes has been reported in several cancers [34–36]. It has been demonstrated that co-blockade of the LAG-3 and PD-1 has positive effects on lymphocyte function and in controlling viral infections or tumors [36–39]. A study demonstrated that administration of blocking antibodies against the LAG-3 accompanied by immunization using an immunodominant epitope can restore virus-specific $CD8^+$ T cell functions in herpes simplex virus type 1 (HSV-1) infection [40].

2.6 CD244

CD244 (2B4, SLAMF4) is a member of the signaling lymphocytic activation molecule (SLAM) family receptor. It was first defined on mouse NK cells as a regulator of NK cell cytotoxicity and antiviral immunity. CD244 is also expressed on T cells, monocytes, basophils, DCs, and myeloid-derived suppressor cells (MDSCs). It is upregulated during chronic viral infections or tumors, especially in $CD8^+$ T cells [41–43]. CD48 acts as CD244 ligand and it also belongs to the SLAM family. CD244 is composed of an extracellular part containing IgV and Ig constant 2-like (IgC2) domains, a transmembrane segment, and a cytoplasmic domain with ITSM [41, 44]. The ITSMs interact with adaptor molecules including SLAM-associated protein (SAP), Ewing sarcoma-activated transcript 2 (EAT2), and phosphatases. Intracellular signaling of CD244 can be activating or inhibitory. Interaction of the ITSMs with the adaptor molecules defines the signal outcome [41, 44]. SAP is a very important adaptive molecule that initiates intracellular signaling by binding to ITSMs upon CD244–CD48 interaction. When sufficient concentration of SAP is available, the activation signal will be triggered. If there is no adequate level of intracellular functional SAP, the phosphatases (including SHP-1, SHP-2), EAT2, and C-Terminal Src Kinase (CsK) recruit to the ITSMs and trigger inhibitory signals [41]. X-linked lymphoproliferative (XLP1) disease is an example of a CD244 signaling defect. The *SH2D1A* gene, which encodes the SAP protein, is mutated in these patients. One of the prominent features of this disease is Epstein-Barr virus (EBV) infection. These patients are susceptible to EBV infection due to NK and $CD8^+$ T cells dysfunctions. CD244 in NK cells and T cells is not able to induce the activation signal and they cannot eliminate virus-infected B cells [43, 45, 46]. Furthermore, the expression level of CD244 on the cells and the balance between CD244 and SAP can influence the signaling. It has been shown that during normal physiologic conditions, the CD244 level is low and intracellular SAP is at the normal level; therefore, it induces activation signals. Pathologic situations such as chronic infection and tumor induce CD244 expression. In this situation, SAP concentration is not sufficient to bind all ITSMs; as a result, recruiting phosphatases triggers inhibitory signals [41]. It has been demonstrated that blocking of CD244–CD48 interaction with specific antibodies can increase the cytotoxicity and cytokine expression capacity of exhausted NK cells [41]. An increase in IFN-γ, TNF-α, and perforin production from virus-specific $CD8^+$ T cells has been shown using anti-CD244 blocking antibodies [41, 43].

2.7 CD160

CD160 initially was identified on NK cells. There are two types of CD160 molecules; the major isoform (CD160-GPI) is a glycosylphosphatidylinositol (GPI)-anchored molecule with an Ig-like domain that is expressed on NK cells, natural killer T cells (NKT), and T cells such as intestinal intraepithelial $CD8^+$ T cells, subsets of $CD4^+$ T cells, and γδT cells [47–49]. CD160 molecules can be cleaved by phosphatidylinositol-specific phospholipase C (PIPLC), GPI-specific phospholipase D (GPI-PLD) as well as metalloprotease enzymes and released from the cell surface [47]. The other isoform (CD160-TM) contains a transmembrane section and a cytoplasmic tail and it is expressed in activated peripheral blood NK cells and NK cell lines [47–49]. The cytoplasmic tail can initiate intracellular signaling via Lck and ERK1/2 [47].

CD160 can bind to human leukocyte antigen C (HLA-C), soluble HLA-G, and to a lesser degree to HLA-A2, HLA-B7, and HLA-E. These interactions lead to NK and T cell activation. However, CD160 also can interact with the herpesvirus entry mediator (HVEM). HVEM belongs to the TNF receptor superfamily (TNFRSF14) and is first described as a receptor for the gD protein of HSV-1. It is expressed in many organs such as lung, liver, kidney, heart, skeletal muscles, and also several immune cell types including T cells, B cells, NK cells, DCs, monocytes, and neutrophils [47]. The other HVEM ligands include lymphotoxin-α (LTα) and LIGHT, which induce activation signals, and BTLA, which promotes inhibitory signal upon binding to HVEM [47]. The extracellular domain of HVEM contains four repeats of cysteine-rich domain (CRD). LIGHT and LTα interact with cysteine-rich domain 2

(CRD2) and CRD3, whereas BTLA and CD160 bind to CRD1. The binding affinity of HVEM to BTLA is higher than to CD160 [47, 50]. CD160 can induce activation or inhibitory signals in different situations. It has been shown that the interaction of CD160 with MHC-I or cross-linking antibodies causes NK cell activation, increased cytotoxicity and cytokine production [51, 52]. Furthermore, CD160 has been considered as an exhaustion marker [53, 54]. CD160-HVEM interaction can hinder T cells activation and function [55]. HCV-specific $CD8^+$ T cells have elevated CD160 expression and show exhausted phenotype [56]. CD160 has been implicated in different clinical conditions such as cancer, chronic viral infection, malaria, autoimmunity, and skin inflammation. Upregulation of CD160 has been reported in several cancers including chronic lymphocytic leukemia (CLL), colorectal cancer (CRC), and melanoma as well as viral infections such as HIV, HCV, EBV, and cytomegalovirus (CMV). CD160 also plays a key role in autoimmune diseases. Impaired signaling pathway or abnormal CD160 expression in acquired plastic anemia, rheumatoid arthritis, Graves' disease, and Crohn's disease indicate the role of this molecule in the pathogenesis of the autoimmune disorders [50].

2.8 BTLA

B and T-lymphocyte attenuator (BTLA, CD272), discovered in 2003, belongs to the CD28 family and structurally resembles CTLA-4 and PD-1 [57]. BTLA is mainly expressed on T and B cells, as well as NK cells, splenic macrophages, and bone marrow-derived DCs [57, 58]. It is a type I transmembrane glycoprotein that contains extracellular, transmembrane, and cytoplasmic domains [57]. The cytoplasmic domain consists of growth factor receptor bound protein-2 (Grb-2) association motif, ITIM, and ITSM. BTLA binds to HVEM and induces cell signaling. Following BTLA–HVEM interaction, tyrosine phosphatases SHP-1 and SHP-2 are recruited to ITIM and initiate the inhibitory signal. BTLA potentially can induce proliferation and survival signals through binding Grb-2 association motif and subsequent activation of the PI3K pathway [59]. BTLA–HVEM complexes can form in *trans* or *cis*. In a state of homeostasis, *cis* interaction between BTLA and HVEM of the same cell leads to an inhibitory signal and hinders the interaction of co-stimulatory molecule LIGHT with HVEM. In *trans* interaction, BTLA on one cell binds to HVEM on another cell. T cell activation leads to internalization of HVEM and *trans* interaction of BTLA–HVEM is facilitated [60, 61]. BTLA is involved in the maintenance of peripheral tolerance of T cells. In BTLA-deficient mice, T cells have uncontrolled proliferation. Upregulation of BTLA has been shown in different types of cancers and chronic infections, for example in pulmonary tuberculosis, CMV, and HBV infections [61–64]. Downregulation of BTLA can enhance the antitumor activity of NKT cells in mice [65]. It has been reported that tumor-specific $CD8^+$ T cells expressed a high level of BTLA in melanoma patients [63]. A study showed that blocking BTLA along with PD-1 and TIM-3 using specific antibodies reactivates the exhausted T cells and enhances the anti-HIV immune response [62]. Therefore, targeting BTLA signaling can be helpful in the treatment of such diseases [66].

2.9 TIGIT

TIGIT (also known as WUCAM, Vstm3, and VSIG9) was discovered in 2009 as an inhibitory receptor in T cells and NK cells. It belongs to the Ig superfamily and is expressed on NK and T cells including activated T cells, memory T cells, and Tregs. TIGIT structure consists of an extracellular domain, a transmembrane region, and a cytoplasmic tail with an ITIM and an immunoglobulin tail tyrosine (ITT)-like motif for inhibitory signal induction [18, 67]. Phosphorylation of these inhibitory motifs recruits SHIP1 to interrupt the PI3K/MAPK signaling pathways and nuclear factor-κB (NF-κB) activation. Furthermore, TIGIT signaling can reduce NK cell

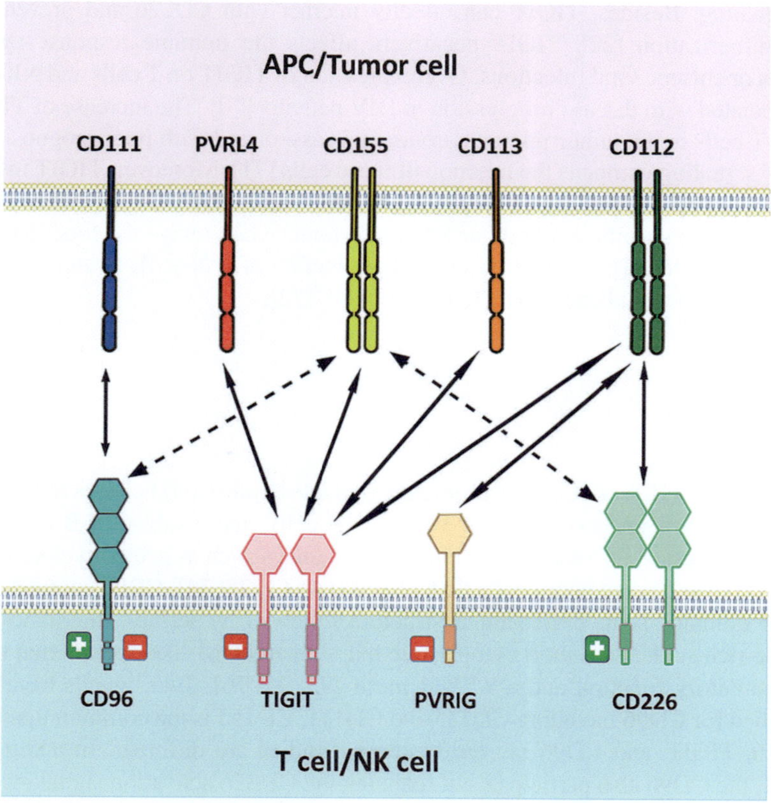

Fig. 2.2 TIGIT/PVR interaction. TIGIT/PVRIG/CD96 form an axis that induce inhibitory signals and suppress T cell activation. poliovirus receptor (PVR) family members include CD155 (PVR), CD112 (PVRL2), CD226, CD113 (PVRL3), PVRL4 and poliovirus receptor-related immunoglobulin domain-containing (PVRIG). TIGIT is an inhibitory receptor expressed on T cells. TIGIT interacts with CD155, CD112, CD113 and PVRL4 on APCs or tumor cells. CD226 is a co-stimulatory receptor which also binds to CD155 and CD112. The TIGIT binding affinity for CD155 is higher than that of CD226 and can competitively inhibit CD226 signaling. CD96 also binds to CD155 and CD111. High-affinity CD96-CD155 interaction attenuates CD226 signaling; however, a co-stimulatory role for CD96 has also been suggested. PVRIG is another inhibitory receptor expressed on T cells and CD112 serves as a common ligand for both PVRIG and CD226. Created using elements from Servier Medical Art (https://smart.servier.com), licensed under CC BY 4.0 (https://creativecommons.org/licenses/by/4.0/), and from NIAID NIH BioArt Source (bioart.niaid.nih.gov)

cytotoxicity by inhibiting the phosphorylation of ERK1/2 and ZAP70/Syk [18, 68, 69]. The ligands that interact with the TIGIT include CD155 (poliovirus receptor or PVR), CD112 (poliovirus receptor-related 2 or PVRL2, nectin-2), CD113 (PVRL3), and PVRL4 (nectin-4), a newly discovered ligand that is exclusive to TIGIT (Fig. 2.2). The TIGIT binding affinity for CD155 is higher than for CD112. These ligands are expressed on APCs, T cells, and a wide range of non-hematopoietic cells [22, 67, 69]. CD226 or DNAX accessory molecule-1 (DNAM-1) is a co-stimulatory receptor that is expressed on NK cells, T cells, and monocytes and has a stimulatory effect on cytotoxicity and cytokine production ability of these cells. CD226 also binds to CD155 and CD112 [67]. TIGIT binds to CD155 with higher affinity than CD226; thus, it can compete with CD226 for the interaction with CD155 and block its signaling. Besides, TIGIT can directly interact with CD226 and prevents its homodimerization [22]. TIGIT negatively affects the immune response against tumors or chronic viral infections. Overexpression of TIGIT on T cells and NK cells is associated with disease progression in HIV patients [70]. The increase of $TIGIT^+$ $CD8^+$ T cells in the tumor microenvironment is associated with poor prognosis and TIGIT signaling dampens the function of these cells [71]. Moreover, TIGIT intensifies the suppressive activity of Tregs [69]. Several studies have shown that blockade of TIGIT with specific antibody or RNA interference can revive the functions of T cells and NK cells [67]. Cytotoxicity and production of IFN-γ, IL-6, and TNF-α of these cells can be enhanced by TIGIT inhibitors [72].

2.10 CD96

CD96 or TACTILE (T cell activation increased late expression) belongs to Ig superfamily receptors and expresses on T cells, NK cells, and a subset of B cells. It is broadly expressed in some hematologic malignancies such as acute myeloid leukemia (AML) and acute lymphoblastic leukemia (ALL) [73, 74]. CD96 contains three Ig-like domains in its extracellular structure followed by serine-, threonine-, and proline-rich stalk and a short cytoplasmic tail with an ITIM-like domain that mediates inhibitory function and a YXXM motif [73, 75, 76]. Two ligands have been identified for CD96 including CD155 and CD111. CD155 is the common ligand for CD226, TIGIT, and CD96 but the binding affinities are different. In addition to TIGIT, the CD96 also participates in reducing the CD226 activation signal by competing for CD155 binding [73, 74]. The CD226/TIGIT/CD96 combination is similar to the interaction of CD28 and CTLA-4 with B7 ligands that exert co-stimulatory and co-inhibitory signals in the T cell, respectively. TIGIT has the highest affinity (1–3 $nmol/L^2$), also CD96 has a higher affinity (37.6 $nmol/L^2$) in comparison to activation receptor CD226 (114–119 $nmol/L^2$) for binding to CD155 [73]. CD226 is important for NK cell adhesion, cytotoxicity, and secretion of inflammatory cytokines [77, 78]. Based on a study, tumor growth and metastasis were more restricted in CD96-deficient (*Cd96*$^{-/-}$) mice. CD96 reduced IFN-γ production by NK cells and these mice were more susceptible to the hyperinflammatory response induced by lipopolysaccharide (LPS) [79]. A study of human hepatocellular carcinoma (HCC) revealed that CD96 expression had increased in intratumoral NK cells. These cells were functionally exhausted and had low IFN-γ and TNF-α secretion following activation with phorbol myristate acetate (PMA)/ionomycin. Interestingly, the CD96 blockade increased the cytotoxicity potency of the NK cells [80]. CD96 can induce an activation signal under certain conditions. Chiang et al. showed that CD96 acts as a co-stimulatory receptor in $CD8^+$ T cells [81].

2.11 PVRIG

Poliovirus receptor (PVR)-like proteins are a group of surface molecules that share PVR signature motifs in their first IgV domain. PVR family members include CD155 (PVR), CD112 (PVRL2), CD226, CD113 (PVRL3), PVRL4, and poliovirus receptor-related immunoglobulin domain-containing (PVRIG). PVRIG or CD112R was discovered in 2016 and act as an inhibitory molecule in human and mouse [82, 83]. PVRIG is a 36-kDa protein with an extracellular IgV domain. There are two tyrosine residues in the intracellular domain of PVRIG, one of them is located in an ITIM-like motif and can recruit phosphatases. T cells, especially $CD8^+$ T and NK cells, express PVRIG and it is overexpressed on activated T cells. CD112 is the ligand of PVRIG that is expressed by DCs and tumor cells [82, 84]. TIGIT/PVRIG/CD96 pathways exert inhibitory signals and suppress NK and T cell functions. PVRIG only interacts with CD112. Furthermore, CD226 also binds to CD112 and CD155 and initiates activation signal. Thus, the balance between inhibitory and activation signals determines the fate of the immune cell expressing these molecules, particularly in the tumor context [74]. It has been demonstrated that NK cells expressing CD112R in breast cancer have lower cytotoxicity and IFN-γ production. CD112R blockers increase T cell function by disrupting CD112R–CD112 interaction [84].

2.12 B7 Family

B7 family molecules belong to the Ig superfamily and have important roles in immune regulation. There are several molecules in this category including B7-1 (CD80) and B7–2 (CD86), B7-H1 (PD-L1), B7-DC (PD-L2), B7-H2 (ICOSL), B7-H3 (CD276), B7-H4 (Vtcn1), B7-H5, B7-H6 (NCR3LG1), and B7-H7 [85]. B7-1 and B7-2 are the ligands of two well-known receptors, CD28 and CTLA-4 on T cells. PD-L1 and PD-L2 are the PD-1 ligands. B7-H5 and B7-H4 have an inhibitory function, while B7-H6 is an activation receptor. For B7-H3 and B7-H7, both inhibition and activation functions have been described [86].

2.12.1 B7-H3

B7-H3 or CD276 is a B7 family member that contributes to immunomodulation. B7-H3 mRNA is found in a wide range of normal cells, but B7-H3 protein expression is more limited. It can be expressed on different immune cells including myeloid cells and lymphocytes. The receptors of B7-H3 have not been fully identified, but some putative receptors are assumed on tumor-associated macrophages (TAMs) and tumor-infiltrating lymphocytes (TILs). So far, triggering receptor expressed on myeloid cell-like transcript 2 (TLT-2) and interleukin-20 receptor subunit alpha (IL-20RA) are considered as receptors of this molecule. The B7-H3 gene is located on chromosome 15 and has two isoforms, including 2IgB7-H3 and 4IgB7-H3. The soluble form of B7-H3 is also released through the enzymatic cleavage of B7-H3 on the cell surface. Soluble B7-H3 induces proliferation and activation of T lymphocytes [87, 88]. B7-H3 was firstly defined as a stimulatory molecule on T cells [89, 90]. It has been shown that adenoviral expression of B7-H3 (Ad-B7-H3-GFP) in mice reduced tumor growth. The treated group had a higher frequency of tumor-specific $CD8^+$ CTL and higher IL-12 levels [91]. In contrast, numerous studies indicate the inhibitory role of B7-H3 in immune responses. B7-H3 is overexpressed in several malignancies and is associated with poorer clinical outcomes [92]. B7-H3 role in allergic and autoimmune diseases has been proven. In an animal model of asthma, blocking this molecule inhibited the Th2 response. Moreover, in the experimental autoimmune encephalomyelitis (EAE), deletion of B7-H3 was associated with more severe disease [87].

2.12.2 B7-H4

B7-H4 (B7x, B7-S1, and Vtcn1) contains an IgV and IgC-like domain in the extracellular region and has no signaling motif in its short cytoplasmic domain. It acts as a negative regulatory molecule in adaptive and innate immune responses. B7-H4 suppresses T cell functions including cytokine secretion or cytotoxicity and arrests cell cycle [93, 94]. B7-H4 mRNA has been detected in many tissues such as lung, liver, pancreas, spleen, and thymus; however, the B7-H4 protein expression is mainly restricted to epithelial tissues [93–95]. No certain receptor for B7-H4 has been identified yet. Nrp1 has been proposed as B7-H4 receptor on thymus-derived Tregs [93]. The regulatory function of B7-H4 in autoimmune responses and inflammation has been proven. Interaction of B7-H4 with its receptor inhibits T cell proliferation and function [96]. Overexpression of B7-H4 induces anti-inflammatory effects. A study found that B7-H4 deleted mice were more susceptible to diabetes and B7-H4 overexpression was protective and could inhibit autoimmunity. In the EAE model, B7-H4 blockade decreased T cell infiltration and limited disease progression [93, 97]. B7-H4 signaling is also important in infections. B7-H4 KO mice are more resistant to *Leishmania*, *Listeria*, or pneumonia infections [94].

2.12.3 VISTA

V-domain immunoglobulin suppressor of T cell activation (VISTA), also known as B7-H5, PD-1H, c10orf54, DD1a, Dies1, is a novel immune checkpoint molecule that belongs to type I transmembrane proteins [98, 99]. Phylogenetic analysis revealed that VISTA is highly similar to PD-1 [98]. This 279 amino acids protein is encoded on chromosome 10 and contains an N-terminal IgV domain followed by a 30 amino acids stalk, a transmembrane region, and a cytoplasmic tail [98, 100]. The cytoplasmic domain lacks any classic ITIM, ITAM, or ITSM. Instead, it has one SH-2 binding motif and three C-terminal SH3-binding domains that participate in signal transduction [98, 100]. VISTA is expressed on T cells, macrophages, DCs, monocytes, and neutrophils [92, 98]. It is also expressed in several tumors and is correlated with disease progression [101]. It can overexpress in chronic viral infections. Increased expression of VISTA has been reported on $CD4^+$ and $CD8^+$ T cells of HIV positive individuals [102]. To date, two confirmed ligands have been identified for VISTA including V-Set and immunoglobulin domain containing 3 (VSIG-3) and P-selectin glycoprotein ligand 1 (PSGL1). VSIG-3 interacts with VISTA on activated T cells and inhibits their proliferation and cytokine production. PSGL-1 also suppresses T cell function [103]. VISTA acts as a co-inhibitory receptor on $CD4^+$ T cells and also as a co-inhibitory ligand on APCs for suppressing T cells [92]. VISTA plays a key role in T cell homeostasis. VISTA-deficient mice show an accumulation of activated T cells and have elevated inflammatory cytokines production [104]. The association of VISTA with autoimmune diseases has been observed in several studies, and its deletion can cause autoimmune reactions. The specific expression of VISTA in placental tissues indicates the importance of this molecule in immune tolerance in pregnancy [103].

2.12.4 B7-H7

Human endogenous retro virus-H long terminal repeat associating-2 (HHLA2) or B7-H7 is another member of the B7 family that has three extracellular Ig domains, including an Ig constant-like domain and two IgV domains in its structure [105]. The B7-H7 gene is located on chromosome 3q13.13 [106]. Two receptors are identified for B7-H7, including transmembrane and Ig domain-containing 2 (TMIGD2) and killer cell immunoglobulin-like receptor, three Ig domains and long cytoplasmic Tail 3 (KIR3DL3). TMIGD2/CD28H is a glycoprotein of Ig superfamily that is encoded on chromosome 19q13.3. KIR3DL3 belongs to the KIR family, which contains an ITIM in its cytoplasmic tail [106]. Both of them express on different subsets of T and NK cells and bind to B7-H7 on different sites. Although TMIGD2 acts as a stimulatory receptor, KIR3DL3 has more potent inhibitory activity, which suppresses the function of immune cells [106]. B7-H7 mainly expresses on macrophages, monocytes, and activated lymphocytes. It is also found in some tissues such as intestine, placenta, breast, kidney, and gallbladder. Like B7-H7, both co-stimulatory and co-inhibitory effects on T cells function have been described for B7-H7 [105]. It has been reported that HHLA2/TMIGD2 signaling induces T cell proliferation and cytokine production during interaction with APC. Nevertheless, the inhibitory role B7-H7 is dominant. B7-H7 can suppress T cells proliferation and cytokine production [106, 107]. It has been shown that stimulation of T cells with anti-CD3/28 antibodies induced B7-H7 expression on T cells. The activated T cells had higher level of B7-H7 and blocking HHLA2/TMIGD2 signaling resulted in higher proliferation of T cells. TNF-α and IFN-γ secretion were decreased in B7-H7$^+$ T cells. Furthermore, the co-expression of PD-1 and LAG along with B7-H7 on activated T cells suggests that it can be considered as one of the exhausted T cells markers [108]. Metastatic tumors show high level expression of B7-H7 and deletion of this gene suppresses tumor proliferation, migration, and invasion [106].

2.13 Purinergic System

The purinergic system plays an important role in immune response regulation. Adenosine triphosphate (ATP) is the major source of energy in the cells. ATP also releases into extracellular space (eATP) during necrosis and apoptosis or other conditions such as inflammation and hypoxia [109, 110]. eATP as a signaling molecule participates in the regulation of cellular metabolism. eATP signaling shows pro-inflammatory effects. ATP signaling results in T cell activation and inhibition of Tregs, while adenosine derived from eATP degradation by ectonucleotidases causes immunosuppression [109, 111]. Ectonucleotidase family includes several enzymes such as ectonucleoside triphosphate phosphohydrolase (ENTPDase) CD39, ecto-nucleotide pyrophosphatases/phosphodiesterases 1 (ENPP1) or CD203a, 5′-ecto-nucleotidase CD73, and CD38/NADase [109, 112]. ATP signaling is mediated through P2 purinergic receptors (P2X and P2Y families) [110], whereas adenosine interacts with P1 receptors on the cell surface. P1 comprises four members including A1R, A2AR, A2BR, and A3R [113]. Targeting of adenosine receptors, especially A2AR and A2BR, can enhance the antitumor immune response [114].

CD39 is a membrane protein that consists of an extracellular hydrophobic domain with five conserved domains, two transmembrane domains, followed by a small cytoplasmic domain [110]. It is expressed on immune cells including monocytes/macrophages, DCs, B cells, NK cells, Tregs, and neutrophils. CD39 dephosphorylates ATP to AMP and CD73 converts the AMP derived from the enzymatic activity of CD39 into adenosine. CD39/CD73 pathway causes the accumulation of adenosine molecules and converts the inflammatory milieu to an anti-inflammatory state that can limit inflammation [109, 110, 112]. CD73 is a homodimer of two identical subunits that are anchored to the cell membrane by a GPI. It is expressed on different tissues and leukocytes [110, 115]. CD39 and CD73 are strongly expressed on Tregs and boost the suppressive activity of these cells [110]. CD39 expression is increased in chronic infections and cancers and it is involved in the tumor progression. Therefore, CD39 is considered as an exhaustion marker [110, 112]. CD39/CD73 axis contributes to tumor immune escape by inhibiting functions of T cells, NK cells, and DCs. In this regard, CD39 and CD73 inhibitors can be effective in the treatment of cancers by enhancing the antitumor immune response [110, 111, 116]. Besides the CD39/CD73 pathway, there is an alternative pathway for producing adenosine consisting of CD38/CD203a/CD73 molecules. CD38 generates ADP Ribose (ADPR) from nicotinamide adenine dinucleotide (NAD^+), or by the degradation of cyclic ADPR, and then CD203a metabolizes ADPR to AMP, which, in turn, is converted to adenosine by CD73. CD203 can directly produce AMP from ATP [117–119]. In addition to CD38, it has been demonstrated that CD157 can convert NAD^+ to ADPR [120].

2.14 KLRG1

Killer-cell lectin-like receptor G1 (KLRG1) is an immune checkpoint with a C-type lectin-like domain (CTLD) in the extracellular region and an ITIM motif in the cytoplasmic domain. KLRG1 is known as a senescence marker and also can participate in T cell exhaustion. It belongs to the lectin family and is detected on NK cells, $CD8^+$ T cells, $CD4^+$ T cells, and group 2 innate lymphoid cells (ILC2). KLRG1 is highly expressed on terminally differentiated T cells. In addition, KLRG1 is expressed on a subset of $CD4^+$ $Foxp3^+$ Tregs [121–124]. KLRG1 can interact with cadherin receptors including E-, N-, and R-cadherin. N- and R-cadherin are found in the nervous system, whereas E-cadherin is mainly expressed on epithelial cells [122]. Interaction of soluble E-cadherin with KLRG1 reduces cytokine production and cytotoxicity of T cells. KLRG1 is upregulated during chronic infections such as CMV and HIV [121, 125]. Expression of KLRG1 along with TIGIT and CD160 has been demonstrated on partially exhausted $CD8^+$ T cells [126]. Li MH et al. showed that KLRG1 expression was increased on NK cells during HBV infection and could reduce the production of IFN-γ in NK cells [127]. Overexpression of KLRG1 has been reported on $CD4^+$ T cells of active tuberculosis patients. Interestingly, these cells had higher IL-2 and IFN-γ production than KLRG-negative T cells but had a higher apoptosis rate and shorter lifespan. Secretion of IL-2 and IFN-γ were increased following KLRG1 blocking. It seems that tuberculosis infection caused an increase in short-lived terminally differentiated $KLRG1^+$ T cells [123]. $KLRG1^+$ Tregs are terminally differentiated cells. This subset has higher expression of CTLA-4 and CD39 and shows more potent suppressive properties. The association of $KLRG1^+$ Tregs with autoimmune diseases and cancers has been documented: for example, the correlation of the increase of these cells with the severity of autoimmune EAE and the increase of $KLRG1^+$ $CD103^+$ Tregs in the case of lung tumor. Considering the importance of $KLRG1^+$ T cells and NK cells in some tumors and infections, blocking this immune checkpoint can helpful in these diseases [124].

2.15 SIRPα–CD47 Axis

The signal regulatory protein (SIRP) family includes SIRPα (CD172a), SIRPβ (CD172b), and SIRPγ (CD172g) molecules. SIRPβ is an activation receptor, whereas SIRPα is an inhibitory receptor. SIRPα is an immune checkpoint found on myeloid cells including monocytes, dendritic cells, granulocytes, and hematopoietic stem cells [128, 129]. CD47 is the ligand of SIRPα expressed on a variety of normal cells. CD47 is known as a "don't eat me" molecule [130]. It has ITIM motifs in its cytoplasmic domain and can promote inhibitory signals via recruiting SH2, SHP-1, and SHP-2 that leads to the disruption of phagocyte cells functions. SIRPα–CD47 signaling can suppress non-muscle myosin IIA function, a molecule that contributes to phagocytosis [131]. In cancers, CD47 is overexpressed and macrophages are defective in phagocytosis. Overexpression of CD47 has been reported in many cancers such as ovarian, breast, bladder, and colon cancers and it is involved in the tumor immune escape. CD47 blocking antibodies can enhance the clearance of cancer cells by phagocytes as well as the induction of antibody-dependent cellular cytotoxicity (ADCC) by NK cells. They can also increase the cross-presentation of tumor antigen by DCs to $CD8^{+}$ T cells [130, 132]. Therefore, blocking of SIRPα–CD47 axis is promising to restore macrophages functions and enhance antitumor immune response. So far, several blocking agents targeting CD47 and SIRPα have been developed [120, 131].

2.16 LILRB

Leucocyte immunoglobulin-like receptors (LILR) are important immunoregulatory receptors. The LILRB family is located on chromosome 19q13.4 [133]. They are divided into two subfamilies: LILRA1-A6 (known as LIR6, ILT1, ILT6, ILT7, ILT11, and ILT8) subfamily that have ITAM and exert activation signals and LILRB1-B5 (known as ILT2, ILT4, ILT5, ILT3, and LIR8) subfamily that promote inhibitory signals through ITIMs. LILR is expressed on monocytes, DCs, B cells, and subsets of NK and T cells and serves as immune checkpoints [134–136].

2.16.1 LILRB1

LILRB1 (ILT2, CD85J) structure includes four extracellular Ig domains and four ITIMs. Upregulation of LILRB1 on immune cells has been reported in different diseases such as viral infection, cancer, and rheumatoid arthritis [137]. It can bind to a wide variety of classical and nonclassical MHC-I molecules (HLA-A, HLAB, HLA-C, HLA-E, HLA-F, and HLA-G) with a high affinity for HLA-G. It can also bind to the UL18 molecule of CMV. LILRB1 interacts with the a3 domain and β2 microglobulin (β2m) subunit of MHC-I. This interaction suppresses macrophage phagocytosis function, thus like CD47, the β2m can be considered as another "don't eat me" molecule [134, 135]. In B cells, LILRB1 signaling causes inhibition of activation, proliferation, and antibody production [135]. LILRB1$^+$ NK cells are increased in cancer. HLA-G, a LILRB1 ligand, also is overexpressed in several cancer types. LILRB1–HLA-G interaction can negatively regulate the activation and cytotoxicity of NK cells [138]. Blockade of LILRB1 can recover NK cell cytotoxicity [139]. LILRB1 expression increases in tumor-associated macrophages [134, 135] LILRB1 signaling during DC differentiation dampens their cytokine production [139]. LILRB1 also can suppress T cell function. It is often co-expressed with senescence marker CD57. Gustafson et al. showed that virus-specific CD8$^+$ T cells expressing LILRB1 are senescent rather than exhausted and LILRB1 blockade can enhance the function of the T cells [138].

2.16.2 LILRB2

LILRB2 (ILT4, CD85D), another member of LILRs, contains three ITIM in the cytoplasmic tail for promoting inhibitory signals. It is expressed on a variety of immune cells including monocytes, DCs, neutrophils, basophils, and activates T cells [137]. LILRB2 ligands include MHC I molecules, nonclassical MHCs, CD1d, and β-amyloid. Interaction of LILRB2 with MHC can occur in a β2m-independent manner. LILRB2 can suppress immune cells such as T cell, B cell, monocyte, and DC [135, 136, 140]. LILRB2 plays a suppressive role in physiological conditions such as pregnancy and pathological conditions including viral and bacterial infections and cancers. Upregulation of LILRB2 induces tolerogenic DCs and inhibits neutrophils phagocytosis [137].

2.16.3 LILRB3

LILRB3 (ILT5 or LIR3 or CD85a) is a protein of the LILR family that has four ITIMs in its cytoplasmic domain. It is expressed on monocytes, DCs, neutrophils, and basophils [137]. LILRB3 inhibits Fc receptor-mediated phagocytosis and antimicrobial functions of neutrophils [141]. Yeboah et al. demonstrated that function of T cells is suppressed following the engagement of LILRB3 on myeloid cells. Furthermore, LILRB3 ligation on monocytes induces immune suppressive features similar to M2 macrophages in these cells [133]. Ming et al. showed that LILRB3 was upregulated on monocytes of sepsis patients. In *Pseudomonas aeruginosa*-infected mice, the function of macrophages expressing LILRB3 including reactive oxygen species (ROS) and nitric oxide (NO) production was suppressed and silencing of this molecule boosted bacterial killing activity and cytokine production of macrophages [142]. The apolipoprotein E (APOE) family is involved in lipid transportation as well as immune regulation. There are three isoforms of APOE including APOE2, APOE3, and APOE4. Among those, APOE4 has been described as a ligand for LILRB3. It strongly interacts with the extracellular domain of LILRB3. Furthermore, APOE3 can weakly bind to LILRB3 [143].

2.16.4 LILRB4

LILRB4 (ILT3, LIR5, CD85K, or HM18) contains two extracellular Ig-like domains and three ITIM in the intracellular tail that recruit phosphatases and inhibit ITAM containing receptors signaling. LILRB4 is expressed on monocytes, macrophages, and lymphocytes but is mainly expressed on monocytic cells. LILRB4 in macrophages attenuates Fc-gamma receptor 1 (FcγRI) signaling and suppresses their phagocytosis and TNF-α production. LILRB4 can be overexpressed on tolerogenic DCs (tDCs) and is involved in the suppression of $CD4^+$ Th cells and induction of Treg cells by tDCs [144]. APOE is defined as an activator ligand of LILRB4. Integrin $\alpha V\beta 3$ is another ligand that binds to gp49B (mouse homolog of LILRB4) [145, 146]. It has been suggested that CD166/activated leukocyte cell adhesion molecule (ALCAM) can bind to LILRB4. CD166 is expressed on myeloid progenitors and activates T cells and several tumor types [147]. Expression of LILRB4 on immune cells has been reported in tumor microenvironment and causes immunosuppression in cancer. LILRB4 is expressed on MDSCs and is associated with poor prognosis in non-small-cell lung cancer (NSCLC). Blocking of LILRB4 can attenuate the suppressive ability of MDSCs [144].

2.16.5 LILRB5

LILRB5 (CD85C, LIR8), the last member of human LILRBs, has two ITIMs in its cytoplasmic tail [137]. It is expressed on immune cells such as monocyte, T cell, NK cell, and mast cell. HLA-B27 and HLA-B7 heavy chains have been suggested as LILRB5 ligands [148]. Although there are limited studies on this molecule, some data indicate the role of LILRB5 in bacterial infection as well as the regulation of mast cell function [137].

2.17 Siglecs

Sialic acid-binding immunoglobulin-like lectins (Siglecs) are molecules that bind to sialic acid-containing glycans (syaloglycans). To date, several different Siglec receptors have been described that are classified into two groups. The first group of Siglecs is conserved in all mammals including Siglec-1, -2, -4, -15. The second group is known as CD33-related Siglecs, which differs between species. The latter group in human includes Siglec-3 (CD33), -5, -6, -7, -8, -9, -10, -11, -14, and Siglec-16 [149, 150]. Sialic acids, the ligands of Siglecs, form the glycocalyx and are broadly found in mammalian cells. They are linked to terminal sequences of glycans in glycoproteins and glycolipids of the cells. Sialoglycans can be abnormally expressed on tumor cells [151–153]. Siglecs can mediate inhibitory or activating signals based on their cytoplasmic domain's structure. Siglec-5 to Siglec-11 are inhibitory Siglecs and contain ITIM and/or ITIM-like motifs that recruit tyrosine phosphatases. Siglec-14, -15, -16 are activating receptors and signal through DAP10/12, an adaptor protein containing ITAM motifs, that leads to transcription of pro-inflammatory cytokines genes [150, 154] Siglec-1 and Siglec-4 do not have inhibitory or activation motifs. It seems that they contribute to cell–cell interaction [154].

Siglecs are mainly expressed by hematopoietic cells; however, they can be present in other cells, for example, Siglec-4 is a myelin-associated glycoprotein [154]. Monocytes, macrophages, and DCs express Siglec-1, -3, -7, -9 (and also some other Siglecs depending on cell type) on their surface [150]. Siglec-9 can bind to sialylated glycophorin A on erythrocytes and dampen the neutrophil activation [149]. Furthermore, it has been shown that Siglec-9 interacts with high molecular weight hyaluronan (HMW-HA) and prevents oxidative burst and neutrophil extracellular trap (NET) formation [155]. Antibody targeting Siglec-7 induces the secretion of pro-inflammatory cytokines from monocytes [156]. Eosinophils, basophils, and mast cells display Siglec-7 and Siglec-8 on the cell membrane [149]. Siglec-7 engagement limits IgE-mediated mast cell and basophil activation [157]. Siglec-7 crosslinking reduces peroxidase secretion from GM-CSF-activated eosinophils [158]. NK cells highly express Siglec-7. They also express Siglec-9 and -3. Interactions of Siglec-7 and -9 with sialoglycans of tumor cells suppresses NK cells cytotoxicity. Blocking Siglec-7 and -9 can recover NK cells activity. In T cells, expression of Siglec-7 and -9 has been reported and is upregulated in activated T cells. Siglec-9 is highly expressed on $CD8^{+}$ TILs in several cancers along with other inhibitory receptors such as PD-1 and TIM-3 [149, 153, 159]. Engagement of siglec-9 by its ligands or a specific antibody leads to reduction of cytotoxicity and cytokine production of T cells [160]. DCs may express Siglec-3, -5, -7, and -9, which are all inhibitory and negatively modulate DC function. Siglec-14, -15, and -16 are activating and can be expressed on human myeloid cells. However, an inhibitory role of Siglec-15 has been reported in TILs. The binding of CD24 on tumor cells to Siglec-10 on TAMs induces a "don't eat me" signal and inhibits the phagocytic function of these cells. Blocking of CD24–Siglec-10 interaction enhances the phagocytosis ability of macrophages [153, 161]. Siglec-2 (CD22) is the major Siglec present on the B cell surface. CD22 has ITIM domains for induction inhibitory signal. CD22 signaling induces tolerance in B cells and suppresses its functions [162]. Mice lacking CD22 are prone to develop autoimmune disease [149]. Moreover, CD22 can recruit Grb2 and Shc, which regulate cell survival through the activation of the MAP kinase pathway [162].

2.18 CD200R

CD200 receptor (CD200R) belongs to the Ig superfamily. Five types of CD200 receptors have been identified (including CD200R1-R5), of which the CD200R1 has the highest affinity for binding to the CD200 and is mainly expressed on myeloid cells as well as lymphoid cells such as NK and T cells [163]. Its ligand, CD200 (OX2), is also a member of the Ig superfamily, which has been found in a wide range of cells including epithelial cells, endothelial cells, fibroblasts, and tumor cells. CD200 is especially overexpressed in hematological malignancies such as AML. CD200R signaling inhibits the immune functions of NK and T cells [161, 164]. It has been demonstrated that overexpression of CD200R in *Salmonella* and *Schistosoma* infections in animal models is associated with impaired T cell function [165]. It can also inhibit inflammatory macrophage activity and cytokine production [163]. Furthermore, CD200 expression can cause expansion of Tregs and MDSCs populations in tumors [166]. The signaling pathway of CD200R is different from other inhibitory molecules. It has no ITIM motif in its intracellular tail, and signal transduction is carried by recruiting tyrosine kinase 1 (DOK1) and DOK2 adaptor proteins and finally inhibition of the MAPK pathway [161, 167].

2.19 LAIR-1

Leukocyte-associated Ig-like receptor (LAIR)-1 or CD305 is an inhibitory immune checkpoint that belongs to the Ig superfamily and is encoded on chromosome 19 [168]. LAIR-1 contains two ITIMs in its cytoplasmic domain that can recruit SHP-1. It can be expressed on immune cells including T cells, B cells, NK cells, eosinophils, basophils, and especially on monocytes, macrophages, and DCs [168, 169]. Collagens (particularly Collagen XVII) and collagen-containing proteins such as collagenous C-type lectin and C1q are the ligands of LAIR-1 [169–171]. This interaction occurs through the conserved Gly-Pro-Hyp repeats of the collagen [170]. Interestingly, some tumors increase collagen production, which acts as a LAIR-1 ligand to reduce the antitumor immune responses [172]. Expression of LAIR-1 is increased on macrophages and DCs during inflammation and engagement of this receptor can inhibit activation of these cells, which indicates the regulatory role of this molecule in inflammation [169]. In neutrophils, LAIR-1 signaling inhibits ROS production [171]. Furthermore, it has been shown that LAIR-1 cross-linking can disrupt TCR signaling and T cell activation as well as BCR-mediated signaling in B cells and inhibits NK-mediated cytotoxicity [172–174].

2.20 CD300

The CD300 family genes consist of seven members in alphabetical order "a to g," located on chromosome 7 in humans. In mice, these genes consist of nine members that are located on chromosome 11. Among the CD300 family, CD300a and CD300f are inhibitory molecules and have ITIMs in their cytoplasmic tails. CD300a expression has been reported on NK cells, T cells, B cells, monocytes, DCs, and granulocytes. It has been demonstrated that triggering CD300a signaling by cross-linking antibodies inhibits NK cell cytotoxicity, activates B and T cell, blocks IgE-mediated mediators release from mast cell, and reduces eosinophil migration and survival. CD300f is expressed on monocytes, DCs, and granulocytes [175]. Stimulation with anti-CD3 and anti-CD28 antibodies can increase the expression of CD300a on $CD4^+$ T cells. Hypoxia condition or the presence of LPS and IFN-γ have a positive effect on the CD300a expression on monocytes. CD300a binds to apoptotic or dead cells. Phosphatidylserine (PtdSer) and phosphatidylethanolamine (PE), which are exposed on the outer leaflet of apoptotic cell membranes act as an eat-signal for phagocytes. CD300a expressed on macrophages binds to these two ligands and inhibits the engulfment of apoptotic/dead cells [176]. It has also been shown that tumor cells inhibit the cytotoxicity of NK through the CD300a–PtdSer interaction [177]. The role of these inhibitory molecules in viral infections has also been investigated [178]. Vitallé et al. showed that $CD300a^+$ $CD4^+$ T cells were associated with disease progression in HIV-infected individuals. They also reported the expansion of $CD300a^+$ $PD1^+$ $CD38^+$ $CD4^+$ T cells in these patients [179]. Furthermore, increased expression of CD300f is also associated with the expansion of HIV infection [180]. Recently, it has been revealed that overexpression of CD300a on NK cells suppressed the cytotoxic activity and downregulated cytokine production of these cells in HIV infection [181].

2.21 CD101

CD101 (IGSF-2, EWI-101, V7) is a type I integral membrane protein expressed on activated T cells, Tregs, memory T cells, monocytes, granulocytes, and intraepithelial lymphocytes (IELs) of the gut. This protein contains seven extracellular Ig-like domains, a 25 residues transmembrane section, and a 42 residues cytoplasmic domain. So far, no ligand has been identified for CD101 [182, 183]. It can inhibit T cell TCR/CD3-induced proliferation. CD101 signaling suppresses IL-2 expression in T cells through the inhibition of tyrosine kinases and stopping nuclear factor of activated T cells (NFAT) translocation to the nucleus. It can also suppress IL-2RA expression on the surface of T cells [184–186]. It has been found that CD101 molecules on cutaneous DC can inhibit T cell proliferation via induction of IL-10 production in DCs [187]. A study of mouse Tregs has demonstrated that the suppressive property of $CD101^{high}$ Tregs is more than $CD101^{low}$ Tregs [185]. CD101 plays an important anti-inflammatory role in the gut. In the IBD patients, a decrease of CD101 on T cells and monocytes was correlated with higher IL-17 levels and disease severity. In the animal model of chronic colitis, the transfer of $CD101^{-/-}$ T cells led to an increase of Th17 cells and severe colitis [183, 188]. Finally, it has been shown that the expression of CD38 and CD101 is increased on $PD-1^+$ $CD8^+$ T cells in ovarian cancer. Therefore, $PD-1^+$ $CD38^+$ $CD101^+$ $CD8^+$ T cells population can be considered as a biomarker for cancer diagnosis and treatment [189].

2.22 Stabilin-1

Stabilin-1 (also known as CLEVER-1 or FEEL-1) is another receptor for PtdSer and participates in apoptotic cells clearance (Fig. 2.2). Stabilin-1 is expressed on various cells, including anti-inflammatory M2 macrophages, sinusoidal endothelial cells of liver, spleen, and lymph nodes. Besides, other functions have been defined for Stabilin-1, such as leukocyte trafficking and endocytosis of lipoproteins [190]. Stabilin-1 is considered as a cancer biomarker. Various studies have shown that increased expression of Stabilin-1 is associated with metastasis and poor prognosis of cancer [191]. $Stabilin-1^+$ TAMs suppress Th1 response. Stabilin-1 gene knockdown can increase the secretion of a pro-inflammatory cytokine from macrophages and also IFN-γ synthesis in T cells [192]. Virtakoivu et al. showed that a Stabilin-1 blocker (FP-1305) is effective in inhibiting the growth of solid tumors. They found that the Stabilin-1 inhibitor increases the cross-presentation of tumor antigens by macrophages and enhances the activation of $CD8^+$ T cells [193].

2.23 CLEC12A

C-type lectin domain family 12 member A (CLEC12A) or myeloid inhibitory C-type lectin-like receptor (MICL) belongs to C-type lectin receptors (CLRs) with an extracellular CTLD and one ITIM in its intracellular region, which can recruit SHP-1 and SHP-2 and induces inhibitory signaling. It is expressed on myeloid cells, especially neutrophils and monocytes [194, 195]. Monosodium urate crystals (MSU), an etiological agent of gout, acts as a ligand for CLEC12A. In addition, CLEC12A can bind to pathogen-derived ligands such as hemozoin crystals of *Plasmodium*. Decreased expression of CLEC12A on neutrophils following exposure to MSU is one of the first evidence indicating the role of CLEC12A in inflammatory diseases. Stimulation of monocytes by TLR ligands diminishes the CLEC12A on the cell surface. A study of CLEC12A KO mice revealed the regulatory function of this receptor. The TNF-α level in CLEC12A KO mice was higher during the inflammatory response. In addition, MSU-stimulated CLEC12A KO neutrophils produced a higher amount of ROS and had more migration activity. The correlation of CLEC12A expression levels with disease activity and neutrophil function has been shown in several inflammatory situations including gouty arthritis, rheumatoid arthritis (RA), Crohn's disease, SLE, and Behcet's disease. For example, low expression of CLEC12A in SLE is associated with more active and severe disease. CLEC12A expression regulates the neutrophils functions. In mice with collagen antibody-induced arthritis (CAIA) that were CLEC12A KO, the neutrophil activity and the severity of joint inflammation were greater than in wild-type mice [194].

2.24 DCIR

C-lectin receptor dendritic cell immunoreceptor (DCIR) is another inhibitory receptor of the C-type lectin family that is expressed on myeloid cells and has a common structure with CLEC12A particularly in CTLD and ITIM. DCIR can bond to endogenous ligands including asialo-N-glycans on myeloid cells and exogenous ligands such as gp120 and gp140 proteins of HIV-1 [194]. Negative regulation of TLR responses in myeloid cells by DCIR has been proven. In peritoneal macrophages of mice with high expression of DCIR, TLR9 activation using CpG oligodeoxynucleotides (CpG-ODN) is suppressed and knocking down of DCIR expression can revive TLR9-dependent MAPK signaling and pro-inflammatory cytokine production [196]. DCIR is an important regulatory molecule in immune responses. DCs of DCIR KO mice are more proliferative and they are prone to develop autoimmunity such as experimental EAE and autoimmune sialadenitis [194]. Furthermore, DCIR has a regulatory role in bone metabolism. It has been shown that osteoclasts and DCs can bind to asialo-biantennary N-glycan (NA2) on bone cells via their surface DCIR. This interaction can inhibit osteoclastogenesis [197].

2.25 SIRL-1

SIRL-1 is an inhibitory receptor belonging to the Ig superfamily, which contains two ITIMs for recruiting SHP-1 and SHP-2. It is expressed on myeloid cells such as neutrophils and monocytes. SIRL-1 ligation and signaling using anti-SIRL-1 antibodies can suppress FcR-mediated ROS production in neutrophils or monocytes and NET formation in response to specific stimuli-like MSU [198]. S100 proteins are a family of similar proteins that includes 21 members. Some of the S100 proteins are released during cell damage and act as damage-associated molecular patterns (DAMPs). It has been showed that SIRL-1 binds to S100 proteins. Blocking of this interaction in neutrophils increases ROS production [199]. Staphylococcal α-helical peptides, known as staphylococcal α-type phenol-soluble modulins (PSMs), act as SIRL-1 ligand. Furthermore, anti-microbial peptide cathelicidin LL-37, which is similar to PSMs in terms of structure and function, is considered as an endogenous ligand for SIRL-1 [200].

2.26 Butyrophilins

Butyrophilin (BTN) and butyrophilin-like (BTNL) protein families belong to Ig superfamily receptors and are involved in immune response regulation. BTNs are structurally related to the B7 family proteins. BTNs have IgV and IgC domains in the extracellular structure, without any conventional motifs in the intracellular region; instead, there are B30.2 domains (PRYSPRY) in this region. In humans, the gene loci of these molecules have been identified, including the BTN cluster (consisting of seven genes: BTN3A2, BTN2A2, BTN3A1, BTN2A3ps, BTN3A3, BTN2A1, BTN1A1) and a BTNL (BTNL2), which are located on chromosome 6p22.1 and also a BTNL cluster (consisting of three genes: BTNL8, BTNL3, BTNL9) located on chromosome 5q35. BTNs and BTNLs are expressed on a wide range of immune cells such as B cells, macrophages, and DCs as well as tumors [201–203].

Both activation and inhibitory functions have been reported for BTNs. γδ T cells are a subset of T cells that lack the classic alpha/beta TCR and their TCR consists of gamma and delta chains. These cells are considered innate like T lymphocytes. Skint1 (a mouse BTN) is involved in the thymic selection and homing of Vγ5Vδ1 intraepithelial lymphocytes (IELs). Human BTN3A1 plays an important role in the activation of Vγ9Vδ2 T cells by phosphoantigens (pAgs). pAgs are phosphorylated nonprotein molecules. Bacterial hydroxy-methyl-butyl-pyrophosphate (HMBPP) and endogenous isopentenyl pyrophosphate (IPP) are examples of phosphoproteins. A study of BTN3A-pAg sensing mechanism has shown that pAgs interact with the intracellular B30.2 domain of BTN3A1. BTN3A1 transmits activation signals to γδ T cells. The direct binding of γδTCR and BTN3A1 has not been identified, but the interaction of BTN2A1 with the Vγ9 domain of the TCR has been elucidated. Recent findings show that BTN2A1, together with BNT3A1, may contribute to the $V\gamma9V\delta2^{+}$ TCR engagement and γδT cells activation [201, 204].

The immunomodulatory effects of BTNs have been demonstrated in several studies. Btn2a2 KO mice had more active Th1 and Th2 cells in response to immunization. These mice also showed an increased antitumor response following the administration of an antitumor vaccine (B16-OVA). Mog-induced EAE is more severe in Btn2a2-deficient mice due to boosted Th1 and Th17 responses. On the other hand, it has been found that Btnl1 blocking antibodies in mice worsen the autoimmune disease by enhancing the T cell response. These findings indicate that BTNs can act as a negative regulator of T cell function. In vitro studies have shown that BTN3A positive cells inhibit the proliferation and production of IL-2 and IFN-γ cytokines in T cells. Similar inhibitory functions have been depicted for mouse Btn1a1 and Btnl2 [201]. The γ9δ2T cells are important components of the immune system in TME. Marabelle et al. demonstrated that anti-BTN3A agonist antibody increases the infiltration, proliferation, and activation of $V\gamma9V\delta2^{+}$ T cells in patients with advanced stage cancers [205]. Another study has shown that anti-BTN3A antibodies, in addition to γδ T cells activation, prevent the inhibition of αβ T cells induced by cancer cells. BTN3A1 can inhibit the function of αβ T cells through binding to CD45 N-mannosylated residues. Therefore, targeting this immune checkpoint can be useful in cancer immunotherapy [206].

2.27 Conclusion

The immune system's intricate balance between activation and regulation is crucial for maintaining health and combating pathogens. This chapter has explored the structure, function, and expression of various immune checkpoint molecules and highlighted their critical role in modulating immune responses. Immune checkpoints, such as CTLA-4, PD-1, TIM-3, LAG-3, and others, serve as key regulators of T cell function. These molecules interact with their respective ligands to generate inhibitory signals that prevent excessive immune activation and maintain self-tolerance. However, in the context of chronic infections and cancer, the overexpression of these checkpoints can lead to T cell exhaustion, compromising the immune system's ability to effectively combat pathogens and tumors. The chapter has also highlighted the complexity of immune checkpoint interactions, with many molecules having multiple ligands and some checkpoints exhibiting both inhibitory and stimulatory functions depending on the context. This complexity features the need for a nuanced understanding of these pathways in developing effective immunotherapies. Recent advances in cancer immunotherapy, particularly the success of checkpoint inhibitors targeting CTLA-4 and PD-1/PD-L1, have demonstrated the therapeutic potential of manipulating these pathways. However, the emergence of resistance to single-agent therapies and the heterogeneity of immune checkpoint expression across different cancers and patients highlight the need for combination approaches and personalized strategies. As research in this field progresses, a deeper understanding of the interplay between various immune checkpoints, their regulation in different disease states, and their impact on diverse immune cell populations will be crucial. This knowledge will pave the way for more effective and targeted immunotherapies, not only in cancer but also potentially in chronic infections, autoimmune diseases, and other immune-related disorders.

Acknowledgments The authors gratefully acknowledge the valuable assistance provided by Maryam Sadr.

References

1. Marhelava K, Pilch Z, Bajor M, Graczyk-Jarzynka A, Zagozdzon R. Targeting negative and positive immune checkpoints with monoclonal antibodies in therapy of cancer. Cancer. 2019;11(11):1756.
2. Paluch C, Santos AM, Anzilotti C, Cornall RJ, Davis SJ. Immune checkpoints as therapeutic targets in autoimmunity. Front Immunol. 2018;9:2306.

3. Catakovic K, Klieser E, Neureiter D, Geisberger R. T cell exhaustion: from pathophysiological basics to tumor immunotherapy. Cell Commun Signal. 2017;15(1):1–16.
4. Saeidi A, Zandi K, Cheok YY, Saeidi H, Wong WF, Lee CYQ, et al. T-cell exhaustion in chronic infections: reversing the state of exhaustion and reinvigorating optimal protective immune responses. Front Immunol. 2018;9:2569.
5. Rowshanravan B, Halliday N, Sansom DM. CTLA-4: a moving target in immunotherapy. Blood. 2018;131(1):58–67.
6. Hossen MM, Ma Y, Yin Z, Xia Y, Du J, Huang JY, et al. Current understanding of CTLA-4: from mechanism to autoimmune diseases. Front Immunol. 2023;14:1198365.
7. Lingel H, Brunner-Weinzierl MC. CTLA-4 (CD152): a versatile receptor for immune-based therapy. Semin Immunol. 2019;42:101298.
8. Buchbinder EI, Desai A. CTLA-4 and PD-1 pathways: similarities, differences, and implications of their inhibition. Am J Clin Oncol. 2016;39(1):98–106.
9. Finn PW, He H, Wang Y, Wang Z, Guan G, Listman J, et al. Synergistic induction of CTLA-4 expression by costimulation with TCR plus CD28 signals mediated by increased transcription and messenger ribonucleic acid stability. J Immunol (Baltimore, Md: 1950). 1997;158(9):4074–81.
10. Tivol EA, Borriello F, Schweitzer AN, Lynch WP, Bluestone JA, Sharpe AH. Loss of CTLA-4 leads to massive lymphoproliferation and fatal multiorgan tissue destruction, revealing a critical negative regulatory role of CTLA-4. Immunity. 1995;3(5):541–7.
11. Zhang H, Mi J, Xin Q, Cao W, Song C, Zhang N, et al. Recent research and clinical progress of CTLA-4-based immunotherapy for breast cancer. Front Oncol. 2023;13:1256360.
12. Bardhan K, Anagnostou T, Boussiotis VA. The PD1:PD-L1/2 pathway from discovery to clinical implementation. Front Immunol. 2016;7:550.
13. Keir ME, Butte MJ, Freeman GJ, Sharpe AH. PD-1 and its ligands in tolerance and immunity. Annu Rev Immunol. 2008;26:677–704.
14. Freeman GJ. Structures of PD-1 with its ligands: sideways and dancing cheek to cheek. Proc Natl Acad Sci USA. 2008;105(30):10275–6.
15. Chen RY, Zhu Y, Shen YY, Xu QY, Tang HY, Cui NX, et al. The role of PD-1 signaling in health and immune-related diseases. Front Immunol. 2023;14:1163633.
16. Jubel JM, Barbati ZR, Burger C, Wirtz DC, Schildberg FA. The role of PD-1 in acute and chronic infection. Front Immunol. 2020;11:487.
17. Yi M, Zheng X, Niu M, Zhu S, Ge H, Wu K. Combination strategies with PD-1/PD-L1 blockade: current advances and future directions. Mol Cancer. 2022;21(1):28.
18. Joller N, Kuchroo VK. Tim-3, Lag-3, and TIGIT. Curr Top Microbiol Immunol. 2017;410:127–56.
19. Das M, Zhu C, Kuchroo VK. Tim-3 and its role in regulating anti-tumor immunity. Immunol Rev. 2017;276(1):97–111.
20. Sauer N, Janicka N, Szlasa W, Skinderowicz B, Kołodzińska K, Dwernicka W, et al. TIM-3 as a promising target for cancer immunotherapy in a wide range of tumors. Cancer Immunol Immunother. 2023;72(11):3405–25.
21. van de Weyer PS, Muehlfeit M, Klose C, Bonventre JV, Walz G, Kuehn EW. A highly conserved tyrosine of Tim-3 is phosphorylated upon stimulation by its ligand galectin-9. Biochem Biophys Res Commun. 2006;351(2):571–6.
22. Anderson AC, Joller N, Kuchroo VK. Lag-3, Tim-3, and TIGIT: co-inhibitory receptors with specialized functions in immune regulation. Immunity. 2016;44(5):989–1004.
23. Zhu C, Anderson AC, Schubart A, Xiong H, Imitola J, Khoury SJ, et al. The Tim-3 ligand galectin-9 negatively regulates T helper type 1 immunity. Nat Immunol. 2005;6(12):1245–52.
24. Acharya N, Sabatos-Peyton C, Anderson AC. Tim-3 finds its place in the cancer immunotherapy landscape. J Immunother Cancer. 2020;8(1)
25. Huang YH, Zhu C, Kondo Y, Anderson AC, Gandhi A, Russell A, et al. CEACAM1 regulates TIM-3-mediated tolerance and exhaustion. Nature. 2015;517(7534):386–90.

26. Tang D, Lotze MT. Tumor immunity times out: TIM-3 and HMGB1. Nat Immunol. 2012;13(9):808–10.
27. Segawa K, Nagata S. An apoptotic 'eat me' signal: phosphatidylserine exposure. Trends Cell Biol. 2015;25(11):639–50.
28. Zhu C, Anderson AC, Kuchroo VK. TIM-3 and its regulatory role in immune responses. Curr Top Microbiol Immunol. 2011;350:1–15.
29. Andrews LP, Marciscano AE, Drake CG, Vignali DA. LAG3 (CD223) as a cancer immunotherapy target. Immunol Rev. 2017;276(1):80–96.
30. Aggarwal V, Workman CJ, Vignali DAA. LAG-3 as the third checkpoint inhibitor. Nat Immunol. 2023;24(9):1415–22.
31. Elia AR, Caputo S, Bellone M. Immune checkpoint-mediated interactions between cancer and immune cells in prostate adenocarcinoma and melanoma. Front Immunol. 2018;9:1786.
32. Wang J, Sanmamed MF, Datar I, Su TT, Ji L, Sun J, et al. Fibrinogen-like protein 1 is a major immune inhibitory ligand of LAG-3. Cell. 2019;176(1–2):334–47.e12.
33. Long L, Zhang X, Chen F, Pan Q, Phiphatwatchara P, Zeng Y, et al. The promising immune checkpoint LAG-3: from tumor microenvironment to cancer immunotherapy. Genes Cancer. 2018;9(5–6):176–89.
34. Lichtenegger FS, Rothe M, Schnorfeil FM, Deiser K, Krupka C, Augsberger C, et al. Targeting LAG-3 and PD-1 to enhance T cell activation by antigen-presenting cells. Front Immunol. 2018;9:385.
35. Dashnamoorthy R, Chen B, Galera P, Chang H, Beheshti A, Ghosh S, et al. The immune checkpoint receptors PD-1, PD-L1, TIM-3 and LAG-3 in lymphoma: tumor cell and tumor infiltrating lymphocyte (TIL) expression, patient prognostication, and identification of rational therapeutic targets. Blood. 2017;130(Suppl 1):2750.
36. Blackburn SD, Shin H, Haining WN, Zou T, Workman CJ, Polley A, et al. Coregulation of $CD8^+$ T cell exhaustion by multiple inhibitory receptors during chronic viral infection. Nat Immunol. 2009;10(1):29–37.
37. Wierz M, Pierson S, Guyonnet L, Viry E, Lequeux A, Oudin A, et al. Dual PD1/LAG3 immune checkpoint blockade limits tumor development in a murine model of chronic lymphocytic leukemia. Blood. 2018;131(14):1617–21.
38. Woo S-R, Turnis ME, Goldberg MV, Bankoti J, Selby M, Nirschl CJ, et al. Immune inhibitory molecules LAG-3 and PD-1 synergistically regulate T-cell function to promote Tumoral immune escape. Cancer Res. 2012;72(4):917–27.
39. Du H, Yi Z, Wang L, Li Z, Niu B, Ren G. The co-expression characteristics of LAG3 and PD-1 on the T cells of patients with breast cancer reveal a new therapeutic strategy. Int Immunopharmacol. 2020;78:106113.
40. Roy S, Coulon P-G, Srivastava R, Vahed H, Kim GJ, Walia SS, et al. Blockade of LAG-3 immune checkpoint combined with therapeutic vaccination restore the function of tissue-resident anti-viral $CD8^+$ T cells and protect against recurrent ocular herpes simplex infection and disease. Front Immunol. 2018;9:2922.
41. Agresta L, Hoebe KHN, Janssen EM. The emerging role of CD244 signaling in immune cells of the tumor microenvironment. Front Immunol. 2018;9:2809.
42. Eissmann P, Beauchamp L, Wooters J, Tilton JC, Long EO, Watzl C. Molecular basis for positive and negative signaling by the natural killer cell receptor 2B4 (CD244). Blood. 2005;105(12):4722–9.
43. Waggoner SN, Kumar V. Evolving role of 2B4/CD244 in T and NK cell responses during virus infection. Front Immunol. 2012;3:377.
44. Pahima H, Puzzovio PG, Levi-Schaffer F. 2B4 and CD48: a powerful couple of the immune system. Clinical Immunol (Orlando, Fla). 2019;204:64–8.
45. Sun L, Gang X, Li Z, Zhao X, Zhou T, Zhang S, et al. Advances in understanding the roles of CD244 (SLAMF4) in immune regulation and associated diseases. Front Immunol. 2021;12:648182.

46. Booth C, Gilmour KC, Veys P, Gennery AR, Slatter MA, Chapel H, et al. X-linked lymphoproliferative disease due to SAP/SH2D1A deficiency: a multicenter study on the manifestations, management and outcome of the disease. Blood. 2011;117(1):53–62.
47. Cai G, Freeman GJ. The CD160, BTLA, LIGHT/HVEM pathway: a bidirectional switch regulating T-cell activation. Immunol Rev. 2009;229(1):244–58.
48. Liu W, Garrett SC, Fedorov EV, Ramagopal UA, Garforth SJ, Bonanno JB, et al. Structural Basis of CD160:HVEM Recognition. Structure (London, England: 1993). 2019;27(8):1286–95.e4.
49. Le Bouteiller P, Tabiasco J, Polgar B, Kozma N, Giustiniani J, Siewiera J, et al. CD160: a unique activating NK cell receptor. Immunol Lett. 2011;138(2):93–6.
50. Piotrowska M, Spodzieja M, Kuncewicz K, Rodziewicz-Motowidło S, Orlikowska M. CD160 protein as a new therapeutic target in a battle against autoimmune, infectious and lifestyle diseases. Analysis of the structure, interactions and functions. Eur J Med Chem. 2021;224:113694.
51. Barakonyi A, Rabot M, Marie-Cardine A, Aguerre-Girr M, Polgar B, Schiavon V, et al. Cutting edge: engagement of CD160 by its HLA-C physiological ligand triggers a unique cytokine profile secretion in the cytotoxic peripheral blood NK cell subset. J Immunol (Baltimore, Md: 1950). 2004;173(9):5349–54.
52. Bensussan A, Gluckman E, el Marsafy S, Schiavon V, Mansur IG, Dausset J, et al. BY55 monoclonal antibody delineates within human cord blood and bone marrow lymphocytes distinct cell subsets mediating cytotoxic activity. Proc Natl Acad Sci USA. 1994;91(19):9136–40.
53. Chibueze CE, Yoshimitsu M, Arima N. CD160 expression defines a uniquely exhausted subset of T lymphocytes in HTLV-1 infection. Biochem Biophys Res Commun. 2014;453(3):379–84.
54. Riches JC, Davies JK, McClanahan F, Fatah R, Iqbal S, Agrawal S, et al. T cells from CLL patients exhibit features of T-cell exhaustion but retain capacity for cytokine production. Blood. 2013;121(9):1612–21.
55. Cheung TC, Oborne LM, Steinberg MW, Macauley MG, Fukuyama S, Sanjo H, et al. T cell intrinsic heterodimeric complexes between HVEM and BTLA determine receptivity to the surrounding microenvironment. J Immunol (Baltimore, Md: 1950). 2009;183(11):7286–96.
56. Bengsch B, Seigel B, Ruhl M, Timm J, Kuntz M, Blum HE, et al. Coexpression of PD-1, 2B4, CD160 and KLRG1 on exhausted HCV-specific CD8$^+$ T cells is linked to antigen recognition and T cell differentiation. PLoS Pathog. 2010;6(6):e1000947.
57. Yu X, Zheng Y, Mao R, Su Z, Zhang J. BTLA/HVEM signaling: milestones in research and role in chronic hepatitis B virus infection. Front Immunol. 2019;10:617.
58. Sedy JR, Gavrieli M, Potter KG, Hurchla MA, Lindsley RC, Hildner K, et al. B and T lymphocyte attenuator regulates T cell activation through interaction with herpesvirus entry mediator. Nat Immunol. 2005;6(1):90–8.
59. Gavrieli M, Murphy KM. Association of Grb-2 and PI3K p85 with phosphotyrosile peptides derived from BTLA. Biochem Biophys Res Commun. 2006;345(4):1440–5.
60. Murphy TL, Murphy KM. Slow down and survive: enigmatic immunoregulation by BTLA and HVEM. Annu Rev Immunol. 2010;28:389–411.
61. Ning Z, Liu K, Xiong H. Roles of BTLA in immunity and immune disorders. Front Immunol. 2021;12:654960.
62. Grabmeier-Pfistershammer K, Stecher C, Zettl M, Rosskopf S, Rieger A, Zlabinger GJ, et al. Antibodies targeting BTLA or TIM-3 enhance HIV-1 specific T cell responses in combination with PD-1 blockade. Clin Immunol (Orlando, Fla). 2017;183:167–73.
63. Derré L, Rivals J-P, Jandus C, Pastor S, Rimoldi D, Romero P, et al. BTLA mediates inhibition of human tumor-specific CD8$^+$ T cells that can be partially reversed by vaccination. J Clin Invest. 2010;120(1):157–67.
64. Lan X, Li S, Gao H, Nanding A, Quan L, Yang C, et al. Increased BTLA and HVEM in gastric cancer are associated with progression and poor prognosis. Onco Targets Ther. 2017;10:919–26.

65. Sekar D, Govene L, Del Rio ML, Sirait-Fischer E, Fink AF, Brune B, et al. Downregulation of BTLA on NKT cells promotes tumor immune control in a mouse model of mammary carcinoma. Int J Mol Sci. 2018;19(3)
66. Song J, Wu L. Friend or foe: prognostic and immunotherapy roles of BTLA in colorectal cancer. Front Mol Biosci. 2020;7:148.
67. Solomon BL, Garrido-Laguna I. TIGIT: a novel immunotherapy target moving from bench to bedside. Cancer Immunol Immunother. 2018;67(11):1659–67.
68. Liu S, Zhang H, Li M, Hu D, Li C, Ge B, et al. Recruitment of Grb2 and SHIP1 by the ITT-like motif of TIGIT suppresses granule polarization and cytotoxicity of NK cells. Cell Death Differ. 2013;20(3):456–64.
69. Chiang EY, Mellman I. TIGIT-CD226-PVR axis: advancing immune checkpoint blockade for cancer immunotherapy. J Immunother Cancer. 2022;10(4)
70. Holder KA, Grant MD. TIGIT blockade: a multipronged approach to target the HIV reservoir. Front Cell Infect Microbiol. 2020;10
71. Liu Z, Zhou Q, Wang Z, Zhang H, Zeng H, Huang Q, et al. Intratumoral TIGIT$^+$ CD8$^+$ T-cell infiltration determines poor prognosis and immune evasion in patients with muscle-invasive bladder cancer. J Immunother Cancer. 2020;8(2)
72. Zhang B, Zhao W, Li H, Chen Y, Tian H, Li L, et al. Immunoreceptor TIGIT inhibits the cytotoxicity of human cytokine-induced killer cells by interacting with CD155. Cancer Immunol Immunother. 2016;65(3):305–14.
73. Dougall WC, Kurtulus S, Smyth MJ, Anderson AC. TIGIT and CD96: new checkpoint receptor targets for cancer immunotherapy. Immunol Rev. 2017;276(1):112–20.
74. Sanchez-Correa B, Valhondo I, Hassouneh F, Lopez-Sejas N, Pera A, Bergua JM, et al. DNAM-1 and the TIGIT/PVRIG/TACTILE Axis: novel immune checkpoints for natural killer cell-based cancer immunotherapy. Cancer. 2019;11(6)
75. Fuchs A, Colonna M. The role of NK cell recognition of nectin and nectin-like proteins in tumor immunosurveillance. Semin Cancer Biol. 2006;16(5):359–66.
76. Feng S, Isayev O, Werner J, Bazhin AV. CD96 as a potential immune regulator in cancers. Int J Mol Sci. 2023;24(2)
77. Martinet L, Smyth MJ. Balancing natural killer cell activation through paired receptors. Nat Rev Immunol. 2015;15(4):243–54.
78. Blake SJ, Dougall WC, Miles JJ, Teng MW, Smyth MJ. Molecular pathways: targeting CD96 and TIGIT for cancer immunotherapy. Clin Cancer Res. 2016;22(21):5183–8.
79. Chan CJ, Martinet L, Gilfillan S, Souza-Fonseca-Guimaraes F, Chow MT, Town L, et al. The receptors CD96 and CD226 oppose each other in the regulation of natural killer cell functions. Nat Immunol. 2014;15(5):431–8.
80. Sun H, Huang Q, Huang M, Wen H, Lin R, Zheng M, et al. Human CD96 correlates to natural killer cell exhaustion and predicts the prognosis of human hepatocellular carcinoma. Hepatology (Baltimore, Md). 2019;70(1):168–83.
81. Chiang EY, de Almeida PE, de Almeida Nagata DE, Bowles KH, Du X, Chitre AS, et al. CD96 functions as a co-stimulatory receptor to enhance CD8$^+$ T cell activation and effector responses. Eur J Immunol. 2020;50:891.
82. Zhu Y, Paniccia A, Schulick AC, Chen W, Koenig MR, Byers JT, et al. Identification of CD112R as a novel checkpoint for human T cells. J Exp Med. 2016;213(2):167–76.
83. Murter B, Pan X, Ophir E, Alteber Z, Azulay M, Sen R, et al. Mouse PVRIG has CD8($^+$) T cell-specific Coinhibitory functions and dampens antitumor immunity. Cancer Immunol Res. 2019;7(2):244–56.
84. Wu B, Zhong C, Lang Q, Liang Z, Zhang Y, Zhao X, et al. Poliovirus receptor (PVR)-like protein cosignaling network: new opportunities for cancer immunotherapy. J Exp Clin Cancer Res. 2021;40(1):267.
85. Greaves P, Gribben JG. The role of B7 family molecules in hematologic malignancy. Blood. 2013;121(5):734–44.

86. Ni L, Dong C. New B7 family checkpoints in human cancers. Mol Cancer Ther. 2017;16(7):1203–11.
87. Kanchan RK, Doss D, Khan P, Nasser MW, Mahapatra S. To kill a cancer: targeting the immune inhibitory checkpoint molecule, B7-H3. Biochim Biophys Acta Rev Cancer. 2022;1877(5):188783.
88. Getu AA, Tigabu A, Zhou M, Lu J, Fodstad Ø, Tan M. New frontiers in immune checkpoint B7-H3 (CD276) research and drug development. Mol Cancer. 2023;22(1):43.
89. Flem-Karlsen K, Fodstad O, Tan M, Nunes-Xavier CE. B7-H3 in cancer – beyond immune regulation. Trends Cancer. 2018;4(6):401–4.
90. Yang S, Wei W, Zhao Q. B7-H3, a checkpoint molecule, as a target for cancer immunotherapy. Int J Biol Sci. 2020;16(11):1767.
91. Lupu CM, Eisenbach C, Lupu AD, Kuefner MA, Hoyler B, Stremmel W, et al. Adenoviral B7-H3 therapy induces tumor specific immune responses and reduces secondary metastasis in a murine model of colon cancer. Oncol Rep. 2007;18(3):745–8.
92. Ni L, Dong C. New checkpoints in cancer immunotherapy. Immunol Rev. 2017;276(1):52–65.
93. Kaur G, Janakiram M. B7x—from bench to bedside. ESMO Open. 2019;4(5):e000554.
94. John P, Wei Y, Liu W, Du M, Guan F, Zang X. The B7x immune checkpoint pathway: from discovery to clinical trial. Trends Pharmacol Sci. 2019;40(11):883–96.
95. Smith JB, Stashwick C, Powell DJ. B7-H4 as a potential target for immunotherapy for gynecologic cancers: a closer look. Gynecol Oncol. 2014;134(1):181–9.
96. Wang J-Y, Wang W-P. B7-H4, a promising target for immunotherapy. Cell Immunol. 2020;347:104008.
97. Podojil JR, Miller SD. Potential targeting of B7-H4 for the treatment of cancer. Immunol Rev. 2017;276(1):40–51.
98. Nowak EC, Lines JL, Varn FS, Deng J, Sarde A, Mabaera R, et al. Immunoregulatory functions of VISTA. Immunol Rev. 2017;276(1):66–79.
99. Mehta N, Maddineni S, Mathews II, Andres Parra Sperberg R, Huang P-S, Cochran JR. Structure and functional binding epitope of V-domain Ig suppressor of T cell activation. Cell Rep. 2019;28(10):2509–16.e5.
100. Xu W, Hieu T, Malarkannan S, Wang L. The structure, expression, and multifaceted role of immune-checkpoint protein VISTA as a critical regulator of anti-tumor immunity, autoimmunity, and inflammation. Cell Mol Immunol. 2018;15(5):438–46.
101. ElTanbouly MA, Croteau W, Noelle RJ, Lines JL. VISTA: a novel immunotherapy target for normalizing innate and adaptive immunity. Semin Immunol. 2019;42:101308.
102. Shahbaz S, Dunsmore G, Koleva P, Xu L, Houston S, Elahi S. Galectin-9 and VISTA expression define terminally exhausted T cells in HIV-1 infection. J Immunol. 2020;204(9):2474–91.
103. Zheng M, Zhang Z, Yu L, Wang Z, Dong Y, Tong A, et al. Immune-checkpoint protein VISTA in allergic, autoimmune disease and transplant rejection. Front Immunol. 2023;14:1194421.
104. Wang L, Le Mercier I, Putra J, Chen W, Liu J, Schenk AD, et al. Disruption of the immune-checkpoint VISTA gene imparts a proinflammatory phenotype with predisposition to the development of autoimmunity. Proc Natl Acad Sci USA. 2014;111(41):14846–51.
105. Bolandi N, Derakhshani A, Hemmat N, Baghbanzadeh A, Asadzadeh Z, Afrashteh Nour M, et al. The positive and negative immunoregulatory role of B7 family: promising novel targets in gastric cancer treatment. Int J Mol Sci. 2021;22(19)
106. Li Y, Lv C, Yu Y, Wu B, Zhang Y, Lang Q, et al. KIR3DL3-HHLA2 and TMIGD2-HHLA2 pathways: the dual role of HHLA2 in immune responses and its potential therapeutic approach for cancer immunotherapy. J Adv Res. 2023;47:137–50.
107. Janakiram M, Shah UA, Liu W, Zhao A, Schoenberg MP, Zang X. The third group of the B7-CD28 immune checkpoint family: HHLA2, TMIGD2, B7x, and B7-H3. Immunol Rev. 2017;276(1):26–39.
108. Luu K, Schwarz H, Lundqvist A. B7-H7 is inducible on T cells to regulate their immune response and serves as a marker for exhaustion. Front Immunol. 2021;12:682627.

109. Takenaka MC, Robson S, Quintana FJ. Regulation of the T cell response by CD39. Trends Immunol. 2016;37(7):427–39.
110. Antonioli L, Pacher P, Vizi ES, Hasko G. CD39 and CD73 in immunity and inflammation. Trends Mol Med. 2013;19(6):355–67.
111. Allard B, Longhi MS, Robson SC, Stagg J. The ectonucleotidases CD39 and CD73: novel checkpoint inhibitor targets. Immunol Rev. 2017;276(1):121–44.
112. Canale FP, Ramello MC, Nunez N, Araujo Furlan CL, Bossio SN, Gorosito Serran M, et al. CD39 expression defines cell exhaustion in tumor-infiltrating CD8(+) T cells. Cancer Res. 2018;78(1):115–28.
113. Horenstein AL, Chillemi A, Zini R, Quarona V, Bianchi N, Manfredini R, et al. Cytokine-induced killer cells express CD39, CD38, CD203a, CD73 Ectoenzymes and P1 adenosinergic receptors. Front Pharmacol. 2018;9:196.
114. Allard D, Turcotte M, Stagg J. Targeting A2 adenosine receptors in cancer. Immunol Cell Biol. 2017;95(4):333–9.
115. Allard D, Chrobak P, Allard B, Messaoudi N, Stagg J. Targeting the CD73-adenosine axis in immuno-oncology. Immunol Lett. 2019;205:31–9.
116. Battastini AMO, Figueiró F, Leal DBR, Doleski PH, Schetinger MRC. CD39 and CD73 as promising therapeutic targets: what could be the limitations? Front Pharmacol. 2021;12:633603.
117. Horenstein AL, Chillemi A, Zaccarello G, Bruzzone S, Quarona V, Zito A, et al. A CD38/CD203a/CD73 ectoenzymatic pathway independent of CD39 drives a novel adenosinergic loop in human T lymphocytes. Onco Targets Ther. 2013;2(9):e26246.
118. Ferrero E, Faini AC, Malavasi F. A phylogenetic view of the leukocyte ectonucleotidases. Immunol Lett. 2019;205:51–8.
119. Morandi F, Horenstein A, Rizzo R, Malavasi F. The role of extracellular adenosine generation in the development of autoimmune diseases. Mediat Inflamm. 2018;2018:1–10.
120. Ortolan E, Augeri S, Fissolo G, Musso I, Funaro A. CD157: from immunoregulatory protein to potential therapeutic target. Immunol Lett. 2019;205:59–64.
121. Larsson M, Shankar EM, Che KF, Saeidi A, Ellegard R, Barathan M, et al. Molecular signatures of T-cell inhibition in HIV-1 infection. Retrovirology. 2013;10:31.
122. Henson SM, Akbar AN. KLRG1--more than a marker for T cell senescence. Age (Dordr). 2009;31(4):285–91.
123. Hu Z, Zhao HM, Li CL, Liu XH, Barkan D, Lowrie DB, et al. The role of KLRG1 in human CD4+ T-cell immunity against tuberculosis. J Infect Dis. 2018;217(9):1491–503.
124. Borys SM, Bag AK, Brossay L, Adeegbe DO. The Yin and Yang of targeting KLRG1(+) Tregs and effector cells. Front Immunol. 2022;13:894508.
125. Thimme R, Appay V, Koschella M, Panther E, Roth E, Hislop AD, et al. Increased expression of the NK cell receptor KLRG1 by virus-specific CD8 T cells during persistent antigen stimulation. J Virol. 2005;79(18):12112–6.
126. Long SA, Thorpe J, DeBerg HA, Gersuk V, Eddy J, Harris KM, et al. Partial exhaustion of CD8 T cells and clinical response to teplizumab in new-onset type 1 diabetes. Sci Immunol. 2016;1(5)
127. Li MH, Zhang QF, Yin WW, Zhang DZ, Ren H. Functional effects of killer cell lectin-like receptor subfamily G member 1 on natural killer cells in chronic hepatitis B infection. Zhonghua gan zang bing za zhi = Zhonghua ganzangbing zazhi = Chin J Hepatol. 2018;26(8):585–9.
128. Takahashi S. Molecular functions of SIRPα and its role in cancer. Biomed Rep. 2018;9(1):3–7.
129. Liu X, Kwon H, Li Z, Fu Y-X. Is CD47 an innate immune checkpoint for tumor evasion? J Hematol Oncol. 2017;10(1):12.
130. Hayat SMG, Bianconi V, Pirro M, Jaafari MR, Hatamipour M, Sahebkar A. CD47: role in the immune system and application to cancer therapy. Cell Oncol (Dordr). 2019;43:19.
131. Veillette A, Chen J. SIRPalpha-CD47 immune checkpoint blockade in anticancer therapy. Trends Immunol. 2018;39(3):173–84.

132. Jia X, Yan B, Tian X, Liu Q, Jin J, Shi J, et al. CD47/SIRPα pathway mediates cancer immune escape and immunotherapy. Int J Biol Sci. 2021;17(13):3281–7.
133. Yeboah M, Papagregoriou C, Jones DC, Chan HTC, Hu G, McPartlan JS, et al. LILRB3 (ILT5) is a myeloid cell checkpoint that elicits profound immunomodulation. JCI Insight. 2020;5(18)
134. Zhao J, Zhong S, Niu X, Jiang J, Zhang R, Li Q. The MHC class I-LILRB1 signalling axis as a promising target in cancer therapy. Scand J Immunol. 2019;90(5):e12804.
135. Kang X, Kim J, Deng M, John S, Chen H, Wu G, et al. Inhibitory leukocyte immunoglobulin-like receptors: immune checkpoint proteins and tumor sustaining factors. Cell Cycle (Georgetown, Tex). 2016;15(1):25–40.
136. Wang Q, Song H, Cheng H, Qi J, Nam G, Tan S, et al. Structures of the four Ig-like domain LILRB2 and the four-domain LILRB1 and HLA-G1 complex. Cell Mol Immunol. 2019;17:966.
137. Deng M, Chen H, Liu X, Huang R, He Y, Yoo B, et al. Leukocyte immunoglobulin-like receptor subfamily B: therapeutic targets in cancer. Antibody Ther. 2021;4(1):16–33.
138. Gustafson CE, Qi Q, Hutter-Saunders J, Gupta S, Jadhav R, Newell E, et al. Immune checkpoint function of CD85j in CD8 T cell differentiation and aging. Front Immunol. 2017;8:692.
139. Roberti MP, Julia EP, Rocca YS, Amat M, Bravo AI, Loza J, et al. Overexpression of CD85j in TNBC patients inhibits Cetuximab-mediated NK-cell ADCC but can be restored with CD85j functional blockade. Eur J Immunol. 2015;45(5):1560–9.
140. Fanger NA, Cosman D, Peterson L, Braddy SC, Maliszewski CR, Borges L. The MHC class I binding proteins LIR-1 and LIR-2 inhibit fc receptor-mediated signaling in monocytes. Eur J Immunol. 1998;28(11):3423–34.
141. Zhao Y, van Woudenbergh E, Zhu J, Heck AJR, van Kessel KPM, de Haas CJC, et al. The orphan immune receptor LILRB3 modulates fc receptor-mediated functions of neutrophils. J Immunol (Baltimore, Md: 1950). 2020;204(4):954–66.
142. Ming S, Li M, Wu M, Zhang J, Zhong H, Chen J, et al. Immunoglobulin-like transcript 5 inhibits macrophage-mediated bacterial killing and antigen presentation during sepsis. J Infect Dis. 2019;220(10):1688–99.
143. Zhou J, Wang Y, Huang G, Yang M, Zhu Y, Jin C, et al. LilrB3 is a putative cell surface receptor of APOE4. Cell Res. 2023;33(2):116–30.
144. Yang T, Qian Y, Liang X, Wu J, Zou M, Deng M. LILRB4, an immune checkpoint on myeloid cells. Blood Sci (Baltimore, Md). 2022;4(2):49–56.
145. Deng M, Gui X, Kim J, Xie L, Chen W, Li Z, et al. LILRB4 signalling in leukaemia cells mediates T cell suppression and tumour infiltration. Nature. 2018;562(7728):605–9.
146. Sharma N, Atolagbe OT, Ge Z, Allison JP. LILRB4 suppresses immunity in solid tumors and is a potential target for immunotherapy. J Exp Med. 2021;218(7):e20201811.
147. Xu Z, Chang CC, Li M, Zhang QY, Vasilescu EM, D'Agati V, et al. ILT3.Fc-CD166 interaction induces inactivation of p70 S6 kinase and inhibits tumor cell growth. J Immunol (Baltimore, Md: 1950). 2018;200(3):1207–19.
148. Zhang Z, Hatano H, Shaw J, Olde Nordkamp M, Jiang G, Li D, et al. The leukocyte immunoglobulin-like receptor family member LILRB5 binds to HLA-class I heavy chains. PLoS One. 2015;10(6):e0129063.
149. Barenwaldt A, Laubli H. The sialoglycan-Siglec glyco-immune checkpoint – a target for improving innate and adaptive anti-cancer immunity. Expert Opin Ther Targets. 2019;23(10):839–53.
150. Lubbers J, Rodriguez E, van Kooyk Y. Modulation of immune tolerance via Siglec-sialic acid interactions. Front Immunol. 2018;9:2807.
151. Laubli H, Varki A. Sialic acid-binding immunoglobulin-like lectins (Siglecs) detect self-associated molecular patterns to regulate immune responses. Cell Mol Life Sci. 2019;77:593.
152. Crocker PR, Paulson JC, Varki A. Siglecs and their roles in the immune system. Nat Rev Immunol. 2007;7(4):255–66.

153. van de Wall S, Santegoets KC, van Houtum EJ, Büll C, Adema GJ. Sialoglycans and siglecs can shape the tumor immune microenvironment. Trends Immunol. 2020;41(4):274–85.
154. Bornhöfft KF, Goldammer T, Rebl A, Galuska SP. Siglecs: a journey through the evolution of sialic acid-binding immunoglobulin-type lectins. Dev Compar Immunol. 2018;86:219–31.
155. Secundino I, Lizcano A, Roupe KM, Wang X, Cole JN, Olson J, et al. Host and pathogen hyaluronan signal through human siglec-9 to suppress neutrophil activation. J Mol Med (Berl). 2016;94(2):219–33.
156. Varchetta S, Brunetta E, Roberto A, Mikulak J, Hudspeth KL, Mondelli MU, et al. Engagement of Siglec-7 receptor induces a pro-inflammatory response selectively in monocytes. PLoS One. 2012;7(9):e45821.
157. Mizrahi S, Gibbs BF, Karra L, Ben-Zimra M, Levi-Schaffer F. Siglec-7 is an inhibitory receptor on human mast cells and basophils. J Allergy Clin Immunol. 2014;134(1):230–3.
158. Legrand F, Landolina N, Zaffran I, Emeh RO, Chen E, Klion AD, et al. Siglec-7 on peripheral blood eosinophils: surface expression and function. Allergy. 2019;74(7):1257–65.
159. Jandus C, Boligan KF, Chijioke O, Liu H, Dahlhaus M, Demoulins T, et al. Interactions between Siglec-7/9 receptors and ligands influence NK cell-dependent tumor immunosurveillance. J Clin Invest. 2014;124(4):1810–20.
160. Haas Q, Boligan KF, Jandus C, Schneider C, Simillion C, Stanczak MA, et al. Siglec-9 regulates an effector memory CD8(+) T-cell subset that congregates in the melanoma tumor microenvironment. Cancer Immunol Res. 2019;7(5):707–18.
161. Moon SY, Han M, Ryu G, Shin SA, Lee JH, Lee CS. Emerging immune checkpoint molecules on cancer cells: CD24 and CD200. Int J Mol Sci. 2023;24(20)
162. Clark EA, Giltiay NV. CD22: a regulator of innate and adaptive B cell responses and autoimmunity. Front Immunol. 2018;9:2235.
163. Li D, Wang Y, Tang L, Jin X, Xia C, Xu H, et al. CD200-CD200R1 signalling attenuates imiquimod-induced psoriatic inflammation by inhibiting the activation of skin inflammatory macrophages. Int Immunopharmacol. 2020;78:106046.
164. Norde WJ, Hobo W, van der Voort R, Dolstra H. Coinhibitory molecules in hematologic malignancies: targets for therapeutic intervention. Blood. 2012;120(4):728–36.
165. Gannavaram S, Bhattacharya P, Ismail N, Kaul A, Singh R, Nakhasi HL. Modulation of innate immune mechanisms to enhance Leishmania vaccine-induced immunity: role of coinhibitory molecules. Front Immunol. 2016;7:187.
166. Xiong Z, Mesias EA, Pluhar GE, Rathe SK, Largaespada DA, Sham YY, et al. CD200 checkpoint reversal: a novel approach to immunotherapy. Clin Cancer Res. 2020;26(1):232–41.
167. Hatherley D, Lea SM, Johnson S, Barclay AN. Structures of CD200/CD200 receptor family and implications for topology, regulation, and evolution. Structure (London, England: 1993). 2013;21(5):820–32.
168. Meyaard L. The inhibitory collagen receptor LAIR-1 (CD305). J Leukoc Biol. 2008;83(4):799–803.
169. Carvalheiro T, Garcia S, Pascoal Ramos MI, Giovannone B, Radstake TR, Marut W, et al. Leukocyte associated immunoglobulin like receptor 1 regulation and function on monocytes and dendritic cells during inflammation. Front Immunol. 2020;11:1793.
170. Lebbink RJ, de Ruiter T, Adelmeijer J, Brenkman AB, van Helvoort JM, Koch M, et al. Collagens are functional, high affinity ligands for the inhibitory immune receptor LAIR-1. J Exp Med. 2006;203(6):1419–25.
171. Olde Nordkamp MJ, van Eijk M, Urbanus RT, Bont L, Haagsman HP, Meyaard L. Leukocyte-associated Ig-like receptor-1 is a novel inhibitory receptor for surfactant protein D. J Leukoc Biol. 2014;96(1):105–11.
172. Rygiel TP, Stolte EH, de Ruiter T, van de Weijer ML, Meyaard L. Tumor-expressed collagens can modulate immune cell function through the inhibitory collagen receptor LAIR-1. Mol Immunol. 2011;49(1–2):402–6.

173. Maasho K, Masilamani M, Valas R, Basu S, Coligan JE, Borrego F. The inhibitory leukocyte-associated Ig-like receptor-1 (LAIR-1) is expressed at high levels by human naive T cells and inhibits TCR mediated activation. Mol Immunol. 2005;42(12):1521–30.
174. der Vuurst V, de Vries AR, Clevers H, Logtenberg T, Meyaard L. Leukocyte-associated immunoglobulin-like receptor-1 (LAIR-1) is differentially expressed during human B cell differentiation and inhibits B cell receptor-mediated signaling. Eur J Immunol. 1999;29(10):3160–7.
175. Borrego F. The CD300 molecules: an emerging family of regulators of the immune system. Blood. 2013;121(11):1951–60.
176. Zenarruzabeitia O, Vitallé J, Eguizabal C, Simhadri VR, Borrego F. The biology and disease relevance of CD300a, an inhibitory receptor for phosphatidylserine and phosphatidylethanolamine. J Immunol. 2015;194(11):5053–60.
177. Lankry D, Rovis TL, Jonjic S, Mandelboim O. The interaction between CD 300a and phosphatidylserine inhibits tumor cell killing by NK cells. Eur J Immunol. 2013;43(8):2151–61.
178. Vitallé J, Terrén I, Orrantia A, Zenarruzabeitia O, Borrego F. CD300 receptor family in viral infections. Eur J Immunol. 2019;49(3):364–74.
179. Vitallé J, Terrén I, Gamboa-Urquijo L, Orrantia A, Tarancón-Díez L, Genebat M, et al. Altered expression of CD300a inhibitory receptor on CD4+ T cells from human immunodeficiency virus-1-infected patients: association with disease progression markers. Front Immunol. 2018;9:1709.
180. Vitallé J, Zenarruzabeitia O, Terrén I, Plana M, Guardo AC, Leal L, et al. Monocytes phenotype and cytokine production in human immunodeficiency virus-1 infected patients receiving a modified vaccinia Ankara-based HIV-1 vaccine: relationship to CD300 molecules expression. Front Immunol. 2017;8:836.
181. Vitallé J, Terrén I, Orrantia A, Pérez-Garay R, Vidal F, Iribarren JA, et al. CD300a inhibits CD16-mediated NK cell effector functions in HIV-1-infected patients. Cell Mol Immunol. 2019;16(12):940–2.
182. Ruegg CL, Rivas A, Madani ND, Zeitung J, Laus R, Engleman EG. V7, a novel leukocyte surface protein that participates in T cell activation. II. Molecular cloning and characterization of the V7 gene. J Immunol (Baltimore, Md: 1950). 1995;154(9):4434–43.
183. Wrage M, Kaltwasser J, Menge S, Mattner J. CD101 as an indicator molecule for pathological changes at the interface of host-microbiota interactions. Int J Med Microbiol. 2021;311(4):151497.
184. Rivas A, Ruegg CL, Zeitung J, Laus R, Warnke R, Benike C, et al. V7, a novel leukocyte surface protein that participates in T cell activation. I. Tissue distribution and functional studies. J Immunol (Baltimore, Md: 1950). 1995;154(9):4423–33.
185. Soares LR, Tsavaler L, Rivas A, Engleman EG. V7 (CD101) ligation inhibits TCR/CD3-induced IL-2 production by blocking $Ca2^{+}$ flux and nuclear factor of activated T cell nuclear translocation. J Immunol (Baltimore, Md: 1950). 1998;161(1):209–17.
186. Fernandez I, Zeiser R, Karsunky H, Kambham N, Beilhack A, Soderstrom K, et al. CD101 surface expression discriminates potency among murine $FoxP3^{+}$ regulatory T cells. J Immunol (Baltimore, Md: 1950). 2007;179(5):2808–14.
187. Bouloc A, Bagot M, Delaire S, Bensussan A, Boumsell L. Triggering CD101 molecule on human cutaneous dendritic cells inhibits T cell proliferation via IL-10 production. Eur J Immunol. 2000;30(11):3132–9.
188. Schey R, Dornhoff H, Baier JL, Purtak M, Opoka R, Koller AK, et al. CD101 inhibits the expansion of colitogenic T cells. Mucosal Immunol. 2016;9(5):1205–17.
189. Zhou J, Wang W, Liang Z, Ni B, He W, Wang D. Clinical significance of CD38 and CD101 expression in PD-1^{+} $CD8^{+}$ T cells in patients with epithelial ovarian cancer. Oncol Lett. 2020;20(1):724–32.
190. Park S-Y, Kim I-S. Stabilin receptors: role as phosphatidylserine receptors. Biomolecules. 2019;9(8):387.

191. Hollmén M, Figueiredo CR, Jalkanen S. New tools to prevent cancer growth and spread: a 'Clever' approach. Br J Cancer. 2020;123:1–9.
192. Palani S, Elima K, Ekholm E, Jalkanen S, Salmi M. Monocyte stabilin-1 suppresses the activation of Th1 lymphocytes. J Immunol. 2016;196(1):115–23.
193. Virtakoivu R, Rannikko JH, Viitala M, Vaura F, Takeda A, Lönnberg T, et al. Systemic blockade of Clever-1 elicits lymphocyte activation alongside checkpoint molecule downregulation in patients with solid tumors: results from a phase I/II clinical trial. Clin Cancer Res. 2021;27(15):4205–20.
194. McLeish KR, Fernandes MJ. Understanding inhibitory receptor function in neutrophils through the lens of CLEC12A. Immunol Rev. 2023;314(1):50–68.
195. Fischer S, Stegmann F, Gnanapragassam VS, Lepenies B. From structure to function – ligand recognition by myeloid C-type lectin receptors. Comput Struct Biotechnol J. 2022;20:5790–812.
196. Zhao X, Shen Y, Hu W, Chen J, Wu T, Sun X, et al. DCIR negatively regulates CpG-ODN-induced IL-1β and IL-6 production. Mol Immunol. 2015;68(2 Pt C):641–7.
197. Kaifu T, Yabe R, Maruhashi T, Chung S-H, Tateno H, Fujikado N, et al. DCIR and its ligand asialo-biantennary N-glycan regulate DC function and osteoclastogenesis. J Exp Med. 2021;218(12)
198. Fernandes MJ, Naccache PH. The role of inhibitory receptors in monosodium urate crystal-induced inflammation. Front Immunol. 2018;9:1883.
199. Rumpret M, von Richthofen HJ, van der Linden M, Westerlaken GHA, Talavera Ormeño C, Low TY, et al. Recognition of S100 proteins by signal inhibitory receptor on Leukocytes-1 negatively regulates human neutrophils. Eur J Immunol. 2021;51(9):2210–7.
200. Rumpret M, von Richthofen HJ, van der Linden M, Westerlaken GHA, Talavera Ormeño C, van Strijp JAG, et al. Signal inhibitory receptor on leukocytes-1 recognizes bacterial and endogenous amphipathic α-helical peptides. FASEB J. 2021;35(10):e21875.
201. Rhodes DA, Reith W, Trowsdale J. Regulation of immunity by Butyrophilins. Annu Rev Immunol. 2016;34:151–72.
202. Abeler-Dörner L, Swamy M, Williams G, Hayday AC, Bas A. Butyrophilins: an emerging family of immune regulators. Trends Immunol. 2012;33(1):34–41.
203. Kumari R, Hosseini ES, Warrington KE, Milonas T, Payne KK. Butyrophilins: dynamic regulators of protective T cell immunity in cancer. Int J Mol Sci. 2023;24(10)
204. Rigau M, Uldrich AP, Behren A. Targeting butyrophilins for cancer immunotherapy. Trends Immunol. 2021;42(8):670–80.
205. Marabelle A, Jungels C, Bono JD, Vey N, Wermke M, Garralda E, et al. 316 EVICTION study: preliminary results in solid tumor patients with ICT01, a first-in-class, gamma9 delta2 T cell activating antibody targeting butyrophilin-3A. J Immunother Cancer. 2020;8(Suppl 3):A194–A5.
206. Payne KK, Mine JA, Biswas S, Chaurio RA, Perales-Puchalt A, Anadon CM, et al. BTN3A1 governs antitumor responses by coordinating αβ and γδ T cells. Science (New York, NY). 2020;369(6506):942–9.

Chapter 3
Genetic and Epigenetic Regulation of Immune Checkpoints

3.1 Introduction

During acute infection, the activation and clonal expansion of T cells lead to the elimination of the pathogen but in chronic infections and cancers, persistent activation leads to T cells hyporesponsiveness. These cells are defective in the proliferation and effector functions such as cytokine production and cytotoxicity and express a range of immune checkpoints on their surface. This status is called T cell exhaustion. Epigenetic remodeling plays an important role in regulating T cell exhaustion. Epigenetic modifications can control cell activities independently of DNA sequence changes. By regulating the access of transcription factors to DNA, epigenetic mechanisms can determine the silencing or activation of genes. Epigenetic modifications are affected by environmental factors, diseases, and drugs. DNA methylation and chromatin remodeling by histone modification (such as histone acetylation and histone methylation) are among the epigenetic mechanisms. The role of transcription factors and epigenetic modifications in determining the immune checkpoint expression profile of lymphocytes has been demonstrated in numerous studies [1, 2]. PD-1 is an important inhibitory molecule under physiological and pathological conditions. The PD-1/PD-L1 axis is essential for regulating T cell responses and controlling inflammation or preventing autoimmunity. Increased expression of PD-1 on tumor-infiltrating $CD4^+$ T cells is associated with cancer progression and poor prognosis. In chronic infections such as lymphocytic choriomeningitis virus (LCMV), the role of PD-1 in suppressing the immune response against the pathogen has been identified [3, 4]. In this chapter, the structure of the PD-1 gene and the regulatory region of its promoter and the important transcription factors in regulating the expression of PD-1 as a main immune checkpoint are explained. In the following, the effects of DNA methylation and histone methylation in the expression of various immune checkpoints are discussed.

L. Tayebi, M. Abdolmaleki, *Immune System Regulation*,
https://doi.org/10.1007/978-981-95-8026-2_3

3.2 PD-1 Gene Structure

The expression of PD-1 has been reported on various immune cells, including T cells, B cells, natural killer (NK) cells, macrophages, and dendritic cells (DCs). Overexpression of PD-1 is a prominent feature of exhausted T cells. PD-1 is a protein belonging to the immunoglobulin family encoded by the PD-1 gene (PDCD1). The PDCD1 gene is located on chromosome 2 in humans and on chromosome 1 in mice. This gene contains five exons with exon 1 produces the signal sequence and exon 2 encodes the extracellular IgV-like domain of PD-1 protein. The stalk and the transmembrane domain are encoded by exon 3, and the cytoplasmic domain and a long 3′-UTR are encoded by exons 4 and 5, respectively. Various regulatory regions have been identified in the PDCD1 gene that control its transcription. Conserved region B (CR-B) and conserved region C (CR-C) are among the first identified regulatory regions that are located at 0.1 Kb and 1.1 Kb upstream of the transcription start site (TSS) of the PDCD1 gene, respectively. CR-B interacts with activator protein 1 (AP-1), while CR-C provides binding sites for various transcription factors such as interferon-stimulated response element (ISRE), nuclear factor-κB (NF-κB), nuclear factor of activated T cells (NFAT), forkhead box protein O1 (FoxO1), and p65; therefore, it plays an important role in regulating PDCD1 gene transcription. There are other regulatory sites near CR-B and CR-C that contain binding sites for RBP-Jκ, B lymphocyte-induced maturation protein 1 (Blimp-1), and T-bet. In addition, there are two enhancers at −3.7 kb and +17.1 kb of PDCD1, which contain STAT-binding sites [5, 6].

3.3 Transcriptional Factors Regulating Immune Checkpoint Expression

Several transcription factors bind to *cis*-regulatory elements at the PDCD1 gene, including NFAT, AP-1 subunit c-Fos, FoxO1, NF-κB, Blimp-1, T-bet, IRF4, and NR4A [7]. Some of the important transcription regulators of PDCD1 gene are discussed in this section.

3.3.1 NFAT

NFAT is an important transcription factor that participates in the transcription of different genes in different cell types. The NFAT family includes five members and some of them are particularly important in immune cells, e.g., NFATc1, which is an effective regulator of T cell activation. Following T cell receptor (TCR) engagement in T cells, NFATc1 becomes activated through the calcineurin pathway and enters the nucleus. NFAT by binding to various transcription factors, including AP-1 in T helper or FoxP3 in Treg, induces the expression of several genes. It has been revealed that NFAT is not only involved in the activation of T cells but also can induce T cell hyporesponsiveness [8, 9]. NFAT can bind to regulatory regions in the promoter of various immune checkpoint genes such as PD-1 and TIM-3 and increases their expression in exhausted CD8⁺ T cells. The NFAT-AP-1 complex plays a critical role in gene expression induced after T cell activation; however, this is not the only pathway of NFAT action. Using CA-RIT-NFAT1 (an engineered type of NFAT1 with constant activity that cannot bind to AP-1) demonstrated that NFAT can bind to the regulatory regions of anergy or exhaustion-related genes independently of AP1. These cells had impaired effector functions and produced low levels of IL-2, while CA-RIT-NFAT1 increased the expression of inhibitory molecules PD-1, TIM-3, and LAG-3. Activation of NFAT is dependent on Ca^{2+}-calcineurin signaling. Inhibitors of this pathway, such as cyclosporin A, limit NFAT activity [9, 10].

3.3.2 Blimp-1

Blimp-1 promotes the differentiation of B cells into plasma cells in the germinal center. The effect of Blimp-1 in the differentiation of other hematopoietic cells has also been proven. Blimp-1 positively regulates the function of effector $CD8^+$ T cells or memory T cells. It has been observed that during chronic viral infection in mice, Blimp-1 was upregulated in exhausted $CD8^+$ T cells. The elevated activity of Blimp-1 in these cells increased the expression of PD-1. Deletion of Blimp-1 was associated with the downregulation of inhibitory receptors. Collectively, the increased levels of Blimp-1 are associated with overexpression of inhibitory molecules in exhausted T cells, while low levels of Blimp-1 contribute to the physiological function of T cells [11]. Zhu et al. showed that Blimp-1 expression is increased in T cells of acute myeloid leukemia (AML) patients. The upregulation of Blimp-1 was related to the increase of inhibitory molecules, especially PD-1 and TIGIT, on $CD4^+$ and $CD8^+$ T cells. After in vitro stimulation, these cells were defective in the production of IFN-γ and IL-2 cytokines, as well as the ability to produce perforin and granzyme B was decreased in Blimp-1^+ $CD8^+$ T cells. Interestingly, Blimp-1 knockdown decreased PD-1 and TIGIT mRNA levels in T cells. In these patients, the majority of T cells expressing Blimp-1 were antigen-experienced cells, while most of Blimp-1^- T cells were naïve cells [12]. Similar results have been reported in the mouse model of chronic toxoplasmosis. Toxoplasma-specific $CD4^+$ T cells were exhausted. PD-1 expression was increased in these cells and they had high levels of Blimp-1. Conditional deletion of Blimp-1 decreased the expression of PD-1, LAG-3, 2B4, and CD160 and restored the function of exhausted T cells [13].

3.3.3 Notch

Notch proteins are membrane receptors and four members of the Notch family have been identified so far. The expression of Notch family proteins on lymphoid progenitors shows that they contribute in lymphoid ontogeny. Notch is involved in the development of lymphoid progenitors into T lymphocytes. In addition, it has been found that Notch activation causes NF-kB activation, proliferation of T cells, and production of cytokines such as IFN-γ. In addition, Notch enhances the cytolytic activity of $CD8^+$ T cells. Notch can be activated after TCR/CD28 signaling in $CD4^+$ and $CD8^+$ T cells. After activation, Notch intracellular domain (NICD) is cleaved by gamma-secretase. NCID enters the nucleus and binds to the recombination signal binding protein (RBP-Jκ), which, along with MAML1 (Mastermind-like 1), forms a coactivator complex. The Notch complex recruits the acetyltransferase p300 and increases histone acetylation, thereby facilitating target gene transcription [14–17]. However, it has been found that the Notch pathway participates in the regulation of PD-1 expression in T cells. A study showed that Notch increases the expression of PD-1 on immune cells during sepsis-induced immunosuppression [18]. In $CD8^+$ T lymphocytes, Notch signaling enhances the expression of PD-1. NICD/RBP-Jκ complex binds to the relative regulatory regions in Pdcd1 and activates the PD-1 transcription [19].

3.3.4 TOX

TOX (thymocyte selection-associated HMG BOX protein) is a member of the DNA-binding protein family that is involved in the development of the immune system. TOX was first identified as a regulator of thymic positive selection of T cells. It has been demonstrated that TOX is crucial for the development and function of $CD4^+$ T cells and NK cells, and the formation of lymph nodes and Peyer's patches [20]. The role of TOX in T cell exhaustion has been indicated by Khan et al. They showed that TOX is a key regulator of T cell exhaustion, including the expression of inhibitory molecules, impaired function and the expression of various transcription factors. Virus-specific $CD8^+$ T cells in LCMV-infected mice had a high level of TOX expression. PD-1, TIGIT, LAG-3, and CD160 was overexpressed in TOX^+ lymphocytes. In addition, TOX knockout cells expressed lower levels of inhibitory receptors. They also showed that calcineurin-NFAT signaling is necessary for TOX expression, but after the establishment of T cell exhaustion, the production and function of TOX in these cells are independent of NFAT. Based on these findings, TOX promotes and sustains T cell exhaustion [21]. In chronic infections such as cytomegalovirus (CMV), Epstein–Barr virus (EBV), and human immunodeficiency virus (HIV), TOX expression is not limited to exhausted $CD8^+$ T cells and effector memory $CD8^+$ T cells also express this transcription factor [22]. A study of TOX in a mouse model of chronic viral infection has shown that removing the DNA-binding domain of TOX reduces the expression of PD-1 and increases the function of exhausted T cells [23]. In addition, the role of TOX in reducing the hyporesponsiveness of $CD4^+$ and $CD8^+$ T cells in the tumor microenvironment has been observed [24]. TOX has been reported to increase the expression of PD-1, TIM-3, and CTLA-4 in intratumoral $CD8^+$ T cells and suppress the antitumor immune response in cancers such as melanoma, non-small cell lung cancer (NSCLC), and hepatocellular carcinoma. It has also been found that the expression of immune checkpoints in TOX knockdown $CD8^+$ T cells reduced the tumor-infiltrated $CD8^+$ T cells. TOX downregulation led to the boosting of cytotoxic T cells antitumor response [25, 26].

3.3.5 STAT

The JAK-STAT pathway is a fundamental signaling pathway in innate and adaptive immune responses. Several cytokines act through STATs and thereby regulate the metabolism of T cells [27]. STATs also affect PD-1 expression. A study showed that stimulation of mouse $CD8^+$ T cells with anti-CD3/CD28, along with the adding of IFNα, IL-6, and IL-12 to the culture, increased the PD-1 expression. IL-6 through STAT3 and IL-12 through STAT4 enhance PDCD1 gene transcription. Further investigations revealed that STAT3 and STAT4 bind to the −3.7 and +17.1 regulatory regions of the PDCD1 gene, respectively, and upregulate the PD-1 expression in CD8 T cells [28]. A recent study by Liang et al. revealed that the expression of PD-1 was directly related to the levels of IFNB1 (interferon beta1) and IFNAR1 (interferon-alpha/beta receptor 1) in myeloid cells of colorectal cancer patients. Treatment of myeloid cells with IFNβ significantly increased PD-1 levels. Deletion of IFNAR1, in addition to PD-1 downregulation, strongly suppressed IFNβ-induced PD-1 expression. They found that IFN-I exerts its effect through IRFs (interferon regulatory factors). IRFs are activated following the JAK-STAT signaling pathway. They found that IFNβ increases the transcription of PDCD1 through the STAT1-IRF2 axis. Activation of STAT1 by IFNβ subsequently activates IRF2 gene expression. IRF2 can increase the PD-1 expression by binding to the PDCD1 promoter [29]. IFN-stimulated gene factor 3 (ISGF3) is a complex consisting of STAT1, STAT2, and IRF9, which is activated by type I-IFNs and binds to IFN-stimulated response element (ISRE) elements in target genes and promotes their transcription [30]. In vitro studies have shown that IFNα can also upregulate PD-1 expression. IFNα mediates the binding of ISGF to the ISRE in the PD-1 gene promoter [31]. In addition, the relationship of IRF4 with the expression of various inhibitory molecules in exhausted T cells during LCMV infection has been determined. The decrease expression of IRF4 is associated with the upregulation of immune checkpoints on the cell surface and an improvement in the function of T cells [32].

3.3.6 Other Transcription Factors

It has been found that FoxO1 maintains the continuous transcriptional expression of the PDCD1 gene in $CD8^+$ T cells during chronic LCMV infection. The interaction of this transcription factor with the CR-C initiates gene transcription [33]. In the tumor environment, activator protein 1 (AP-1) plays an important role in the induction of PDCD1 gene transcription in exhausted T cells. AP-1 binds to the AP-1-binding site in CR-B through the c-Fos subunit and induces the PD-1 expression [34]. NR4A family is also one of the transcription factors involved in T cell exhaustion. The increased expression of NR4A in PD-1^{hi}TIM-3^{hi} $CD8^+$ T cells of melanoma mice indicates the role of this factor in T cell exhaustion. In addition, the transfer of NR4A to $CD8^+$ T cells inhibits the expression of PD-1, TIM-3, LAG-3, 2B4, and increases TIGIT [35, 36].

3.4 Epigenetic Regulation of Immune Checkpoints

Epigenetic mechanisms can regulate gene expression without changing the DNA sequence. DNA methylation and histone modifications are among the most important mechanisms of gene expression regulation. The relationship between epigenetic modifications and expression of immune checkpoints has been reported in various studies, which indicates the importance of epigenetic mechanisms in the regulation of T cell exhaustion.

3.4.1 DNA Methylation

DNA methylation is an important process in the regulation of gene expression, during which a methyl group from S-adenosylmethionine is added by DNA methyltransferases (DNMTs) to the 5′ position of cytosines in CpG sites scattered in the genome. CqG islands are frequent in gene promoters. DNA methylation of these regions is associated with gene expression silencing [37]. The relationship between methylation of CTLA-4, PD-1, PD-L1, and PD-L2 genes with infiltration of immune cells to the tumor and overall survival has been demonstrated in several cancers including breast cancer, papillary thyroid carcinoma, Merkel cell carcinoma, and head and neck squamous cell carcinoma (HNSCC) [38–41]. Hypomethylation of the promoters of inhibitory molecules such as CTLA-4, TIM-3, LAG-3, and TIGIT is positively related to their expression in the tumor [42, 43]. PD-1 promoter methylation has been suggested as a valuable prognostic marker in many cancers. The correlation of methylation of immune checkpoint genes with lower-grade gliomas (LGG) has also been reported. According to this study, methylation of CTLA-4, PD-1, PD-L1, and PD-L2 promoters was lower in LGG patients with isocitrate dehydrogenase (IDH) mutations compared to other subgroups. PDCD1 methylation is a potential prognostic factor in these patients [44]. Evaluation of the methylation status of PD-1 and LAG-3 in colorectal cancer (CRC) patients showed that hypermethylation of these immune checkpoints is associated with a decrease in the risk of CRC [45]. In addition, a cohort study of 498 prostate cancer patients revealed that PD-1 promoter hypermethylation is inversely related to PD-1 mRNA expression. PD-1 methylation in these patients significantly was correlated with preoperative prostate-specific antigen (PSA) [46]. The study of non-small cell lung cancer tissue samples showed that the methylation of CTLA-4 and PD-1 genes in cancer tissues was lower compared to tumor-free tissues of patients and their expression was increased by hypomethylation [47]. Hypomethylating agents (HMAs) such as 5-azacytidine (5-aza) are effective treatments for improving the outcome of myelodysplastic syndromes (MDS). It has been assumed that activation of tumor suppressor genes and increased expression of tumor antigens are among the effector mechanisms of HMAs. However, some MDS patients become resistant to HMAs treatment [8, 9]. Ørskov et al. found that 5-aza reduced PD-1 promoter methylation. A large percentage of MDS/AML patients treated with 5-aza had PDCD1 demethylation in their T lymphocytes, which was associated with a poorer clinical response. The overall response rate (ORR) was significantly higher in the group of patients without PDCD1 demethylation. PDCD1 demethylation increased the expression of PD-1 on T cells. They concluded that upregulation of PD-1 expression and development of T cell exhaustion are possible mechanisms of resistance to 5-aza [48].

In addition to cancer, the correlation of methylation of immune checkpoints and their expression has been studied in infections. Youngblood et al. indicated that in the mouse model of LCMV infection, the expression of PD-1 in antigen-specific $CD8^+$ T cells increased at the beginning of the infection but PD-1 was downregulated by the clearance of the virus. DNA methylation analysis showed that CpG sites in CR-C and CR-B of the PD-1 gene were transiently demethylated in CD8 T cells but became remethylated again after clearance of the infection. In contrast, PDCD1 demethylation in antigen-specific $CD8^+$ T cells was persistent during chronic infection and was associated with long-term upregulation of PD-1 expression. In addition, it was found that in chronic human CMV and EBV infections, virus-specific $PD1^{hi}$ $CD8^+$ T cells were fully demethylated in PDCD1. These findings show that persistent demethylation in PDCD1 promoter is one of the characteristics of exhausted T cells during chronic infection [49]. In chronic hepatitis B infection, PDCD1 methylation in $CD8^+$ T cells of patients was lower compared to healthy individuals and was related to increased expression of PD-1 on these cells [50]. Similar findings have been observed in HIV infection. During acute HIV infection with a high viral load, PD-1 was upregulated on virus-specific CD8 T cells and PDCD1 was completely demethylated. In the chronic stage of the disease and before highly active antiretroviral therapy (HAART) therapy, HIV-specific $CD8^+$ T cells had unmethylated PDCD1. Notably, despite the low levels of viral load after long-term HAART therapy, PD-1 promoter remained unmethylated. HIV-specific $CD8^+$ T cells showed a decrease in PD-1 expression after treatment, although the transcription of the gene was not completely silenced [51].

3.4.2 Histone Modification

Histone modifications by changing the promoters and enhancers accessibility play a key role in regulating gene expression. Histone modifications can occur in the forms of methylation, acetylation, phosphorylation, and ubiquitination. During histone acetylation, histone acetyltransferases (HATs) add an acetyl group to the side chain of lysine in histone; as a result, the charge of the histone changes and its binding to DNA reduces. Histone deacetylases (HDACs) are another group of enzymes that act opposite to HATs and are involved in the control of histone acetylation. Histone acetylation is related to the activation of gene transcription. Histone methyltransferases and histone demethylases are the main regulators of the histone methylation process. Methyltransferases add methyl groups to arginine and lysine residues of histones. Although histone methylation is often associated with the suppression of gene expression, such as trimethylation of histone H3 at lysine 9 (H3K9me3), methylation of other sites such as (H3K4m3) can lead to activation of transcription [52, 53]. Histone methylation at the promoters of immune checkpoint genes has been investigated in several studies. Nair et al. showed that the expression of PD-1, CTLA-4, TIM-3, and LAG-3 was increased in tumor tissues of breast cancer patients compared to normal tissues. They also found that the binding of two repressive histones including H3K9me3 and H3K27me3 at the LAG-3 promoter of tumor tissues was lower than in normal tissues. The binding of H3K9me3 to PD-1 promoters and CTLA-4 and the binding of H3K27me3 to TIM-3 promoter were reduced [43]. Another study revealed that the binding of H3K27me3 to CTLA-4 promoter and H3K9me3 to PD-1 and TIGIT promoters were lower in tumor tissues of colorectal cancer patients compared to normal tissues. In TIM-3 promoter, both H3K9me3 and H3K27me3 binding was reduced in tumor tissues. These results were consistent with the increased expression of these inhibitory molecules in the tumor tissues [42]. H3K4m3, an activating histone, is also effective in the expression pattern of immune checkpoints in cancer. It has been found that in lung adenocarcinoma patients with high levels of H3K3me3, the expression of CTLA-4, TIGIT, PD-L2, PD-L1, PD-1, and LAG-3 was increased. In addition, high H3K3me3 was associated with the activation of $CD4^+$ and $CD8^+$ T cells and better overall survival [54]. It has also been shown that in colorectal cancer, H3K9me3 was lower in PD-L1 and TOX2 genes, while histone H3K4m3 was upregulated [55]. These findings show that histone modifications are involved in the regulation of immune checkpoints expression in tumors.

3.4.3 MicroRNAs

Noncoding RNAs (ncRNAs) comprise the majority of the genome and do not encode proteins. This family of RNAs can be classified into two main categories including small (less than 200 nucleotides) and long (more than 200 nucleotides) RNAs. In terms of their function, ncRNAs are divided into infrastructural (such as small nucleolar RNAs and ribosomal RNAs) and regulatory subsets (such as microRNAs and long noncoding RNAs) [56, 57]. MicroRNAs (miRNA) are a type of ncRNAs that constitute about 1–5% of the human genome, but they play an important role in regulating gene expression and homeostasis of different cells. It is estimated that miRNAs regulate the expression of 30% of genes. MiRNAs are single-stranded, noncoding RNA molecules with a short length that by binding to the target mRNA stop the production of the protein. This binding can cause mRNA degradation or inhibit the translation process. In summary, the transcription of the miRNA gene leads to the production of primary miRNA. After cleavage and processing, primary miRNA is assembled into RNA-induced silencing complex (RISC) and makes an effector complex that interacts with mRNA [58]. MiRNAs mainly exert their effect by binding to the 3′-untranslated region (3′-UTR) of the target mRNA, although there are exceptions, such as miR-10, which binds to the 5′-UTR, or miR-155, which binds to coding regions. A single miRNA can bind to different mRNA, thereby controlling the expression of several genes. Each tissue has its specific miRNA expression profile. The change of miRNA expression patterns in various diseases such as cancer and infections or autoimmunity indicates their involvement in these diseases. In cancers, the expression of miRNAs is deregulated. Many studies have reported the role of miRNAs in tumor development, growth, metastasis, and resistance to cancer treatment [56, 59].

The relationship of miRNAs with the expression of immune checkpoints in cancer has been demonstrated in numerous studies. For example, miR-200, miR-140, miR-34a, miR-424, miR-214, miR-142-5p, and miR-497-5p can regulate PD-L1 expression [4, 60–66]. Evaluating the expression pattern of miRNAs in cutaneous T cell lymphoma (CTCL) revealed that several miRNAs were related to the upregulation of PD-1, PD-L1, CTLA-4, LAG-3, and TIM-3 immune checkpoints. MiR-146 had the highest correlation among these miRNAs [67]. A study of miR-424-3p expression in specimens of 535 prostate cancer patients showed that this miRNA was related to the clinical outcome of the cancer. A significant correlation between miR-424-3p and CTLA-4 expression was observed. Lower levels of miR-424-3p were associated with worse free survival [68]. It has been found that miR-424 reduces PD-L1 and CD80 expression in ovarian cancer. High levels of miR-424 were inversely related to the expression of PD-L1 and CD80. Upregulated miR-424 was positively associated with progression-free survival (PFS). In addition, in syngeneic ovarian cancer model with stable overexpression of miR-424, the effect of cisplatin treatment was enhanced. In mice with miR-424 overexpressing tumors, survival was longer and the frequency of $CD8^+$ T cells producing IFN-γ significantly increased [69]. These findings indicate the modulatory effect of this miRNA on PD-1/PD-L1 and CD80/CTLA-4 pathways, which play an important role in suppression of the tumor-specific T cell response.

$CD4^+$ T cells with miR-138 expressing vector had lower expression levels of CTLA-4, PD-1, and FoxP3. In addition, treatment of GL261 glioma mice with miR-138 decreased tumor growth, and the expression of CTLA-4 and PD-1 was decreased in both effector T cells ($CD4^+$ $FoxP3^-$) and Tregs ($CD4^+$ $FoxP3^+$) populations. By deletion of $CD4^+$ or $CD8^+$ T cells in mice, the effect of miR-138 on tumor suppression was lost, which implies that miR-138 has a regulatory effect on the antitumor response of T cells [70]. Li et al. found that in B16F10 melanoma mouse model, T cells were exhausted and the expression of immune checkpoints was increased on their surface. MiRNA expression analysis showed that miR-28, miR-150, and miR-151-5p were downregulated in $CD4^+$ $PD1^+$ T cells of tumor-bearing mice. Among them, miR-28 could bind to the 3′-UTR of PD-1, TIM-3, and BTLA. In vitro studies showed that transfection of T cells isolated from melanoma mice with miR-28 mimic downregulated the expression of PD-1 and increased the frequency of $PD1^+$ $CD4^+$ T cells and $PD1^+$ $CD8^+$ T cells, while miR-28 inhibitor expression upregulated the PD-1, TIM-3, and BTLA expression. In addition, $PD1^+$ Treg and TIM-3^+ Treg cells were reduced in miR-28 mimic group. In contrast, miR-28 inhibitor was associated with the increased frequency of these cells. The production of IL-2 and TNF-α from T cells was increased in the presence of miR-28 mimic [71]. Overall, these findings show that miR-28 can be useful in restoring the activity of exhausted T cells against tumor. MiR-125a-3p and miR-133a-5p have been reported to silence TIM-3 transcription. Transfecting AML cell line (HL-60) with miR-125a-3p and miR-133a-5p decreased TIM-3 expression [72, 73]. According to a study, the expression of miR-32 was reduced in ovarian cancer tissues. In addition, ovarian cancer cell line (SKOV3) transfected with miR-32 had suppressed proliferation, migration, and invasion. It was found that the antitumor effect of miR-32 is partly related to its regulatory effect on BTLA. MiR-32 can bind to the 3′-UTR of the BTLA gene. MiR-32 mimic decreased BTLA expression on SKOV3 cells, while BTLA was upregulated in cells transfected with miR-32 inhibitor. Overexpression of BTLA was associated with increased proliferation and migration of the cells [74]. CD276 is an immune checkpoint of the B7 family that is overexpressed in cancer and is involved in tumor cell proliferation and cancer progression [75]. MiR-1253 has antitumor properties in medulloblastoma. miR-1253 upregulation inhibits the proliferation of tumor cells. It has been found that one of the target genes of miR-1253 is B7-H3 (CD276) and miR-1253 can downregulate its expression [76]. MiR-29 and miR-187 are other miRNAs that inhibit tumor cell proliferation through downregulation of B7-H3 expression [77, 78]. CD47 inhibits macrophage phagocytosis by binding to its ligand SIRPα. CD47 is overexpressed in many cancers and is involved in the development and progression of tumor [79]. The regulatory effect of miR-200a, miR-133a, and miR-708 in CD47 expression and inhibiting tumorigenesis has been investigated. MiR-200a inhibits the phagocytosis of nasopharyngeal carcinoma cells by macrophages and promotes proliferation, migration, and invasion of tumor cells by downregulating CD47 expression [80]. MiR-708 is inversely related to CD47 expression in T cell acute lymphoblastic leukemia (T-ALL). MiR-708 can modulate CD47 expression by binding to the 3′-UTR of the CD47 gene [81]. Decreased miR-133a expression levels have been reported in esophageal squamous cell carcinoma. It has been found that miR-133a can inhibit the proliferation of tumor cells by reducing the expression of CD47 [82]. Similar findings have been reported regarding the association of miR-340 with CD47 modulation [83]. MiRNAs involving in immune checkpoints expression in cancer are listed in Table 3.1.

Table 3.1 List of miRNAs regulating the immune checkpoints in cancer

Immune checkpoint	MicroRNA	Cancer type	Ref.
CTLA-4	miR-138	Glioma	[70]
	miR-155	Melanoma	[84]
	miR-424-3p	Prostate cancer	[68]
PD-1	miR-138	Glioma	[70]
	miR-28	Melanoma	[71]
	miR-374b	Liver cancer	[85]
	miR-33a	Lung cancer	[86]
	miR-4717	Hepatocellular carcinoma	[87]
PD-L1	miR-34	Acute myeloid leukemia	[88, 89]
	miR-138-5p	Colorectal cancer	[90]
	miR-200	Lung cancer, osteosarcoma	[91, 92]
	miR-424	Ovarian cancer	[69]
	miR-195	Prostate cancer	[93]
	miR-15	Malignant pleural mesothelioma	[94]
	miR-16	Prostate cancer, malignant pleural mesothelioma	[93, 94]
	miR-570	Gastric adenocarcinoma	[95]
	miR-152	Gastric carcinoma	[96]
	miR-197	Non-small cell lung cancer	[97]
	miR-570-3p	Breast cancer	[98]
	miR-873	Breast cancer	[99]
	miR-497-5p	Renal cell carcinoma	[100]
	miR-3609	Breast cancer	[101]
	miR-93	Pancreatic cancer	[102]
	miR-106b	Pancreatic cancer	[102]
	miR-142-5p	Pancreatic cancer	[103]
	miRNA-148a-3p	Colorectal cancer	[104]
	miR-214	Diffuse large B-cell lymphoma	[105]
	miR-140	Non-small cell lung cancer	[106]
	miR-23a-3p	Liver cancer	[107]
	miR-27a-3p	Breast cancer	[108]
	miR-145	Ovarian carcinoma	[109]
TIM-3	miR-28	Melanoma	[71]
	miR-125a-3p	Acute myeloid leukemia	[73]
	miR-133a-5p	Acute myeloid leukemia	[72]
BTLA	miR-28	Melanoma	[71]
	miR-32	Ovarian cancer	[74]

(continued)

Table 3.1 (continued)

Immune checkpoint	MicroRNA	Cancer type	Ref.
B7-H3	miR-1253	Medulloblastoma	[76]
	miR-187	Colorectal cancer	[78]
	miR-29	Solid tumors	[77]
CD47	miR-708	T cell acute lymphoblastic leukemia	[81]
	miR-133a	Esophageal squamous cell carcinoma	[82]
	miR-200a	Nasopharyngeal carcinoma	[80]
	miR-340	Pancreatic ductal adenocarcinoma	[83]

3.5 Conclusion

The regulation of immune checkpoint expression involves complex interplay between genetic and epigenetic mechanisms. This chapter has explored the key transcriptional and epigenetic factors that control the expression of immune checkpoints, with a particular focus on PD-1 as a model. Transcription factors such as NFAT, Blimp-1, Notch, TOX, and STATs play crucial roles in modulating immune checkpoint gene expression in response to various stimuli. These factors can bind to regulatory regions in checkpoint gene promoters and enhancers to activate or repress transcription. Notably, many of these transcription factors are involved in both T cell activation and exhaustion pathways, highlighting the delicate balance in immune regulation. Epigenetic modifications, including DNA methylation and histone modifications, add another layer of control. DNA methylation generally represses checkpoint gene expression, while certain histone modifications such as H3K27ac are associated with active transcription. The dynamic nature of these epigenetic marks allows for rapid and reversible changes in checkpoint expression in response to environmental cues. Importantly, the epigenetic landscape of exhausted T cells appears to be distinct from that of effector or memory T cells. This unique epigenetic profile contributes to the stable exhausted phenotype and may explain why some exhausted T cells are resistant to reinvigoration by checkpoint blockade therapy. These regulatory mechanisms provide valuable insights into the development of T cell exhaustion and offers potential targets for therapeutic intervention. Strategies aimed at modulating the epigenetic state or targeting specific transcription factors could complement existing checkpoint blockade approaches and lead to more effective immunotherapies for cancer and chronic infections. As research in this field progresses, integrating genomic, epigenomic, and functional data will be crucial for developing a comprehensive understanding of immune checkpoint regulation and translating this knowledge into clinical applications.

Acknowledgments The authors gratefully acknowledge the valuable assistance provided by Maryam Sadr.

References

1. Vezzani B, Carinci M, Previati M, Giacovazzi S, Della Sala M, Gafà R, et al. Epigenetic regulation: a link between inflammation and carcinogenesis. Cancer. 2022;14(5)
2. Belk JA, Daniel B, Satpathy AT. Epigenetic regulation of T cell exhaustion. Nat Immunol. 2022;23(6):848–60.
3. Laba S, Mallett G, Amarnath S. The depths of PD-1 function within the tumor microenvironment beyond CD8(+) T cells. Semin Cancer Biol. 2022;86(Pt 2):1045–55.
4. Hudson K, Cross N, Jordan-Mahy N, Leyland R. The extrinsic and intrinsic roles of PD-L1 and its receptor PD-1: implications for immunotherapy treatment. Front Immunol. 2020;11:568931.
5. Chi Z, Lu Y, Yang Y, Li B, Lu P. Transcriptional and epigenetic regulation of PD-1 expression. Cell Mol Life Sci. 2021;78(7):3239–46.
6. Mishra A, Verma M. Epigenetic and genetic regulation of PDCD1 gene in cancer immunology. Methods Mol Biol (Clifton, NJ). 2018;1856:247–54.
7. Curdy N, Lanvin O, Laurent C, Fournié J-J, Franchini D-M. Regulatory mechanisms of inhibitory immune checkpoint receptors expression. Trends Cell Biol. 2019;29(10):777–90.
8. Oestreich KJ, Yoon H, Ahmed R, Boss JM. NFATc1 regulates PD-1 expression upon T cell activation. J Immunol (Baltimore, Md: 1950). 2008;181(7):4832–9.
9. Martinez GJ, Pereira RM, Äijö T, Kim EY, Marangoni F, Pipkin ME, et al. The transcription factor NFAT promotes exhaustion of activated CD8+ T cells. Immunity. 2015;42(2):265–78.
10. Hogan PG. Calcium-NFAT transcriptional signalling in T cell activation and T cell exhaustion. Cell Calcium. 2017;63:66–9.
11. Shin H, Blackburn SD, Intlekofer AM, Kao C, Angelosanto JM, Reiner SL, et al. A role for the transcriptional repressor Blimp-1 in CD8(+) T cell exhaustion during chronic viral infection. Immunity. 2009;31(2):309–20.
12. Zhu L, Kong Y, Zhang J, Claxton DF, Ehmann WC, Rybka WB, et al. Blimp-1 impairs T cell function via upregulation of TIGIT and PD-1 in patients with acute myeloid leukemia. J Hematol Oncol. 2017;10(1):124.
13. Hwang S, Cobb DA, Bhadra R, Youngblood B, Khan IA. Blimp-1-mediated CD4 T cell exhaustion causes CD8 T cell dysfunction during chronic toxoplasmosis. J Exp Med. 2016;213(9):1799–818.
14. Palaga T, Miele L, Golde TE, Osborne BA. TCR-mediated notch signaling regulates proliferation and IFN-gamma production in peripheral T cells. J Immunol. (Baltimore, Md : 1950). 2003;171(6):3019–24.
15. Cho OH, Shin HM, Miele L, Golde TE, Fauq A, Minter LM, et al. Notch regulates cytolytic effector function in CD8+ T cells. J Immunol (Baltimore, Md: 1950). 2009;182(6):3380–9.
16. Maekawa Y, Minato Y, Ishifune C, Kurihara T, Kitamura A, Kojima H, et al. Notch2 integrates signaling by the transcription factors RBP-J and CREB1 to promote T cell cytotoxicity. Nat Immunol. 2008;9(10):1140–7.
17. Borggrefe T, Lauth M, Zwijsen A, Huylebroeck D, Oswald F, Giaimo BD. The Notch intracellular domain integrates signals from Wnt, Hedgehog, TGFβ/BMP and hypoxia pathways. Biochim Biophys Acta. 2016;1863(2):303–13.
18. Pan T, Liu Z, Yin J, Zhou T, Liu J, Qu H. Notch signaling pathway was involved in regulating programmed cell death 1 expression during sepsis-induced immunosuppression. Mediators Inflamm. 2015;2015:539841.
19. Mathieu M, Cotta-Grand N, Daudelin JF, Thébault P, Labrecque N. Notch signaling regulates PD-1 expression during CD8(+) T-cell activation. Immunol Cell Biol. 2013;91(1):82–8.
20. Aliahmad P, Seksenyan A, Kaye J. The many roles of TOX in the immune system. Curr Opin Immunol. 2012;24(2):173–7.
21. Khan O, Giles JR, McDonald S, Manne S, Ngiow SF, Patel KP, et al. TOX transcriptionally and epigenetically programs CD8(+) T cell exhaustion. Nature. 2019;571(7764):211–8.

22. Sekine T, Perez-Potti A, Nguyen S, Gorin JB, Wu VH, Gostick E, et al. TOX is expressed by exhausted and polyfunctional human effector memory CD8(+) T cells. Sci Immunol. 2020;5(49)
23. Alfei F, Kanev K, Hofmann M, Wu M, Ghoneim HE, Roelli P, et al. TOX reinforces the phenotype and longevity of exhausted T cells in chronic viral infection. Nature. 2019;571(7764):265–9.
24. Niu H, Wang H. TOX regulates T lymphocytes differentiation and its function in tumor. Front Immunol. 2023;14:990419.
25. Kim K, Park S, Park SY, Kim G, Park SM, Cho JW, et al. Single-cell transcriptome analysis reveals TOX as a promoting factor for T cell exhaustion and a predictor for anti-PD-1 responses in human cancer. Genome Med. 2020;12(1):22.
26. Wang X, He Q, Shen H, Xia A, Tian W, Yu W, et al. TOX promotes the exhaustion of antitumor CD8(+) T cells by preventing PD1 degradation in hepatocellular carcinoma. J Hepatol. 2019;71(4):731–41.
27. Villarino AV. Transcriptional programing of T cell metabolism by STAT family transcription factors. Eur J Immunol. 2023;53(6):e2048825.
28. Austin JW, Lu P, Majumder P, Ahmed R, Boss JM. STAT3, STAT4, NFATc1, and CTCF regulate PD-1 through multiple novel regulatory regions in murine T cells. J Immunol (Baltimore, Md: 1950). 2014;192(10):4876–86.
29. Liang L, Yang Y, Deng K, Wu Y, Li Y, Bai L, et al. Type I interferon activates PD-1 expression through activation of the STAT1-IRF2 pathway in myeloid cells. Cells. 2024;13(13)
30. Platanitis E, Demiroz D, Schneller A, Fischer K, Capelle C, Hartl M, et al. A molecular switch from STAT2-IRF9 to ISGF3 underlies interferon-induced gene transcription. Nat Commun. 2019;10(1):2921.
31. Terawaki S, Chikuma S, Shibayama S, Hayashi T, Yoshida T, Okazaki T, et al. IFN-α directly promotes programmed cell death-1 transcription and limits the duration of T cell-mediated immunity. J Immunol (Baltimore, Md: 1950). 2011;186(5):2772–9.
32. Man K, Gabriel SS, Liao Y, Gloury R, Preston S, Henstridge DC, et al. Transcription factor IRF4 promotes CD8(+) T cell exhaustion and limits the development of memory-like T cells during chronic infection. Immunity. 2017;47(6):1129–41.e5.
33. Staron MM, Gray SM, Marshall HD, Parish IA, Chen JH, Perry CJ, et al. The transcription factor FoxO1 sustains expression of the inhibitory receptor PD-1 and survival of antiviral CD8(+) T cells during chronic infection. Immunity. 2014;41(5):802–14.
34. Xiao G, Deng A, Liu H, Ge G, Liu X. Activator protein 1 suppresses antitumor T-cell function via the induction of programmed death 1. Proc Natl Acad Sci USA. 2012;109(38):15419–24.
35. Chen J, López-Moyado IF, Seo H, Lio CJ, Hempleman LJ, Sekiya T, et al. NR4A transcription factors limit CAR T cell function in solid tumours. Nature. 2019;567(7749):530–4.
36. Seo H, Chen J, González-Avalos E, Samaniego-Castruita D, Das A, Wang YH, et al. TOX and TOX2 transcription factors cooperate with NR4A transcription factors to impose CD8(+) T cell exhaustion. Proc Natl Acad Sci USA. 2019;116(25):12410–5.
37. Moore LD, Le T, Fan G. DNA methylation and its basic function. Neuropsychopharmacology. 2013;38(1):23–38.
38. Goltz D, Gevensleben H, Dietrich J, Schroeck F, de Vos L, Droege F, et al. PDCD1 (PD-1) promoter methylation predicts outcome in head and neck squamous cell carcinoma patients. Oncotarget. 2017;8(25):41011–20.
39. Ricci C, Morandi L, Righi A, Gibertoni D, Maletta F, Ambrosi F, et al. PD-1 (PDCD1) promoter methylation in Merkel cell carcinoma: prognostic relevance and relationship with clinico-pathological parameters. Mod Pathol. 2019;32(9):1359–72.
40. Ralser DJ, Klümper N, Gevensleben H, Zarbl R, Kaiser C, Landsberg J, et al. Molecular and immune correlates of PDCD1 (PD-1), PD-L1 (CD274), and PD-L2 (PDCD1LG2) DNA methylation in triple negative breast cancer. J Immunother (Hagerstown, Md: 1997). 2021;44(8):319–24.

41. Vos L, Dietrich J, Strieth S, Bootz F, Dietrich D, Franzen A. PD-1, CTLA4, PD-L1 and PD-L2 DNA methylation in papillary thyroid carcinoma. Immunotherapy. 2020;12(12):903–20.
42. Sasidharan Nair V, Toor SM, Taha RZ, Shaath H, Elkord E. DNA methylation and repressive histones in the promoters of PD-1, CTLA-4, TIM-3, LAG-3, TIGIT, PD-L1, and galectin-9 genes in human colorectal cancer. Clin Epigenetics. 2018;10(1):104.
43. Sasidharan Nair V, El Salhat H, Taha RZ, John A, Ali BR, Elkord E. DNA methylation and repressive H3K9 and H3K27 trimethylation in the promoter regions of PD-1, CTLA-4, TIM-3, LAG-3, TIGIT, and PD-L1 genes in human primary breast cancer. Clin Epigenetics. 2018;10:78.
44. Röver LK, Gevensleben H, Dietrich J, Bootz F, Landsberg J, Goltz D, et al. PD-1 (PDCD1) promoter methylation is a prognostic factor in patients with diffuse lower-grade gliomas harboring Isocitrate dehydrogenase (IDH) mutations. EBioMedicine. 2018;28:97–104.
45. Zhang Y, Zhang L, Sun H, Liu Y, Xu J, Huang H, et al. Inhibitory immune checkpoints PDCD-1 and LAG-3 hypermethylation may reduce the risk of colorectal cancer. Mol Med (Cambridge, MA). 2021;27(1):114.
46. Goltz D, Gevensleben H, Dietrich J, Ellinger J, Landsberg J, Kristiansen G, et al. Promoter methylation of the immune checkpoint receptor PD-1 (PDCD1) is an independent prognostic biomarker for biochemical recurrence-free survival in prostate cancer patients following radical prostatectomy. Onco Targets Ther. 2016;5(10):e1221555.
47. Marwitz S, Scheufele S, Perner S, Reck M, Ammerpohl O, Goldmann T. Epigenetic modifications of the immune-checkpoint genes CTLA4 and PDCD1 in non-small cell lung cancer results in increased expression. Clin Epigenetics. 2017;9:51.
48. Ørskov AD, Treppendahl MB, Skovbo A, Holm MS, Friis LS, Hokland M, et al. Hypomethylation and up-regulation of PD-1 in T cells by azacytidine in MDS/AML patients: a rationale for combined targeting of PD-1 and DNA methylation. Oncotarget. 2015;6(11):9612–26.
49. Youngblood B, Oestreich KJ, Ha SJ, Duraiswamy J, Akondy RS, West EE, et al. Chronic virus infection enforces demethylation of the locus that encodes PD-1 in antigen-specific CD8(+) T cells. Immunity. 2011;35(3):400–12.
50. Jiao L, Chen J, Wu X, Cai B, Su Z, Wang L. Correlation of CpG methylation of the Pdcd1 gene with PD-1 expression on CD8(+) T cells and medical laboratory indicators in chronic hepatitis B infection. J Gene Med. 2020;22(2):e3148.
51. Youngblood B, Noto A, Porichis F, Akondy RS, Ndhlovu ZM, Austin JW, et al. Cutting edge: prolonged exposure to HIV reinforces a poised epigenetic program for PD-1 expression in virus-specific CD8 T cells. J Immunol (Baltimore, Md: 1950). 2013;191(2):540–4.
52. Bannister AJ, Kouzarides T. Regulation of chromatin by histone modifications. Cell Res. 2011;21(3):381–95.
53. Kim S, Kaang BK. Epigenetic regulation and chromatin remodeling in learning and memory. Exp Mol Med. 2017;49(1):e281.
54. Fan T, Zhu M, Muhammad S, Xiao C, Li S, Tian H, et al. H3K4me3-related lncRNAs signature and comprehensive analysis of H3K4me3 regulating tumor immunity in lung adenocarcinoma. Respir Res. 2023;24(1):122.
55. Sasidharan Nair V, Saleh R, Toor SM, Taha RZ, Ahmed AA, Kurer MA, et al. Epigenetic regulation of immune checkpoints and T cell exhaustion markers in tumor-infiltrating T cells of colorectal cancer patients. Epigenomics. 2020;12(21):1871–82.
56. Ratti M, Lampis A, Ghidini M, Salati M, Mirchev MB, Valeri N, et al. MicroRNAs (miRNAs) and long non-coding RNAs (lncRNAs) as new tools for cancer therapy: first steps from bench to bedside. Target Oncol. 2020;15(3):261–78.
57. Kaikkonen MU, Lam MT, Glass CK. Non-coding RNAs as regulators of gene expression and epigenetics. Cardiovasc Res. 2011;90(3):430–40.
58. Macfarlane LA, Murphy PR. MicroRNA: biogenesis, function and role in cancer. Curr Genomics. 2010;11(7):537–61.

59. Peng Y, Croce CM. The role of MicroRNAs in human cancer. Signal Transduct Target Ther. 2016;1:15004.
60. Saleh R, Toor SM, Sasidharan Nair V, Elkord E. Role of epigenetic modifications in inhibitory immune checkpoints in cancer development and progression. Front Immunol. 2020;11:1469.
61. Wang Q, Lin W, Tang X, Li S, Guo L, Lin Y, et al. The roles of microRNAs in regulating the expression of PD-1/PD-L1 immune checkpoint. Int J Mol Sci. 2017;18
62. Jiang Y, Zhao L, Wu Y, Deng S, Cao P, Lei X, et al. The role of NcRNAs to regulate immune checkpoints in cancer. Front Immunol. 2022;13:853480.
63. Shadbad MA, Safaei S, Brunetti O, Derakhshani A, Lotfinejad P, Mokhtarzadeh A, et al. A systematic review on the therapeutic potentiality of PD-L1-inhibiting MicroRNAs for triple-negative breast cancer: toward single-cell sequencing-guided biomimetic delivery. Genes. 2021;12(8):1206.
64. Skafi N, Fayyad-Kazan M, Badran B. Immunomodulatory role for MicroRNAs: regulation of PD-1/PD-L1 and CTLA-4 immune checkpoints expression. Gene. 2020;754:144888.
65. Li K, Wang Z. Non-coding RNAs: key players in T cell exhaustion. Front Immunol. 2022;13:959729.
66. Smolle MA, Prinz F, Calin GA, Pichler M. Current concepts of non-coding RNA regulation of immune checkpoints in cancer. Mol Asp Med. 2019;70:117–26.
67. Querfeld C, Wu X, Sanchez JF, Palmer JM, Motevalli A, Zain J, et al. The miRNA profile of cutaneous T cell lymphoma correlates with the dysfunctional Immunophenotype of the disease. Blood. 2016;128(22):4132.
68. Richardsen E, Andersen S, Al-Saad S, Rakaee M, Nordby Y, Pedersen MI, et al. Low expression of miR-424-3p is highly correlated with clinical failure in prostate cancer. Sci Rep. 2019;9(1):10662.
69. Xu S, Tao Z, Hai B, Liang H, Shi Y, Wang T, et al. miR-424(322) reverses chemoresistance via T-cell immune response activation by blocking the PD-L1 immune checkpoint. Nat Commun. 2016;7:11406.
70. Wei J, Nduom EK, Kong LY, Hashimoto Y, Xu S, Gabrusiewicz K, et al. MiR-138 exerts anti-glioma efficacy by targeting immune checkpoints. Neuro-Oncology. 2016;18(5):639–48.
71. Li Q, Johnston N, Zheng X, Wang H, Zhang X, Gao D, et al. miR-28 modulates exhaustive differentiation of T cells through silencing programmed cell death-1 and regulating cytokine secretion. Oncotarget. 2016;7(33):53735–50.
72. Hojati Z, Ganjalikhani-Hakemi M, Ameri M, Alimohammadi-Jelodar SF, Dehbashi M, Mohammad Ganji M, et al. Evaluation of silencing effect of miR-133a-5p mimic on TIM-3 expression in AML (HL-60) cell line. Indian J Clin Biochem. 2020;35(3):359–66.
73. Emamdoost F, Khanahmad H, Ganjalikhani-Hakemi M, Doosti A. The miR-125a-3p inhibits TIM-3 expression in AML cell line HL-60 in vitro. Indian J Hematol Blood Transfus. 2017;33(3):342–7.
74. Zhang RR, Wang LM, Shen JJ. Overexpression of miR-32 inhibits the proliferation and metastasis of ovarian cancer cells by targeting BTLA. Eur Rev Med Pharmacol Sci. 2020;24(9):4671–8.
75. Getu AA, Tigabu A, Zhou M, Lu J, Fodstad Ø, Tan M. New frontiers in immune checkpoint B7-H3 (CD276) research and drug development. Mol Cancer. 2023;22(1):43.
76. Kanchan RK, Perumal N, Atri P, Chirravuri Venkata R, Thapa I, Klinkebiel DL, et al. MiR-1253 exerts tumor-suppressive effects in medulloblastoma via inhibition of CDK6 and CD276 (B7-H3). Brain Pathol (Zurich, Switzerland). 2020;30(4):732–45.
77. Xu H, Cheung IY, Guo HF, Cheung NK. MicroRNA miR-29 modulates expression of immunoinhibitory molecule B7-H3: potential implications for immune based therapy of human solid tumors. Cancer Res. 2009;69(15):6275–81.
78. Wang ZS, Zhong M, Bian YH, Mu YF, Qin SL, Yu MH, et al. MicroRNA-187 inhibits tumor growth and invasion by directly targeting CD276 in colorectal cancer. Oncotarget. 2016;7(28):44266–76.

79. Jiang Z, Sun H, Yu J, Tian W, Song Y. Targeting CD47 for cancer immunotherapy. J Hematol Oncol. 2021;14(1):180.
80. Zhao Y, Yu X, Tang H, Han R, Wang X, Wang J, et al. MicroRNA-200a promotes phagocytosis of macrophages and suppresses cell proliferation, migration, and invasion in nasopharyngeal carcinoma by targeting CD47. Biomed Res Int. 2020;2020:3723781.
81. Huang W, Wang W-T, Fang K, Chen Z-H, Sun Y-M, Han C, et al. MIR-708 promotes phagocytosis to eradicate T-ALL cells by targeting CD47. Mol Cancer. 2018;17(1):12.
82. Suzuki S, Yokobori T, Tanaka N, Sakai M, Sano A, Inose T, et al. CD47 expression regulated by the miR-133a tumor suppressor is a novel prognostic marker in esophageal squamous cell carcinoma. Oncol Rep. 2012;28(2):465–72.
83. Xi Q, Zhang J, Yang G, Zhang L, Chen Y, Wang C, et al. Restoration of miR-340 controls pancreatic cancer cell CD47 expression to promote macrophage phagocytosis and enhance antitumor immunity. J Immunother Cancer. 2020;8(1)
84. Huffaker TB, Lee SH, Tang WW, Wallace JA, Alexander M, Runtsch MC, et al. Antitumor immunity is defective in T cell-specific microRNA-155-deficient mice and is rescued by immune checkpoint blockade. J Biol Chem. 2017;292(45):18530–41.
85. Huang F, Wang B, Zeng J, Sang S, Lei J, Lu Y. MicroRNA-374b inhibits liver cancer progression via down regulating programmed cell death-1 expression on cytokine-induced killer cells. Oncol Lett. 2018;15(4):4797–804.
86. Boldrini L, Giordano M, Niccoli C, Melfi F, Lucchi M, Mussi A, et al. Role of microRNA-33a in regulating the expression of PD-1 in lung adenocarcinoma. Cancer Cell Int. 2017;17:105.
87. Zhang G, Li N, Li Z, Zhu Q, Li F, Yang C, et al. microRNA-4717 differentially interacts with its polymorphic target in the PD1 3′ untranslated region: A mechanism for regulating PD-1 expression and function in HBV-associated liver diseases. Oncotarget. 2015;6(22):18933–44.
88. Cortez MA, Ivan C, Valdecanas D, Wang X, Peltier HJ, Ye Y, et al. PDL1 regulation by p53 via miR-34. J Natl Cancer Inst. 2016;108(1)
89. Wang X, Li J, Dong K, Lin F, Long M, Ouyang Y, et al. Tumor suppressor miR-34a targets PD-L1 and functions as a potential immunotherapeutic target in acute myeloid leukemia. Cell Signal. 2015;27(3):443–52.
90. Zhao L, Yu H, Yi S, Peng X, Su P, Xiao Z, et al. The tumor suppressor miR-138-5p targets PD-L1 in colorectal cancer. Oncotarget. 2016;7(29):45370–84.
91. Chen L, Gibbons DL, Goswami S, Cortez MA, Ahn YH, Byers LA, et al. Metastasis is regulated via microRNA-200/ZEB1 axis control of tumour cell PD-L1 expression and intratumoral immunosuppression. Nat Commun. 2014;5:5241.
92. Liu Z, Wen J, Wu C, Hu C, Wang J, Bao Q, et al. MicroRNA-200a induces immunosuppression by promoting PTEN-mediated PD-L1 upregulation in osteosarcoma. Aging. 2020;12(2):1213–36.
93. Tao Z, Xu S, Ruan H, Wang T, Song W, Qian L, et al. MiR-195/−16 family enhances radiotherapy via T cell activation in the tumor microenvironment by blocking the PD-L1 immune checkpoint. Cell Physiol Biochem. 2018;48(2):801–14.
94. Kao SC, Cheng YY, Williams M, Kirschner MB, Madore J, Lum T, et al. Tumor suppressor microRNAs contribute to the regulation of PD-L1 expression in malignant pleural mesothelioma. J Thorac Oncol. 2017;12(9):1421–33.
95. Wang W, Li F, Mao Y, Zhou H, Sun J, Li R, et al. A miR-570 binding site polymorphism in the B7-H1 gene is associated with the risk of gastric adenocarcinoma. Hum Genet. 2013;132(6):641–8.
96. Wang Y, Wang D, Xie G, Yin Y, Zhao E, Tao K, et al. MicroRNA-152 regulates immune response via targeting B7-H1 in gastric carcinoma. Oncotarget. 2017;8(17):28125–34.
97. Fujita Y, Yagishita S, Hagiwara K, Yoshioka Y, Kosaka N, Takeshita F, et al. The clinical relevance of the miR-197/CKS1B/STAT3-mediated PD-L1 network in chemoresistant non-small-cell lung cancer. Mol Ther. 2015;23(4):717–27.

98. Wang LL, Huang WW, Huang J, Huang RF, Li NN, Hong Y, et al. Protective effect of hsa-miR-570-3p targeting CD274 on triple negative breast cancer by blocking PI3K/AKT/mTOR signaling pathway. Kaohsiung J Med Sci. 2020;36(8):581–91.
99. Gao L, Guo Q, Li X, Yang X, Ni H, Wang T, et al. MiR-873/PD-L1 axis regulates the stemness of breast cancer cells. EBioMedicine. 2019;41:395–407.
100. Qu F, Ye J, Pan X, Wang J, Gan S, Chu C, et al. MicroRNA-497-5p down-regulation increases PD-L1 expression in clear cell renal cell carcinoma. J Drug Target. 2019;27(1):67–74.
101. Li D, Wang X, Yang M, Kan Q, Duan Z. miR3609 sensitizes breast cancer cells to adriamycin by blocking the programmed death-ligand 1 immune checkpoint. Exp Cell Res. 2019;380(1):20–8.
102. Cioffi M, Trabulo SM, Vallespinos M, Raj D, Kheir TB, Lin ML, et al. The miR-25-93-106b cluster regulates tumor metastasis and immune evasion via modulation of CXCL12 and PD-L1. Oncotarget. 2017;8(13):21609–25.
103. Jia L, Xi Q, Wang H, Zhang Z, Liu H, Cheng Y, et al. miR-142-5p regulates tumor cell PD-L1 expression and enhances anti-tumor immunity. Biochem Biophys Res Commun. 2017;488(2):425–31.
104. Ashizawa M, Okayama H, Ishigame T, Thar Min AK, Saito K, Ujiie D, et al. miRNA-148a-3p regulates immunosuppression in DNA mismatch repair-deficient colorectal cancer by targeting PD-L1. Mol Cancer Res. 2019;17(6):1403–13.
105. Sun JR, Zhang X, Zhang Y. MiR-214 prevents the progression of diffuse large B-cell lymphoma by targeting PD-L1. Cell Mol Biol Lett. 2019;24:68.
106. Xie WB, Liang LH, Wu KG, Wang LX, He X, Song C, et al. MiR-140 expression regulates cell proliferation and targets PD-L1 in NSCLC. Cell Physiol Biochem. 2018;46(2):654–63.
107. Liu J, Fan L, Yu H, Zhang J, He Y, Feng D, et al. Endoplasmic reticulum stress causes liver cancer cells to release Exosomal miR-23a-3p and up-regulate programmed death ligand 1 expression in macrophages. Hepatology (Baltimore, Md). 2019;70(1):241–58.
108. Yao X, Tu Y, Xu Y, Guo Y, Yao F, Zhang X. Endoplasmic reticulum stress-induced exosomal miR-27a-3p promotes immune escape in breast cancer via regulating PD-L1 expression in macrophages. J Cell Mol Med. 2020;24(17):9560–73.
109. Sheng Q, Zhang Y, Wang Z, Ding J, Song Y, Zhao W. Cisplatin-mediated down-regulation of miR-145 contributes to up-regulation of PD-L1 via the c-Myc transcription factor in cisplatin-resistant ovarian carcinoma cells. Clin Exp Immunol. 2020;200(1):45–52.

Chapter 4
Immune Checkpoint Expression in Cancer: Mechanisms and Implications for Immunotherapy

4.1 Introduction

Cancer is one of the most important clinical complications in the twenty-first century. Malignancies are among the main causes of death worldwide and the number of affected people is increasing. The immune system has a close interface with cancer from the development of the tumor to the advanced stages of the disease. During cancer immunoediting, the tumor is stabilized in three stages: elimination, equilibrium, and escape. In the elimination phase, tumor cells are removed by immunosurveillance in the initial stages of development. Immune cells recognize tumor neoantigens and molecules related to cellular stress and eliminate transformed cells. Some of these potential cancer cells survive and enter the equilibrium phase. In the equilibrium phase, the tumor variants resistant to immune effectors are selected. Tumor cells can remain dormant for a long time, even decades. Finally, in the escape phase with the proliferation and growth of the tumor cells, cancer clinically appears [1, 2]. There are several immunomodulating elements in the tumor microenvironment (TME) that support tumor growth, including regulatory cells that regulate immune responses in favor of the tumor, such as regulatory T cells (Tregs), myeloid-derived suppressor cells (MDSCs), and tumor-associated macrophages (TAMs), as well as expression of immunosuppressive molecules and mediators [3]. Immune checkpoints are the pivotal components of immune regulation and are considered as a critical tumor escape mechanism. In malignancies, the immune checkpoint arm is overactive and facilitates tumor growth. The expression of immune checkpoints in TME is well established. Exhausted T cells express various inhibitory molecules such as PD-1, CTLA-4, TIM-3, and LAG-3 on their surface, which make them dysfunctional [4]. In this chapter, the characteristics of TME and the expression of immune checkpoints in the tumor are described.

L. Tayebi, M. Abdolmaleki, *Immune System Regulation*,
https://doi.org/10.1007/978-981-95-8026-2_4

4.2 Tumor Microenvironment

TME regulates the survival, growth, and expansion of the tumor. TME is a complex milieu in which different cell types and various factors such as hypoxia, acidic pH conditions, intracellular reactive oxide species (ROS), and extracellular matrix (ECM) proteins are involved. Because of the rapid and excessive growth of the tumor and the limited access to blood vessels, the central cells of the tumor mass become hypoxic. Hypoxia-inducible angiogenic factors such as vascular endothelial growth factor (VEGF) and other mediators such as hypoxia-inducible factor (HIF) promote tumor growth. The acidic pH helps tumor invasion by induction of expression of angiogenic factors [5].

Immune cells are the major part of TME. Different types of adaptive and innate immune cells are present in the TME. Dendritic cells (DCs) are professional antigen presenting cells (APCs) that provide activation signals to T cells. $CD4^+$ T cells are among the main components of adaptive immune response. $CD4^+$ T cells need two signals for activation. The first signal is triggered by the binding of T cell receptor (TCR) to MHC II-peptide (pMHC-II) complex on DCs. The co-stimulatory signal is conducted by the interaction of CD28 molecules on T cells with CD80 and CD86 on DCs. These signals induce T cells activation, proliferation, and differentiation. One of the most important populations of $CD4^+$ T cells is the T helper type 1 (Th1) subset, which plays a critical role in tumor growth inhibition. Th1 cells suppress tumor growth by secreting pro-inflammatory cytokines, especially IFN-γ. The other subset of T lymphocytes are $CD8^+$ T cells. After recognizing the MHC I–peptide (pMHC-I) complex on DCs by TCR, $CD8^+$ T cells become activated and differentiate into cytotoxic T cells (CTLs). In TME, CTLs detect tumor cells and eliminate them through releasing cytotoxic granules containing perforin and granzyme, or by Fas ligand (FasL)-mediated apoptosis. Tumor-specific B cells accumulate in the lymph nodes near the tumor area. B cells exert their antitumor function by the production of tumor-specific antibodies and the secretion of cytokines. Natural killer (NK) cells ($CD3^-$ $CD56^+$ cells) are very important in antitumor immunity. NK cells destroy tumor cells by releasing perforin and granzyme, or induction of apoptosis via TNF-related apoptosis-inducing ligand (TRAIL) and FasL. In addition, NK cells can enhance antitumor immune response through the secretion of inflammatory cytokines such as IFN-γ and TNF-α [5, 6].

The tumor immune microenvironment (TIME) can be classified into three different classes. Infiltrated–excluded (I–E) TIMEs are vastly formed by immune cells but there is low infiltration of CTLs in the tumor core with low secretion of granzyme B and IFN-γ. In the I–E, CTLs are majorly located in the margin of the tumor mass. I–E TIMEs are correlated with epithelial cancers such as melanoma and colorectal carcinoma. It seems that tumors with I–E TIMEs are poorly immunogenic. Infiltrated–inflamed (I–I) TIMEs are populated by PD-1 positive leukocytes, especially $PD\text{-}1^+$ CTLs and these types of tumors are more immunogenic. There is a subdivision of I–I TIMEs that form tertiary lymphoid structures (TLSs) with cellular distribution resembling lymph nodes including naive and activated T cells, B cells, and DCs, which is called TLS-TIME and correlates with positive prognosis. TLSs are found in the margin and stroma of invasive tumors and act as immune activation sites. T cells are the most important immune cells within the TIME for controlling tumor progression. Chronic activation of T cells by tumor antigens leads to T cell exhaustion and expression of a variety of inhibitory receptors that make them dysfunctional [7].

TAMs and MDSCs are important immunosuppressive cells that contribute to the inhibition of the antitumor immune responses by different mechanisms, including the production of suppressive factors such as IL-10, TGF-β, and indoleamine-2,3-dioxygenase (IDO) [2]. Treg cells, known as $CD4^+$ $CD25^+$ $FoxP3^+$ T cells, suppress the activity of T cells by producing IL-10, IL-35, and TGF-β. CTLA-4 expression on Tregs enhances the suppressive properties of these cells. In general, Tregs are associated with poorer survival in multiple tumors. Regulatory B cells (Bregs) cell is a subset of B cells with immunosuppressive entities. The production of IL-10, IL-35, and TGF-β cytokines is the characteristic of these cells. Bregs affect the adaptive response against the tumor, such as the function of CTLs or the production of IFN-γ. The presence of Bregs is related to a worse clinical outcome in the tumor [8].

4.3 Immune Checkpoints in Cancer

4.3.1 CTLA-4

CTLA-4 is a key immune checkpoint for T cell response regulation. The main mechanism of action of CTLA-4 is the competitive inhibition of CD28 co-stimulatory molecule binding to B7 (CD80/86) molecules on the APCs. In addition, following CTLA-4/B7 engagement, the recruitment of SHP-2 and PP2A phosphatases leads to the termination of TCR-induced intracellular signaling. In the tumor context, CTLA-4 expression was first observed in leukemia and lymphoma [9]. CTLA-4 is overexpressed in different types of cancers such as melanoma, breast, lung, Prostate, esophageal, and gastric cancers. Increased expression of this receptor also has been reported in hematological malignancies including acute myeloid leukemia (AML), acute lymphoblastic leukemia (ALL), chronic lymphocytic leukemia (CLL), *chronic myeloid leukemia* (CML), adult T-cell leukemia (ATL), cutaneous T cell lymphoma (CTCL), and mantle cell lymphoma (MCL) [10, 11]. Analysis of CTLA-4 expression in several types of cancer has shown the upregulation of CTLA-4 on tumor-infiltrating lymphocytes (TILs), especially $CD8^+$ T cells. CTLA-4 also has been detected on B cells, NK cells, and monocytes. As expected, co-expression of CTLA-4 with other inhibitory receptors such as BTLA, LAG-3, PD-1, and TIGIT occurs on immune cells in TME [11]. CTLA-4 expression in esophageal carcinoma, glioma, pancreatic adenocarcinoma, melanoma, thymoma, ALL, gastric and nasopharyngeal cancers is associated with worse clinical outcomes. However, in some cancers, including non-small cell lung cancer (NSCLC), mesothelioma, and CLL, CTLA-4 overexpression has been correlated with a better overall survival (OS) [10, 11]. Furthermore, according to a meta-analysis, elevated level of the soluble form of CTLA-4 (sCTLA-4) is associated with a favorable prognosis. sCTLA-4 has complicated modulatory mechanisms. It can inhibit cell surface CTLA-4 signaling by binding to CD80/CD86. In several studies, the correlation between the high levels of sCTLA-4 and the increase in pro-inflammatory cytokine levels has been shown [12]. Effector Tregs ($CD45RA^{+}$ $CD25^{hi}$ $FoxP3^{hi}$) are the most important group of Tregs in cancer. These cells with high expression of CTLA-4 have great suppressive potential. In TME, Tregs suppress the immune response in different ways. They limit the activation of conventional T cells (Tconv) through the binding of their surface CTLA-4 to B7 molecules on APCs. Moreover, Tregs can detach B7 proteins from the membrane of APC cells by trogocytosis and transfer them to their surface or cytoplasm [13, 14]. CTLA-4 blocking antibodies, in addition to directly enhancing the tumor-specific T cell responses, enhance the antitumor response by targeting Tregs. Anti-CTLA-4 antibodies causes the elimination of these cells by Fc-mediated antibody-dependent cellular cytotoxicity (ADCC) and antibody-dependent cellular phagocytosis (ADCP) [13]. Ipilimumab, an anti-CTLA-4 agent, was the first immune checkpoint inhibitor approved by the FDA for the treatment of melanoma. To date, hundreds of clinical trials have been conducted on cancer with CTLA-4 inhibitors [15].

4.3.2 PD-1

The PD-1/PD-L1 axis is crucial in damping the antitumor immune response. Interaction of PD-1 with its ligand inhibits $CD4^{+}$/$CD8^{+}$ TILs and reduces IL-2, IFN-γ, and TNF secretion [16, 17]. PD-1^{+} DCs interrupt $CD8^{+}$ T cell function. Furthermore, DCs expressing PD-L1 are involved in the expansion of Tregs. PD-1^{+} Tregs suppress $CD8^{+}$ T cells function through interaction with PD-L1 on the T cells. PD-1 expression also occurs on Bregs in the TME. PD-1^{+} Bregs can regulate $CD4^{+}$ and $CD8^{+}$ T cells functions. It has been found that the increase of $CD4^{+}$ PD-1^{+} TILs, for example in NSCLC and CLL, is associated with tumor progression. PD-1 can promote the polarization of anti-inflammatory M2 macrophages. The increase of PD-1^{+} macrophages in various tumors such as gastric cancer and esophageal squamous cell carcinomas (ESCC) is associated with poor prognosis. PD-1^{+} NK cells are associated with bad prognosis and disease progression in some cancers such as ESCC and renal cell carcinoma [18]. The upregulation of PD-L1 in solid tumors is associated with poor prognosis and aggressive disease [16]. According to a meta-analysis, overexpression of PD-L1 has been associated with worse 3-year OS for several tumors, including esophageal cancer, gastric cancer, hepatocellular carcinoma, and urothelial cancer [19]. Inhibition of PD-1/PD-L1 interaction by PD-1 and PD-L1 blockers has shown to be effective in inhibiting tumor growth and increasing the T cell-mediated antitumor immune responses. Different types of

PD-1 and PD-L1 inhibitor antibodies have been used in cancer clinical trials. Anti-PD-1 antibodies, including nivolumab and pembrolizumab, as well as atezolizumab, a PD-L1 inhibitor, have been approved by the FDA for the treatment of solid cancers [20].

4.3.3 TIM-3

TIM-3 is overexpressed in a wide range of cancers and dampens $CD4^+$ and $CD8^+$ T cells responses in tumor. TIM-3 expression is associated with reduced OS and poor prognosis in solid cancers such as gastric and ovarian cancers [21, 22]. Guo et al. showed that TIM-3 is highly expressed on tumor and non-tumor cells in glioblastoma [23]. The function of microglia is influenced by TIM-3. TIM-3/Galectin-9 (Gal-9) signaling in brain tumors causes the polarization of macrophages toward the M2-like phenotype, which plays an important role in immune suppression and tumor progression [23, 24]. The upregulation of TIM-3 in renal cell carcinoma was associated with poor prognosis. $PD\text{-}1^+$ $TIM\text{-}3^+$ $CD8^+$ T cells of the patients had suppressed cytotoxicity and IL-2, TNF-α, and IFN-γ production [24–26]. In lung cancer, the presence of $TIM\text{-}3^+$ $CD4^+$ TILs correlates with advanced cancer stage [27]. TIM-3 and CEACAM1 have been detected on tumor and immune cells of head and neck squamous cell carcinoma (HNSCC) patients, which is correlated with tumor size, lymph node metastasis, and poor OS [28]. In gastric cancer, TIM-3 expression along with PD-1 causes dysfunction of $CD8^+$ T cells. Increased expression of this immune checkpoint on NK cells and monocytes/macrophages has been detected in gastric cancer. TIM-3/Gal-9 signaling in macrophages stimulates the production of IL-6, IL-8, and IL-10, which is associated with poor outcomes in gastric cancer patients [24, 29]. In melanoma, increased expression of TIM-3 has been found on NK cells, monocytes, and myeloid dendritic cells (mDCs). In these patients, $TIM\text{-}3^+$ $PD\text{-}1^+$ NYESO-1-specific $CD8^+$ T cells had impaired function [30]. TIM-3 expressing $CCR1^+$ $CD14^+$ monocytes in hepatocellular carcinoma (HCC) patients can be immunosuppressive [11]. In colorectal cancer, Tregs expressing LAG-3 and TIM-3 were more suppressive and produced more TGF-β and IL-10 [31]. TIM-3 is also important in hematological malignancies including CML, ALL, CLL, and myelodysplastic syndromes (MDS). The overexpression of TIM-3 on $CD4^+$ and $CD8^+$ T cells, Tregs, and leukemia stem cells is associated with blasts proliferation. Several clinical trials have been conducted to target TIM-3 by blocking agents in hematological cancers [32, 33]. In the TME, TGF-β can induce the expression of TIM-3 and Gal-9. In mouse model of HCC, induction of TIM-3 expression by TGF-β in TAMs and inhibition of $CD8^+$ T cells response has been observed. The synergistic effect of Gal-9 and TGF-β can lead to the expression of Foxp3 and the development of Tregs. $TIM\text{-}3^+$ Tregs are stronger immunosuppressors and are associated with tumor progression [34]. HMGB1 is a nucleic acid binding protein that can be released from tumor cells. HMGB1 binds to RAGE, TLR4, and TLR2 on the surface of DCs and activates them against tumor. TIM-3 inhibits HMGB1 activation signaling in these cells by competitive binding to tumor-associated DCs [35]. The interaction of TIM-3 on DCs with HMGB1 on the surface of tumor cells causes tumor proliferation [34]. Besides the membrane-bound form, exosomes containing TIM-3 have also been identified in cancers. In NSCLC, the presence of exosomes expressing TIM-3 and Gal-9 (exo-TIM-3 and exo-Gal-9) has been related to tumor size, metastasis, and more severe disease. In addition, the secreted form of TIM-3 (sTIM-3) is also released in cancer through the breakdown of TIM-3 on the cell surface by ADAMs, mainly ADAM10 and ADAM17. The increase of sTIM-3 has been reported in several tumors, and the inhibitory role of sTIM-3 in the antitumor response has been described. The increased level of sTIM-3 was associated with the disease progression in gastric cancer, HCC, osteosarcoma, and renal cell carcinoma (RCC). Therefore, sTIM-3 can be considered as a potential prognostic biomarker in cancers [36].

4.3.4 LAG-3

LAG-3 expression has been reported in NSCLC, melanoma, gastric cancer, colorectal cancer, breast cancer, ovarian cancer, and HCC. LAG-3 overexpression is associated with tumor progression and metastasis [37, 38]. Nevertheless, a meta-analysis has shown that LAG-3 expression is associated with a better clinical outcome in early-stage malignancies [39]. LAG-3 is mainly expressed on lymphocytes and it is co-expressed with other immune checkpoints mainly PD-1 and TIM-3. In numerous cancers such as colorectal cancer, HCC, kidney renal clear cell carcinoma (KIRC), NSCLC, primary central nervous system lymphoma (PCNSL), and diffuse large B cell lymphoma (DLBCL) correlation of LAG-3 levels and poor prognosis has been proved [37, 40]. In hematological malignancies, simultaneous expression of LAG-3 and TIM-3 has been reported. In follicular lymphoma patients, LAG-3 expression is correlated to poor outcomes [37]. It has been shown that melanoma cells bind to LAG-3 on $CD4^+$ T cells through the expression of MHC II and inhibit the antitumor response. Furthermore, this interaction can prevent apoptosis of melanoma cells through MAPK/ErK and PI3K/AKT pathways and increase their survival. LAG-3 is a potential biomarker in breast cancer. The presence of LAG-3^+ TILs is associated with more aggressive disease in these patients [37, 41]. In ovarian cancer and follicular lymphoma, PD-1^+ LAG-3^+ T cells had decreased IFN-γ and IL-2 production. In muscle invasive bladder cancer, a higher level of LAG-3 was related to more inhibitory cytokines such as IL-10 and TGF-β, which favor tumor development [40]. The overexpression of FGL1 has been observed in several tumors. LAG-3/FGL1 interaction in TME suppresses IL-2 production of T cells [40]. According to a study, the soluble form of LAG-3 (sLAG-3) in HNSCC was associated with poor progression-free survival (PFS) and OS [42]. LAG-3 is a suitable target for tumor immunotherapy and the effectiveness of LAG-3 inhibitors has been proven in multiple studies [43].

4.3.5 *TIGIT*

TIGIT overexpression has been reported in several tumors such as melanoma, lung, colorectal, and gastric cancers. In many cases, TIGIT is expressed on TILs along with other immune checkpoints such as LAG-3, CTLA-4, and PD-1. $PD-1^{+}$ $TIGIT^{+}$ $CD8^{+}$ TILs are a common cell population in tumors [44]. In general, TIGIT overexpression in cancer is associated with poorer OS and relapse-free survival (RFS) [45]. A study of colorectal cancer patients has shown that upregulation of TIGIT interferes with proliferation, glucose uptake, glycolytic activity, and antitumor function of T cells [46]. TIGIT has also been found on Tregs and NK cells. In endometrial tumors or AML, $TIGIT^{+}$ NK cells had an exhausted phenotype, and the presence of these cells was associated with more advanced disease and poor prognosis. In some cancers, such as melanoma, the simultaneous expression of TIGIT/CD226 has been observed on $CD8^{+}$ T cells. In gastric cancer, the expression of TIGIT along with PVR and CD112 on $CD8^{+}$ TILs has been associated with poor prognosis [47]. CD155 acts as a common ligand for TIGIT, CD96, and CD226. CD226/CD155 axis increases the cytotoxicity of NK and $CD8^{+}$ T cells by inducing the co-stimulatory signal. The upregulation of CD155 on tumor cells causes CD226 internalization and inhibits the activation of this pathway. On the other hand, the soluble isoforms of CD155 derived from tumor occupy the binding capacity of CD226 and facilitate the suppression of tumor-infiltrating NK and T cells function through membrane CD155. In addition, TIGIT and CD96 also compete with CD226 for binding to CD155 and inhibit its signaling. TIGIT interaction with CD155 on DCs affects their maturation. This pathway prevents the production of pro-inflammatory cytokine IL-12 from these cells [48].

4.3.6 *CD96*

CD155 and CD111 are two ligands of CD96. Animal studies have shown that CD96 signaling inhibits the cytotoxicity of NK cells and $CD8^{+}$ T cells. Blockade of CD96 enhances the activity of NK cells to control metastasis in melanoma mice. The association of increased expression of CD96 in human tumors with poor clinical outcomes has been reported in some studies. On the contrary, a negative correlation between the presence of $CD96^{+}$ NK and metastases has been found in pancreatic cancer [49, 50]. In hepatocellular carcinoma, increased expression of CD96 has been associated with decreased OS, which indicates its inhibitory role in this cancer [51]. In cervical cancer patients receiving anti-PD-1, the expression of CD96 on $CD8^{+}$ TILs was increased. $PD-1^{+}$ $CD96^{+}$ $CD8^{+}$ TILs were increased in these patients and these cells showed an exhausted phenotype [52].

4.3.7 PVRIG

PVRIG is expressed on $CD4^+$ T cells, $CD8^+$ T cells, and NK cells in various cancers. Increased expression of PVRIG has been observed in ovarian, kidney, lung, endometrial, breast, stomach, colorectal, and prostate cancers. $TIGIT^+$ PD-1^+ $CD8^+$ TILs show an exhausted phenotype in prostate cancer [49]. The correlation between PVRIG and the prognosis has been demonstrated in some cancers. In gallbladder cancer, pancreatic ductal adenocarcinomas, and AML, the expression of PVRIG has been associated with poor prognosis and shorter OS. $CD8^+$ and $CD4^+$ TILs and NKs, which express PVRIG, are phenotypically exhausted. PVRIG has a high affinity for CD112 and competes with CD226 for binding to this ligand. PVRIG blockers have been associated with tumor growth control and increased survival in mouse models and human cancers [53].

4.3.8 CD244

The expression of this immune checkpoint on exhausted $CD8^+$ T cells has been found in several tumors, for example, the presence of $CD244^+$ PD-1^+ TIM-3^+ $CD8^+$ TILs in melanoma or the expression of CD244 alongside PD-1, CTLA-4, CD160 on $CD8^+$ T cells of AML patients [54]. In CLL, T cells expressing CD244 have decreased proliferation and cytotoxicity [55]. CD244 is also expressed on tumor-dependent NK cells, MDSCs, and DCs and contributes to suppressing of antitumor immune response. Blocking of CD244 on DCs can be effective in enhancing the activation of T cells and NK cells by these cells [54]. In HCC patients treated with anti-PD-1/anti-PD-L1, increased expression of CD244 along with LAG-3 has been found in T cells [56].

4.3.9 BTLA

HVEM-BTLA is an important axis in T cell dysfunction and tumor immune evasion. HVEM has been found in several cancers such as glioblastoma, HCC, renal carcinoma, esophageal squamous cell carcinoma, breast cancer, and hematological malignancies. The expression of HVEM has been reported to be associated with poorer prognosis in progressive lung cancer, glioma, as well as CLL [57]. The overexpression of BTLA on $CD4^+$ and $CD8^+$ TILs in bladder cancer has been associated with worse outcomes. Additionally, in AML patients, elevated BTLA levels have been associated with poor prognosis and decreased OS [58, 59]. BTLA expression also occurs with other inhibitory molecules. The upregulation of BTLA along with the other immune checkpoints including PD-1, PD-L1, CTLA-4, LAG-3, and VISTA indicates the role of this molecule in regulating the antitumor immune response [57, 60]. In many cases, the elevated expression of HVEM in tumor cells is correlated with increased expression of BTLA on TILs. In gastric cancer, it has been revealed that in HVEM+ tumors, BTLA expression has also increased [57]. The interaction of HVEM+ tumor cells with BTLA+ CD8+ T cells can lead to inhibition of tumor-specific lymphocytes functions [58]. The soluble form of BTLA (sBTLA) has also been reported in the tumor context. The findings show that the elevated levels of sBTLA can be considered as a prognostic marker. The association of increased sBTLA levels with shorter survival and more active disease has been demonstrated in prostate cancer, ovarian cancer, pancreatic adenocarcinoma, clear cell renal cancer, and HCC [58].

4.3.10 B7s

4.3.10.1 B7-H3

B7-H3 (CD276) is overexpressed on a range of immune cells including activated B cells, T cells, NK cells, DC, and macrophages in different malignancies such as gastric, colon, prostate, ovary, pancreas, kidney, and lung cancers. B7-H3 enhances tumor invasion and progression. The association between the B7-H3 expression and the poor prognosis of tumors has been demonstrated by several studies. In gastric cancer, the upregulation of B7-H3 is related to poor survival [17, 61]. Increased expression of B7-H3 in metastatic prostate cancer is associated with an increased mortality rate. B7-H3 facilitates tumor growth through different mechanisms. B7-H3 signaling inhibits CD4+ T and CD8+ TILs functions. In addition, it can induce the polarization of M2 macrophages. B7-H3 signaling causes the proliferation and growth of tumor cells and promotes metastasis and tumor angiogenesis through the stimulation of VEGF production. B7-H3 is involved in the resistance of cancer cells to apoptosis by inducing the expression of antiapoptotic proteins Bcl-2 and Bcl-xl and reducing proapoptotic proteins Bax and caspase-8 in tumor cells. So far, many B7-H3 inhibitory agents have been developed to inhibit tumors [62–64].

4.3.10.2 B7-H4

B7-H4 (B7x) has a limited expression on immune cells under physiological conditions, but upregulation of this immune checkpoint has been observed in several tumors such as lung cancer, colorectal cancer, and RCC. B7-H4 expression is associated with tumor dissemination, poor clinical outcome, and lower survival. In RCC, B7-H4 overexpression correlates with tumor size and advanced disease stage. Simultaneous expression of B7-H3 and B7-H4 is associated with poor prognosis and increased mortality. B7-H4 expression has also been detected on myeloid DCs and plasmacytoid DCs of HCC patients [65]. The upregulation of B7-H4 on APC negatively regulates the function of these cells. In breast cancer, B7-H4 expression is associated with increased infiltration of macrophages, Tregs, and neutrophils into the tumor and diminished antitumor immune response [66].

4.3.10.3 VISTA

VISTA (B7-H5) is overexpressed in several tumors including cholangiocarcinoma, glioblastoma, KIRC, AML, and pancreatic adenocarcinoma. VISTA, by binding to its ligands (PSGL-1 and VSIG-3), contributes to tumor immune escape. In TME, increased expression of VISTA occurs on naive $CD4^+$ T cells, $FoxP3^+$ Tregs, MDSCs, and TAMs as well as tumor cells. The association of VISTA expression with poor prognosis has been described in cancers such as prostate cancer, AML, glioblastoma, melanoma, and ovarian cancer. In NSCLC, VISTA is overexpressed on T cells. It has been shown that after treating prostate cancer with ipilimumab, the expression of VISTA and PD-L1 on $CD68^+$ macrophages was significantly increased [67, 68].

4.3.10.4 B7-H7

B7-H7 (HHLA2) is increased in several cancers and can be considered as a marker of exhausted T cells. The expression of B7-H7 is related to the clinical outcome of various cancers. Increased expression of B7-H7 in NSCLC, gastric cancer, colorectal cancer, liver cancer, renal cell carcinoma, and chondroma is associated with poor prognosis or more advanced disease stage and metastasis, whereas the elevated levels of B7-H7 in pancreatic cancer, cervical cancer, ovarian cancer, glioma, and melanoma are associated with better prognosis or improved survival and higher numbers of $CD8^+$ TILs [69]. B7-H7 can be involved in tumor metabolism. B7-H7/TMIGD2 axis promotes angiogenesis in TME. The direct correlation between METTL3 and B7-H7 has been identified. METTL3 is one of the effective factors in tumor angiogenesis and glycolysis [70].

4.3.11 CD39 and CD73

CD39 and CD73 are expressed on different cell populations in TME including tumor cells and immune cells. There is a high amount of extracellular adenosine triphosphate (ATP) released in TME following inflammation, cell necrosis, and anticancer therapy. The extracellular ATP is hydrolyzed to adenosine monophosphate (AMP) by CD39 and then is converted to adenosine by CD73. The CD38/CD203a/CD73 pathway acts as an alternative pathway for producing adenosine. Adenosine has immunosuppressive properties and can inhibit immune cells functions. The binding of adenosine to its receptors on effector immune cells leads to the increase of intracellular cyclic AMP (cAMP) and subsequently suppression of their proliferation, cytokine production, and cytolysis activity [71, 72]. In the presence of high adenosine concentration, the interaction mainly occurs through A2AR and A2BR. These receptors are expressed on a wide range of immune cells, including $CD4^+$ T cells, $CD8^+$ T cells, Tregs, NK cells, DCs, and TAMs in the TME. A2AR or A2BR expression on DCs affects the antitumor immune response of $CD4^+$ T cells. Adenosine reduces the antigen presentation activity of DCs. Furthermore, adenosine increases the production of tolerogenic factors such as IDO, IL-10, and TGF-β from DCs. Studies have shown that A2AR antagonist can neutralize the effect of adenosine on DCs and increase their activity. The binding of adenosine to A2AR on T cells reduces the proliferation of these cells. The presence of $CD39^+$ Th17 cells in TME correlates with poor clinical outcomes. Adenosine affects $CD8^+$ TILs cells functions. $CD8^+$ T cells expressing CD39 have impaired cytotoxicity. $CD73^+$ $CD8^+$ T cells have less glucose uptake and weaker antitumor response. It has been found that increased expression of CD73 on NK cells is related to tumor size in cancer. Adenosine–A2AR interaction inhibits the cytotoxicity of these cells in the tumor, and CD73 blocking antibodies enhance the antitumor function of NK cells. A2BR antagonists increase the cytotoxic activities and IFN-γ production of NK cells and tumor-specific T cells. Besides, adenosine increases the immune suppressive activity of Tregs and MDSCs. The overexpression of CD39 and CD73 on Tregs strengthens their immunosuppressive activity. A2AR signaling can induce the differentiation of Tregs. Adenosine produced in the TME causes the recruitment of Tregs to the tumor. Additionally, Tregs are involved in suppressing the response of $CD8^+$ and $CD4^+$ T cells by producing adenosine. Increased expression of CD73 and CD39 is associated with poor prognosis and tumor progression [71–73]. The expression of CD39 on tumor-infiltrating immune cells and cancer cells has been reported in several tumor types and it is associated with adverse outcomes. CD73 expression in TME has been considered as a prognostic factor in a range of malignancies including lung, gastric, and pancreatic cancers, pheochromocytoma, thyroid carcinoma, esophageal carcinoma, adenocarcinoma, and glioblastoma. Moreover, upregulation of A2A and A2B has been shown in different tumors such as lung cancer, pheochromocytoma, hepatocellular carcinoma, bladder urothelial carcinoma, cervical squamous cell carcinoma, and gastric adenocarcinoma. The increase of A2BR in lung cancer patients has been associated with worse outcomes. Taken together, CD39/CD73/adenosine–A2AR pathway is related to the immune evasion of tumor cells and poor prognosis of the patients. Inhibitors of this pathway, including CD73, CD39, and adenosine receptor blocking agents, have been effective in controlling tumor growth [73–75].

4.3.12 CD47/SIRPα

CD47/SIRPα axis acts as a “don’t eat me” signal to the phagocytes. CD47 is widely expressed in different types of cancers, including glioblastoma, ovarian, breast, bladder, colon, and hepatocellular carcinoma and is associated with decreased survival [76]. CD47 has been also identified in hematological tumors, including AML, multiple myeloma (MM), and non-Hodgkin lymphoma (NHL). CD47 can bind to SIRPα, thrombospondin-1 (TSP-1), and integrins. SIRPα is expressed on monocytes, macrophages, and DCs [77]. The expression of CD47 on tumor cells inhibits the adaptive antitumor response by binding to SIRPα on APCs. It also affects the function of T cells and NK cells through interaction with TSP-1. CD47 overexpression is associated with poor clinical outcomes or decreased PFS in lung cancer. CD47 plays an important role in the clinical characteristics and outcomes of hematological malignancies including NHL, ALL, AML, MDS, and MM [78]. CD47 expression can be upregulated by various factors including MYC oncogene and HIF-1. The binding of Myc and HIF-1 to CD47 promoter induces its expression [79]. CD47/SIRPα axis is an evasion mechanism from phagocytosis for tumor cells. Inhibitors of the CD47/SIRPα axis limit tumor growth in different ways. These agents can enhance the function of APCs and augment the activation of tumor-specific cytotoxic T cells. CD47/SIRPα axis blockers can increase ADCC activity by inhibiting SIRPα [77]. CD47–SIRPα blockade also increases the cross-presentation of tumor antigens by DCs for priming of $CD8^+$ T cells [76]. Anti-SIRPα antibodies decrease SIRPα on the surface of macrophages. Therefore, these inhibitors, along with anti-CD47 antibodies, participate in the clearance of tumor cells. Induction of phagocytosis of AML leukemic cells following the use of anti-CD47 antibodies has been reported [78, 80].

4.4 Conclusion

The exploration of immune checkpoint expression in cancer presented in this chapter highlights the intricate balance between immune activation and regulation in the tumor microenvironment. The detailed examination of various checkpoint molecules reveals their crucial roles in modulating antitumor immune responses and their potential as prognostic markers and therapeutic targets. The chapter explored the complexity of immune checkpoint interactions, with many molecules exhibiting context-dependent functions and often being co-expressed with other inhibitory receptors.

The success of checkpoint inhibitors targeting CTLA-4 and PD-1/PD-L1 in clinical settings has demonstrated the therapeutic potential of manipulating these pathways. However, the emergence of resistance to single-agent therapies and the heterogeneity of checkpoint expression across different cancers and patients emphasize the need for combination approaches and personalized strategies.

The chapter also sheds light on emerging checkpoint molecules and alternative pathways involved in immune evasion, such as the CD39/CD73/adenosine axis and the CD47/SIRPα pathway. These findings open new avenues for therapeutic interventions and highlight the importance of a comprehensive understanding of the immune landscape in cancer.

As research in this field progresses, integrating genomic, epigenomic, and functional data will be vital for developing a better understanding of immune checkpoint regulation. This knowledge will pave the way for more effective and targeted immunotherapies, not only in cancer but potentially in chronic infections, autoimmune diseases, and other immune-related disorders. The future of cancer immunotherapy lies in harnessing the complex network of immune checkpoints to show the full potential of the immune system against tumors.

Acknowledgments The authors gratefully acknowledge the valuable assistance provided by Maryam Sadr.

References

1. Lasek W. Cancer immunoediting hypothesis: history, clinical implications and controversies. Cent Eur J Immunol. 2022;47(2):168–74.
2. Tang S, Ning Q, Yang L, Mo Z, Tang S. Mechanisms of immune escape in the cancer immune cycle. Int Immunopharmacol. 2020;86:106700.
3. Vinay DS, Ryan EP, Pawelec G, Talib WH, Stagg J, Elkord E, et al. Immune evasion in cancer: mechanistic basis and therapeutic strategies. Semin Cancer Biol. 2015;35(Suppl):S185–s98.
4. Goenka A, Khan F, Verma B, Sinha P, Dmello CC, Jogalekar MP, et al. Tumor microenvironment signaling and therapeutics in cancer progression. Cancer Commun. 2023;43(5):525–61.
5. Sadeghi Rad H, Monkman J, Warkiani ME, Ladwa R, O'Byrne K, Rezaei N, et al. Understanding the tumor microenvironment for effective immunotherapy. Med Res Rev. 2021;41(3):1474–98.
6. Anderson NM, Simon MC. The tumor microenvironment. Curr Biol. 2020;30(16):R921–r5.
7. Binnewies M, Roberts EW, Kersten K, Chan V, Fearon DF, Merad M, et al. Understanding the tumor immune microenvironment (TIME) for effective therapy. Nat Med. 2018;24(5):541–50.
8. Brummel K, Eerkens AL, de Bruyn M, Nijman HW. Tumour-infiltrating lymphocytes: from prognosis to treatment selection. Br J Cancer. 2023;128(3):451–8.
9. Oyewole-Said D, Konduri V, Vazquez-Perez J, Weldon SA, Levitt JM, Decker WK. Beyond T-cells: functional characterization of CTLA-4 expression in immune and non-immune cell types. Front Immunol. 2020;11:608024.
10. Abdulkhaleq F, Larossi N, Ogbonda O, Eid RA, Ward FJ. CTLA-4 expression by human tumor cells and its impact on immunotherapeutic strategies: a systematic review. Immuno-Oncol Insights. 2021;2(3):151–69.
11. Zhang C, Chen J, Song Q, Sun X, Xue M, Yang Z, et al. Comprehensive analysis of CTLA-4 in the tumor immune microenvironment of 33 cancer types. Int Immunopharmacol. 2020;85:106633.
12. Hu P, Liu Q, Deng G, Zhang J, Liang N, Xie J, et al. The prognostic value of cytotoxic T-lymphocyte antigen 4 in cancers: a systematic review and meta-analysis. Sci Rep. 2017;7:42913.
13. Tay C, Tanaka A, Sakaguchi S. Tumor-infiltrating regulatory T cells as targets of cancer immunotherapy. Cancer Cell. 2023;41(3):450–65.
14. Togashi Y, Shitara K, Nishikawa H. Regulatory T cells in cancer immunosuppression - implications for anticancer therapy. Nat Rev Clin Oncol. 2019;16(6):356–71.
15. Basudan AM. The role of immune checkpoint inhibitors in cancer therapy. Clin Pract. 2022;13(1):22–40.
16. Hudson K, Cross N, Jordan-Mahy N, Leyland R. The extrinsic and intrinsic roles of PD-L1 and its receptor PD-1: implications for immunotherapy treatment. Front Immunol. 2020;11:568931.

17. Mansorunov D, Apanovich N, Apanovich P, Kipkeeva F, Muzaffarova T, Kuzevanova A, et al. Expression of immune checkpoints in malignant tumors: therapy targets and biomarkers for the gastric cancer prognosis. Diagnostics (Basel, Switzerland). 2021;11(12)
18. Laba S, Mallett G, Amarnath S. The depths of PD-1 function within the tumor microenvironment beyond CD8(+) T cells. Semin Cancer Biol. 2022;86(Pt 2):1045–55.
19. Wu P, Wu D, Li L, Chai Y, Huang J. PD-L1 and survival in solid tumors: a meta-analysis. PLoS One. 2015;10(6):e0131403.
20. Alsaab HO, Sau S, Alzhrani R, Tatiparti K, Bhise K, Kashaw SK, et al. PD-1 and PD-L1 checkpoint signaling inhibition for cancer immunotherapy: mechanism, combinations, and clinical outcome. Front Pharmacol. 2017;8:561.
21. Zang K, Hui L, Wang M, Huang Y, Zhu X, Yao B. TIM-3 as a prognostic marker and a potential immunotherapy target in human malignant tumors: a meta-analysis and bioinformatics validation. Front Oncol. 2021;11:579351.
22. Qin S, Dong B, Yi M, Chu Q, Wu K. Prognostic values of TIM-3 expression in patients with solid tumors: a meta-analysis and database evaluation. Front Oncol. 2020;10:1288.
23. Guo Q, Shen S, Guan G, Zhu C, Zou C, Cao J, et al. Cancer cell intrinsic TIM-3 induces glioblastoma progression. iScience. 2022;25(11):105329.
24. Sauer N, Janicka N, Szlasa W, Skinderowicz B, Kołodzińska K, Dwernicka W, et al. TIM-3 as a promising target for cancer immunotherapy in a wide range of tumors. Cancer Immunol Immunother. 2023;72(11):3405–25.
25. Yuan J, Jiang B, Zhao H, Huang Q. Prognostic implication of TIM-3 in clear cell renal cell carcinoma. Neoplasma. 2014;61(1):35–40.
26. Cai C, Xu YF, Wu ZJ, Dong Q, Li MY, Olson JC, et al. Tim-3 expression represents dysfunctional tumor infiltrating T cells in renal cell carcinoma. World J Urol. 2016;34(4):561–7.
27. Gao X, Zhu Y, Li G, Huang H, Zhang G, Wang F, et al. TIM-3 expression characterizes regulatory T cells in tumor tissues and is associated with lung cancer progression. PLoS One. 2012;7(2):e30676.
28. Yang F, Zeng Z, Li J, Ren X, Wei F. TIM-3 and CEACAM1 are prognostic factors in head and neck squamous cell carcinoma. Front Mol Biosci. 2021;8:619765.
29. Chen K, Gu Y, Cao Y, Fang H, Lv K, Liu X, et al. TIM3(+) cells in gastric cancer: clinical correlates and association with immune context. Br J Cancer. 2022;126(1):100–8.
30. Fourcade J, Sun Z, Benallaoua M, Guillaume P, Luescher IF, Sander C, et al. Upregulation of Tim-3 and PD-1 expression is associated with tumor antigen-specific CD8+ T cell dysfunction in melanoma patients. J Exp Med. 2010;207(10):2175–86.
31. Solinas C, De Silva P, Bron D, Willard-Gallo K, Sangiolo D. Significance of TIM3 expression in cancer: from biology to the clinic. Semin Oncol. 2019;46(4–5):372–9.
32. Rezaei M, Tan J, Zeng C, Li Y, Ganjalikhani-Hakemi M. TIM-3 in leukemia; immune response and beyond. Front Oncol. 2021;11:11.
33. Tan J, Tan H, Li Y. Targeting TIM-3 for hematological malignancy: latest updates from the 2022 ASH annual meeting. Exp Hematol Oncol. 2023;12(1):62.
34. Zhao L, Cheng S, Fan L, Zhang B, Xu S. TIM-3: an update on immunotherapy. Int Immunopharmacol. 2021;99:107933.
35. Acharya N, Sabatos-Peyton C, Anderson AC. Tim-3 finds its place in the cancer immunotherapy landscape. J Immunother Cancer. 2020;8(1)
36. Bailly C, Thuru X, Goossens L, Goossens JF. Soluble TIM-3 as a biomarker of progression and therapeutic response in cancers and other of human diseases. Biochem Pharmacol. 2023;209:115445.
37. Ibrahim R, Saleh K, Chahine C, Khoury R, Khalife N, Cesne AL. LAG-3 inhibitors: novel immune checkpoint inhibitors changing the landscape of immunotherapy. Biomedicine. 2023;11(7)
38. Li R, Qiu J, Zhang Z, Qu C, Tang Z, Yu W, et al. Prognostic significance of Lymphocyte-activation gene 3 (LAG3) in patients with solid tumors: a systematic review, meta-analysis and pan-cancer analysis. Cancer Cell Int. 2023;23(1):306.

39. Saleh RR, Peinado P, Fuentes-Antrás J, Pérez-Segura P, Pandiella A, Amir E, et al. Prognostic value of lymphocyte-activation gene 3 (LAG3) in cancer: a meta-analysis. Front Oncol. 2019;9:1040.
40. Shi AP, Tang XY, Xiong YL, Zheng KF, Liu YJ, Shi XG, et al. Immune checkpoint LAG3 and its ligand FGL1 in cancer. Front Immunol. 2021;12:785091.
41. Liu Q, Qi Y, Zhai J, Kong X, Wang X, Wang Z, et al. Molecular and clinical characterization of LAG3 in breast cancer through 2994 samples. Front Immunol. 2021;12:12.
42. Botticelli A, Zizzari IG, Scagnoli S, Pomati G, Strigari L, Cirillo A, et al. The role of soluble LAG3 and soluble immune checkpoints profile in advanced head and neck cancer: a pilot study. J Pers Med. 2021;11(7)
43. Li Y, Ju M, Miao Y, Zhao L, Xing L, Wei M. Advancement of anti-LAG-3 in cancer therapy. FASEB J. 2023;37(11):e23236.
44. Annese T, Tamma R, Ribatti D. Update in TIGIT immune-checkpoint role in cancer. Front Oncol. 2022;12:871085.
45. Hosseinkhani N, Shadbad MA, Asghari Jafarabadi M, Karim Ahangar N, Asadzadeh Z, Mohammadi SM, et al. A systematic review and meta-analysis on the significance of TIGIT in solid cancers: dual TIGIT/PD-1 blockade to overcome immune-resistance in solid cancers. Int J Mol Sci. 2021;22(19)
46. Jantz-Naeem N, Böttcher-Loschinski R, Borucki K, Mitchell-Flack M, Böttcher M, Schraven B, et al. TIGIT signaling and its influence on T cell metabolism and immune cell function in the tumor microenvironment. Front Oncol. 2023;13:1060112.
47. Chiang EY, Mellman I. TIGIT-CD226-PVR axis: advancing immune checkpoint blockade for cancer immunotherapy. J Immunother Cancer. 2022;10(4)
48. Paolini R, Molfetta R. CD155 and its receptors as targets for cancer therapy. Int J Mol Sci. 2023;24(16)
49. Jin HS, Park Y. Hitting the complexity of the TIGIT-CD96-CD112R-CD226 axis for next-generation cancer immunotherapy. BMB Rep. 2021;54(1):2–11.
50. Blake SJ, Stannard K, Liu J, Allen S, Yong MC, Mittal D, et al. Suppression of metastases using a new lymphocyte checkpoint target for cancer immunotherapy. Cancer Discov. 2016;6(4):446–59.
51. Feng S, Isayev O, Werner J, Bazhin AV. CD96 as a potential immune regulator in cancers. Int J Mol Sci. 2023;24(2):1303.
52. Wang Y, Wang C, Qiu J, Qu X, Peng J, Lu C, et al. Targeting CD96 overcomes PD-1 blockade resistance by enhancing CD8+ TIL function in cervical cancer. J Immunother Cancer. 2022;10(3)
53. Zeng T, Cao Y, Jin T, Tian Y, Dai C, Xu F. The CD112R/CD112 axis: a breakthrough in cancer immunotherapy. J Exp Clin Cancer Res. 2021;40(1):285.
54. Agresta L, Hoebe KHN, Janssen EM. The emerging role of CD244 signaling in immune cells of the tumor microenvironment. Front Immunol. 2018;9:2809.
55. Sun L, Gang X, Li Z, Zhao X, Zhou T, Zhang S, et al. Advances in understanding the roles of CD244 (SLAMF4) in immune regulation and associated diseases. Front Immunol. 2021;12:648182.
56. Hsu CL, Ou DL, Bai LY, Chen CW, Lin L, Huang SF, et al. Exploring markers of exhausted CD8 T cells to predict response to immune checkpoint inhibitor therapy for hepatocellular carcinoma. Liver Cancer. 2021;10(4):346–59.
57. Demerlé C, Gorvel L, Olive D. BTLA-HVEM couple in health and diseases: insights for immunotherapy in lung cancer. Front Oncol. 2021;11:682007.
58. Sordo-Bahamonde C, Lorenzo-Herrero S, Granda-Díaz R, Martínez-Pérez A, Aguilar-García C, Rodrigo JP, et al. Beyond the anti-PD-1/PD-L1 era: promising role of the BTLA/HVEM axis as a future target for cancer immunotherapy. Mol Cancer. 2023;22(1):142.
59. Radwan SM, Elleboudy NS, Nabih NA, El-kholy A, Kamal AM. The prospective prognostic value of the immune checkpoint BTLA expression in adult acute myeloid leukemia patients. Egypt J Med Human Genet. 2021;22(1):78.

60. Fourcade J, Sun Z, Pagliano O, Guillaume P, Luescher IF, Sander C, et al. CD8(+) T cells specific for tumor antigens can be rendered dysfunctional by the tumor microenvironment through upregulation of the inhibitory receptors BTLA and PD-1. Cancer Res. 2012;72(4):887–96.
61. Ye Z, Zheng Z, Li X, Zhu Y, Zhong Z, Peng L, et al. B7-H3 overexpression predicts poor survival of cancer patients: a meta-analysis. Cell Physiol Biochem. 2016;39(4):1568–80.
62. Zhao B, Li H, Xia Y, Wang Y, Wang Y, Shi Y, et al. Immune checkpoint of B7-H3 in cancer: from immunology to clinical immunotherapy. J Hematol Oncol. 2022;15(1):153.
63. Kanchan RK, Doss D, Khan P, Nasser MW, Mahapatra S. To kill a cancer: targeting the immune inhibitory checkpoint molecule, B7-H3. Biochim Biophys Acta Rev Cancer. 2022;1877(5):188783.
64. Zhou W-T, Jin W-L. B7-H3/CD276: an emerging cancer immunotherapy. Front Immunol. 2021;12:12.
65. Kaur G, Janakiram M. B7x-from bench to bedside. ESMO Open. 2019;4(5):e000554.
66. Mortezaee K. B7x in cancer immunity and immunotherapy. Int Immunopharmacol. 2023;118:110133.
67. Im E, Sim DY, Lee HJ, Park JE, Park WY, Ko S, et al. Immune functions as a ligand or a receptor, cancer prognosis potential, clinical implication of VISTA in cancer immunotherapy. Semin Cancer Biol. 2022;86(Pt 2):1066–75.
68. Martin AS, Molloy M, Ugolkov A, von Roemeling RW, Noelle RJ, Lewis LD, et al. VISTA expression and patient selection for immune-based anticancer therapy. Front Immunol. 2023;14:1086102.
69. Su Q, Du J, Xiong X, Xie X, Wang L. B7-H7: a potential target for cancer immunotherapy. Int Immunopharmacol. 2023;121:110403.
70. Mortezaee K. HHLA2 immune-regulatory roles in cancer. Biomed Pharmacother. 2023;162:114639.
71. Moesta AK, Li XY, Smyth MJ. Targeting CD39 in cancer. Nat Rev Immunol. 2020;20(12):739–55.
72. Xing J, Zhang J, Wang J. The immune regulatory role of adenosine in the tumor microenvironment. Int J Mol Sci. 2023;24(19):14928.
73. Sun C, Wang B, Hao S. Adenosine-A2A receptor pathway in cancer immunotherapy. Front Immunol. 2022;13:837230.
74. Xia C, Yin S, To KKW, Fu L. CD39/CD73/A2AR pathway and cancer immunotherapy. Mol Cancer. 2023;22(1):44.
75. Franco R, Rivas-Santisteban R, Navarro G, Reyes-Resina I. Adenosine receptor antagonists to combat cancer and to boost anti-cancer chemotherapy and immunotherapy. Cells. 2021;10(11)
76. Jia X, Yan B, Tian X, Liu Q, Jin J, Shi J, et al. CD47/SIRPα pathway mediates cancer immune escape and immunotherapy. Int J Biol Sci. 2021;17(13):3281–7.
77. Zhu J, Cai C, Li J, Xiao J, Duan X. CD47-SIRPα axis in cancer therapy: precise delivery of CD47-targeted therapeutics and design of anti-phagocytic drug delivery systems. Med Drug Discov. 2022;15:100139.
78. Jiang Z, Sun H, Yu J, Tian W, Song Y. Targeting CD47 for cancer immunotherapy. J Hematol Oncol. 2021;14(1):180.
79. Maute R, Xu J, Weissman IL. CD47-SIRPα-targeted therapeutics: status and prospects. Immuno-oncol Technol. 2022;13:100070.
80. Chao MP, Takimoto CH, Feng DD, McKenna K, Gip P, Liu J, et al. Therapeutic targeting of the macrophage immune checkpoint CD47 in myeloid malignancies. Front Oncol. 2019;9:1380.

Chapter 5
Cancer Immunotherapy Using Immune Checkpoint Blockade

5.1 Introduction

The immune system plays a pivotal role in preventing tumorigenesis. The immune cells can recognize and eliminate tumor cells in the early stages. This process is known as tumor immune surveillance. However, tumors have several mechanisms to evade the immune response that leads to tumor establishment and development. After the presentation of tumor antigens by APCs, tumor-specific T cells become activated. Lymphocyte response is regulated by immune checkpoints such as CTLA-4 and PD-1. One of the mechanisms of tumor escape is to upregulate the expression of these receptors and their ligands and suppress the antitumor immune response. Blocking the inhibitory checkpoints (ICs) in cancer patients can reactivate immune cells and strengthen the specific antitumor immune response. During the last decade, immunotherapy has made a significant breakthrough in oncology. Cancer treatment using immune checkpoint inhibitors (ICIs) is one of the active and expanding areas in the field of tumor immunotherapy and has brought promising outcomes in the treatment of patients [1, 2]. In this chapter, approved ICIs in cancer treatment and recent achievements in this field as well as predictive biomarkers related to ICI therapy of cancer are discussed.

L. Tayebi, M. Abdolmaleki, *Immune System Regulation*,
https://doi.org/10.1007/978-981-95-8026-2_5

5.2 ICIs in the Preclinical Studies and Clinical Trials

Preclinical studies are the first step in evaluating the efficacy and safety of therapeutic agents, which are carried out on cell lines and animal models. These studies provide valuable information about toxicity, optimal dose, route of administration, and timing of the treatment. Animal cancer models such as rats, zebrafish, dogs, mammals, and macaques are used in ICIs studies, for example, evaluating the safety of anti-PD-1 using nonhuman primates or assessing of the toxicity of anti-PD-1 and anti-CTLA-4 in a macaque cancer model. In other studies, the effects of anti-PD-1 and anti-CTLA-4 antibodies on tumor growth, metastasis, and overall survival (OS) have been assessed in patient-derived xenografts (PDX) mouse models. In addition, genetically engineered mouse models or humanized immune system (HIS) are applicable in this context. Tumor organoids and spheroids, with similar structures to tumors, are great platforms to investigate the ICI response in malignancies such as melanoma, colon cancer, and chondroma. Clinical trials employing various ICIs against cancers have been associated with increased survival and quality of life in many cases. ICIs have a promising perspective in cancer treatment and they can be more effective and safer in the future [1].

By 2022, there have been approximately 5000 active clinical trials in which ICIs have been used alone or in combination with other therapeutic agents to treat various diseases. A major part of these clinical trials is related to cancer therapy. Based on medical records of cancer patients treated at the cancer center of the University Hospital Bern, Switzerland, between January 1, 2017 and June 16, 2021, the percentage of patients receiving ICIs has reached from 8.6% in 2017 to 22.9% in 2021, which indicates ICIs are becoming more common in clinical practice [3]. Some of the latest active clinical trials focusing on ICIs in cancer therapy are described in Table 5.1.

Table 5.1 Ongoing active phase 3 or 4 clinical trials of cancer ICI therapy

NCT number	Interventions	Status	Phase	Conditions	Enrollment	Completion (estimated)
NCT05608291	Fianlimab Cemiplimab Pembrolizumab	Recruiting	3	Melanoma	1530	2030
NCT04082364	Margetuximab Retifanlimab Tebotelimab	Active, not recruiting	2/3	HER2-positive gastric cancer (GC), gastroesophageal junction (GEJ) cancer	82	2023
NCT05352672	Fianlimab Cemiplimab Pembrolizumab	Recruiting	3	Unresectable locally advanced or metastatic melanoma	1590	2031
NCT04746924	Tislelizumab Ociperlimab Pembrolizumab	Recruiting	3	Non-small cell lung cancer	660	2025
NCT04294810	Atezolizumab Tiragolumab	Active, not recruiting	3	Locally advanced unresectable or metastatic PD-L1-selected non-small cell lung cancer	620	2025
NCT04543617	Tiragolumab Atezolizumab Tiragolumab	Active, not recruiting	3	Esophageal squamous cell carcinoma	760	2027
NCT05568095	Atezolizumab	Recruiting	3	Advanced upper gastrointestinal tract adenocarcinoma	970	2027
NCT04736173	Domvanalimab Zimberelimab Carboplatin	Recruiting	3	Locally advanced or metastatic non-small cell lung cancer	750	2027

(continued)

Table 5.1 (continued)

NCT number	Interventions	Status	Phase	Conditions	Enrollment	Completion (estimated)
NCT04866017	Tislelizumab Durvalumab Ociperlimab	Active, not recruiting	3	Non-small cell lung cancer	63	2027
NCT05665595	Pembrolizumab/ Vibostolimab Pembrolizumab	Recruiting	3	Melanoma	1560	2031
NCT05002127	Evorpacept (ALX148) Trastuzumab Ramucirumab Paclitaxel	Recruiting	2/3	Gastric cancer	450	2028
NCT03313544	Nivolumab	Recruiting	4	Melanoma, lung cancer	50	2025
NCT03285763	Atezolizumab	Completed	4	Non-small cell lung cancer	619	2022
NCT03715205	Pembrolizumab	Active, not recruiting	4	Non-small cell lung cancer, melanoma	150	2024
NCT05235737	Pembrolizumab	Recruiting	4	Glioblastoma	36	2026
NCT05587374	Cadonilimab Gemcitabine Cisplatin	Recruiting	3	Nasopharyngeal carcinoma	418	2027
NCT04489888	Pembrolizumab Carboplatin Paclitaxel	Active, not recruiting	4	Recurrent/metastatic head and neck squamous cell carcinoma	101	2024
NCT02542293	Durvalumab + tremelimumab Paclitaxel + carboplatin Gemcitabine + cisplatin	Active, not recruiting	3	Non-small cell lung carcinoma	953	2023
NCT02785952	Ipilimumab Nivolumab	Active, not recruiting	3	Squamous cell lung carcinoma	275	2024

NCT03793166	Cabozantinib Ipilimumab Nivolumab	Recruiting	3	Malignant neoplasm	1046	2024
NCT01274338	Ipilimumab Recombinant interferon alfa	Active, not recruiting	3	High-risk stage III–IV melanoma	1673	2019
NCT04949113	Ipilimumab + nivolumab Nivolumab	Recruiting	3	Stage III melanoma	420	2027
NCT05751928	BCD-217 Anti-PD-1	Recruiting	3	Resectable stage III skin melanoma	410	2027
NCT05732805	BCD-217 BCD-100	Recruiting	3	Unresectable/metastatic melanoma	270	2025
NCT04266301	MBG453 Azacitidine	Active, not recruiting	3	Myelodysplastic syndrome	530	2027
NCT05785767	Fianlimab Cemiplimab	Recruiting	2/3	Advanced non-small cell lung cancer	850	2032
NCT05747794	Eftilagimod alpha Paclitaxel	Recruiting	2/3	Metastatic breast cancer	849	2027
NCT05800015	Fianlimab Cemiplimab Pemetrexed	Recruiting	2/3	Advanced non-small cell lung cancer	950	2031
NCT04256421	Tiragolumab Atezolizumab Carboplatin	Active, not recruiting	3	Extensive-stage small cell lung cancer	490	2026
NCT05660213	Atezolizumab + bevacizumab Camrelizumab + Apatinib Sintilimab + bevacizumab	Not yet recruiting	4	Unresectable hepatocellular carcinoma (uHCC)	600	2023
NCT04078152	Durvalumab	Active, not recruiting	4	Solid tumor	165	2023

5.3 ICIs Development in Cancer Therapy

In 2011, the first ICI was approved by the United States Food and Drug Administration (FDA) for the treatment of advanced melanoma. As a result of important achievements in this field, Cancer Immunotherapy was named 2013 "breakthrough of the year" in oncology. Some of the ICIs are in the first line of the cancer therapy. To date, several immune checkpoints have been discovered and new ICIs have been developed for various cancers [4, 5]. So far, ICIs targeting CTLA-4, PD-1, PD-L1, and LAG-3 including 10 monoclonal antibodies have received the FDA approval for cancer treatment. Furthermore, 11 new ICIs targeting CTLA-4 and PD-1 have been approved by the China National Medical Products Administration (NMPA) [6]. Table 5.2 shows the list of these approved ICIs. In addition, several types of ICIs have been developed that are not yet approved but are being evaluated in clinical trials. These agents are summarized in Table 5.3.

5.3.1 FDA-Approved ICIs

5.3.1.1 CTLA-4 Inhibitors

CTLA-4 is a well-defined negative regulator of T cell activation. CTLA-4 is an inhibitory receptor homologous to CD28 expressed on $CD4^+$ and $CD8^+$ T cells, which interacts with high affinity with CD80 and CD86 on APCs and inhibits T cell function. The effect of CTLA-4 blockade has been proven in various human malignancies. Ipilimumab is a recombinant human IgG1 monoclonal antibody (mAb) that can inhibit CTLA-4 activity (Fig. 5.1) [26, 27]. In 2011, ipilimumab was the first ICI approved for the treatment of unresectable or metastatic melanoma patients, which was associated with increased OS and disease control [7]. It is also used in non-small cell lung cancer (NSCLC), mesothelioma, lymphoma, prostate, ovarian, breast, and urinary cancers [27].

Tremelimumab (IMJUDO, ticilimumab) is another CTLA-4 blocking antibody. It is a fully human IgG2 mAb that was used in a phase III trial for the treatment of patients with advanced melanoma in 2010 [28]. After more than a decade, tremelimumab in October 2022 in combination with durvalumab was first approved for the treatment of unresectable hepatocellular carcinoma (uHCC). Furthermore, in November 2022, tremelimumab–durvalumab combination therapy plus platinum-based chemotherapy was approved for metastatic non-small cell lung cancer (mNSCLC) [8].

Table 5.2 List of approved immune checkpoint inhibitors

Target	Agent	First indication	First approval	References
CTLA-4	Ipilimumab	Melanoma	FDA 2011	[7]
	Tremelimumab (in combination with durvalumab)	Unresectable hepatocellular carcinoma	FDA 2022	[8]
PD-1	Pembrolizumab	Melanoma	FDA 2014	[9]
	Cemiplimab	Cutaneous squamous cell carcinoma	FDA 2018	[10]
	Nivolumab (in combination with relatlimab)	Melanoma	FDA 2022	[11]
	Dostarlimab	Endometrial cancer	FDA 2021	[12]
	Toripalimab	Melanoma	NMPA 2018	[13]
	Sintilimab	Hodgkin lymphoma	NMPA 2018	[14]
	Camrelizumab	Hodgkin lymphoma	NMPA 2019	[15]
	Tislelizumab	Hodgkin lymphoma	NMPA 2019	[16]
	Penpulimab	Hodgkin lymphoma	NMPA 2021	[17]
	Serplulimab	Solid Tumor	NMPA 2022	[18]
	Zimberelimab	Hodgkin lymphoma	NMPA 2021	[19]
	Pucotenlimab	Solid tumors	NMPA 2022	
CTLA-4/ PD-1	Candonilimab	Cervical cancer	NMPA 2022	[20]
PD-L1	Atezolizumab	Urothelial carcinoma	FDA 2016	[21]
	Durvalumab	Urothelial carcinoma	FDA 2017	[22]
	Avelumab	Merkel cell carcinoma	FDA 2017	[23]
	Envafolimab	Solid tumor	NMPA 2021	[24]
	Sugemalimab	Non-small cell lung cancer	NMPA 2021	[25]
LAG-3	Relatlimab (in combination with nivolumab)	Melanoma	FDA 2022	[11]

Table 5.3 List of ICIs developed for cancer clinical studies (not approved by the FDA or NMPA)

Target	Agent	Description
CTLA-4	Quavonlimab (MK-1308)	Humanized IgG1 anti-CTLA-4 monoclonal antibody
	QL1706 (PSB205)	Bifunctional PD-1/CTLA-4 dual blocker (anti-PD-1 IgG4 and anti-CTLA-4 IgG1)
	Nurulimab (BCD-145)	Human IgG1 anti-CTLA-4 monoclonal antibody
	BCD-217 (nurulimab + prolgolimab)	Targets and binds to both PD-1 and CTLA-4
PD-1	Spartalizumab	Humanized IgG4κ anti-PD-1 monoclonal antibody
	Budigalimab (ABBV 181)	Humanized IgG1 anti-PD-1 monoclonal antibody
	MGA012	Humanized IgG4 anti-PD-1 monoclonal antibody
	Prolgolimab (BCD-100)	Anti-IgG1 anti-PD-1 monoclonal antibody
	Sym021	Humanized IgG1 effector-function silenced anti-PD-1 monoclonal antibody
	TSR-042	Humanized IgG4k anti-PD-1 monoclonal antibody
	Ezabenlimab (BI 754091)	Anti-PD-1 monoclonal antibody
PD-L1	Garivulimab (BGB-A333)	Humanized IgG1 anti-PD-L1 monoclonal antibody
	Adebrelimab (SHR-1316)	Humanized IgG4 anti-PD-L1 monoclonal antibody
	Socazolimab (ZKAB001)	Anti-PD-L1 monoclonal antibody
	TQB2450	Humanized anti-PD-L1 monoclonal antibody
	SHR-1701	Bifunctional fusion protein anti-PD-L1 and TGF-β
	LY300054	Anti-PD-L1 monoclonal antibody
LAG-3	Fianlimab (REGN3767)	Anti-LAG-3 human monoclonal antibody
	Tebotelimab (MGD013)	Human IgG4κ bispecific PD-1/LAG-3 monoclonal antibody
	Eftilagimod alpha (IMP321)	Recombinant LAG-3Ig fusion protein
	FS118	Anti-PD-L1 and LAG-3 bispecific antibody
	INCAGN02385	Fc-engineered IgG1κ anti-LAG-3 monoclonal antibody
	TSR-033	Human IgG4 antibody anti-LAG-3
	RO7247669	Anti-PD-1-LAG-3 bispecific antibody
	Sym022	Anti-LAG-3 monoclonal antibody
	GSK2831781 (IMP731)	Depleting anti-LAG antibody
	LAG525 (ieramilimab) (IMP701)	Humanized IgG4 anti-LAG-3 monoclonal antibody
	MK-4280 (favezelimab)	Humanized IgG4 anti-LAG-3 monoclonal antibody
	EMB-02	Anti-LAG-3 and PD-1 bispecific antibody
	IBI323	Recombinant LAG-3/PD-L1 bispecific antibody
	XmAb841	Anti-CTLA-4 and LAG-3 bispecific antibody
	HLX26	Humanized anti-LAG-3 monoclonal antibody
TIM-3	Sabatolimab (MBG453)	Humanized IgG4 anti-TIM-3 monoclonal antibody
	Sym023	Human anti-TIM-3 monoclonal antibody
	Cobolimab (TSR-022)	Anti-TIM-3 monoclonal antibody
	LY3321367	Humanized IgG1λ, Fc-null anti-TIM-3 monoclonal antibody

(continued)

Table 5.3 (continued)

Target	Agent	Description
TIGIT	Domvanalimab	Fc-silent humanized IgG1 anti-TIGIT monoclonal antibody
	M6223	Fully human IgG1 anti-TIGIT monoclonal antibody
	HB0030	Humanized IgG1 anti-TIGIT monoclonal antibody
	EOS884448	Fully human IgG1 anti-TIGIT monoclonal antibody
	AZD2936	Bispecific, humanized IgG1 targeting PD-1 and TIGIT
	Tamgiblimab (IBI939)	Fully human IgG4κ anti-TIGIT monoclonal antibody
	Vibostolimab (MK-7684)	Humanized IgG1 anti-TIGIT monoclonal antibody
	Etigilimab	Human IgG1 anti-TIGIT monoclonal antibody
	Tiragolumab (GO30103, RG6058, MTIG7192A)	Humanized IgG1κ anti-TIGIT monoclonal antibody
	Ociperlimab	Humanized IgG1 monoclonal antibody designed to bind to Fc-intact TIGIT
	AB154	Humanized anti-TIGIT monoclonal antibody
	BMS 986207	Anti-TIGIT monoclonal antibody
	SEA-TGT	Anti-TIGIT monoclonal antibody
	COM902	IgG4 fully human high-affinity monoclonal antibody, inhibitor of TIGIT
	IBI321	Bispecific anti-PD-L1/TIGIT antibody
	AB308	Humanized IgG1 anti-TIGIT monoclonal antibody
	BAT6005	Anti-TIGIT monoclonal antibody
	JS006	Humanized IgG4κ anti-TIGIT monoclonal antibody
	HLX53	Anti-TIGIT Fc fusion protein
B7-H3 B7-H4	MGC018	Anti-B7-H3 monoclonal antibody
	FPA150	Fully human antibody against B7-H4
	XMT-1660	B7-H4-directed dolasynthen antibody drug conjugate
	Enoblituzumab (*MGA271)*	Humanized IgG1κ anti-B7-H3 monoclonal antibody
	Orlotamab (MGD009)	Humanized bispecific CD3/B7-H3 targeting molecule
	DS-7300a	B7-H3 antibody drug conjugate (ADC)
	Alsevalimab (FPA 150)	Afucosylated IgG1 anti-B7-H4 monoclonal antibody
	ABL103	Anti-4-1BB/B7-H4 bispecific antibody

(continued)

Table 5.3 (continued)

Target	Agent	Description
A2aR CD73 CD39	EOS100850	A2A receptor antagonist
	Etrumadenant (AB928)	Dual adenosine receptor (A2aR/A2bR) antagonist
	Imaradenant (AZD4635, HTL1071)	Oral A2A receptor antagonist
	Taminadenant (PBF509/ NIR178)	Orally active adenosine A2A receptor antagonist
	SCH58261	A2A receptor antagonist
	Mupadolimab (CPI-006)	IgG1κ humanized FcγR binding-deficient anti-CD73 monoclonal antibody
	Oleclumab (MEDI9447)	Human IgG1λ anti-CD73 monoclonal antibody
	AK131	Anti-PD-1 and CD73 bispecific antibody
	AK119	Anti-CD73 monoclonal antibody
	IBI325	Anti-CD73 monoclonal antibody
	TJ004309	Anti-CD73 monoclonal antibody
	NZV930 (SRF373)	Fully human anti-CD73 monoclonal antibody
	BMS-986179	Anti-CD73 monoclonal antibody
	LY3475070	Orally bioavailable inhibitor of CD73
	Sym024	Anti-CD73 monoclonal antibody
	HLX23	Fully human IgG2 anti-CD73 monoclonal antibody
	AB680	Selective inhibitor of CD73
	LY3475070	Orally bioavailable inhibitor of CD73
	Dalutrafusp alfa (AGEN-1423, GS-1423)	Bifunctional, humanized, aglycosylated IgG1κ anti-CD73/TGFβ antibody
	SRF617	Fully human IgG4 anti-CD39 monoclonal antibody
	JS019	Fully human anti-CD39 monoclonal antibody
	ES014	Anti-CD39/TGF-β bispecific antibody
	TTX-030	Anti-CD39 antibody monoclonal antibody
	ES002023	Humanized IgG1 anti-CD39 monoclonal antibody
	IPH5201	Anti-CD39 monoclonal antibody
CD47/ SIRPα	CC-90002	Humanized anti-CD47 monoclonal antibody
	Hu5F9-G4 (5F9)	Humanized IgG4 anti-CD47 monoclonal antibody
	Evorpacept (ALX148)	High affinity CD47-blocking fusion protein with an inactive Fc region
	AK117	Humanized IgG4 anti-CD47 monoclonal antibody
	AO-176	Humanized IgG2 anti-CD47 monoclonal antibody
	IBI188	Humanized IgG4 anti-CD47 monoclonal antibody
	SRF231	Humanized IgG4 anti-CD47 monoclonal antibody
	TJC4	Fully human IgG4 anti-CD47 monoclonal antibody
	BI 765063	Humanized IgG4 anti-SIRPα monoclonal antibody
	IMM01	SIRPα–IgG1 fusion protein
	SL-172154	SIRPα–Fc-CD40L fusion protein
	TTI-622	SIRPα–IgG4 Fc fusion protein

(continued)

Table 5.3 (continued)

Target	Agent	Description
VISTA	SNS-101	IgG1 anti-VISTA monoclonal antibody
	JNJ-61610588	Fully human IgG1 anti-VISTA monoclonal antibody
	HMBD-002	IgG4 anti-VISTA monoclonal antibody
	CA-170	Oral small molecule antagonist of PD-L1 and VISTA
	KVA12123	Fully human IgG1 anti-VISTA monoclonal antibody
	CI-8993	Human IgG1 anti-VISTA monoclonal antibody
PVRIG/ PVRL2	COM701	Humanized IgG4 anti-PVRIG monoclonal antibody
CLEVER-1	Bexmarilimab (FP-1305)	Humanized IgG4 anti-CLEVER-1 monoclonal antibody

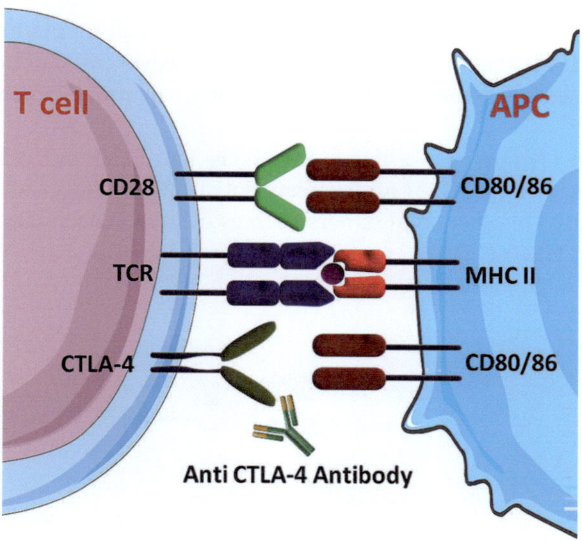

Fig. 5.1 CTLA-4 blocking antibodies in tumor immunotherapy. T cells are activated through engagement of TCR with MHC–peptide complex on antigen presenting cells (APCs). CD28 binds to CD80/86 on the APC and provides the T cell co-stimulatory signal. However, CTLA-4–CD80/86 interaction inhibits CD28 signaling and T cell activation. CTLA-4 blocking antibodies including ipilimumab and tremelimumab keep T cells active against tumor and are effective in cancer treatment. Created using elements from Servier Medical Art (https://smart.servier.com), licensed under CC BY 4.0 (https://creativecommons.org/licenses/by/4.0/)

5.3.1.2 PD-1 Inhibitors

PD-1 is widely expressed on various activated T cells and other immune cells in the tumor microenvironment (TME). The binding of PD-1 to its ligands inhibits T cell responses in peripheral tissues. FDA-approved PD-1 inhibitors include pembrolizumab, nivolumab, cemplimumab, and dostarlimab (Fig. 5.2) [26].

Pembrolizumab (Keytruda) is a humanized IgG4 mAb against PD-1. It was approved in 2014 for the treatment of patients with unresectable or metastatic melanoma [9]. In recent years, it has been used for the treatment of several malignancies such as NSCLC, HNSCC, gastric cancer, cervical cancer, and urothelial carcinoma [26].

Nivolumab is a fully human IgG4 mAb targeting PD-1. In March 2022, a fixed dose combination of nivolumab/relatlimab (Opdualag) was approved for the treatment of unresectable or metastatic melanoma [11]. Nivolumab has been effective in the treatment of NSCLC, renal cell carcinoma, Hodgkin's lymphoma, HNSCC, colorectal cancer, and hepatocellular carcinoma [26].

Cemiplimab (LIBTAYO) is a fully human IgG4 mAb that received the FDA approval for the treatment of cutaneous squamous cell carcinoma (CSCC) in September 2018. It also has been used in NSCLC, basal cell carcinoma, cervical cancer, relapsed/refractory multiple myeloma, ovarian cancer, and lymphoma [10].

Dostarlimab (Jemperli) is a humanized IgG4 anti-PD-1 monoclonal antibody that was approved in April 2021 for the treatment of endometrial cancer. Dostarlimab has been effective in other solid tumors such as ovarian cancer, pancreatic cancer, melanoma, and NSCLC [12].

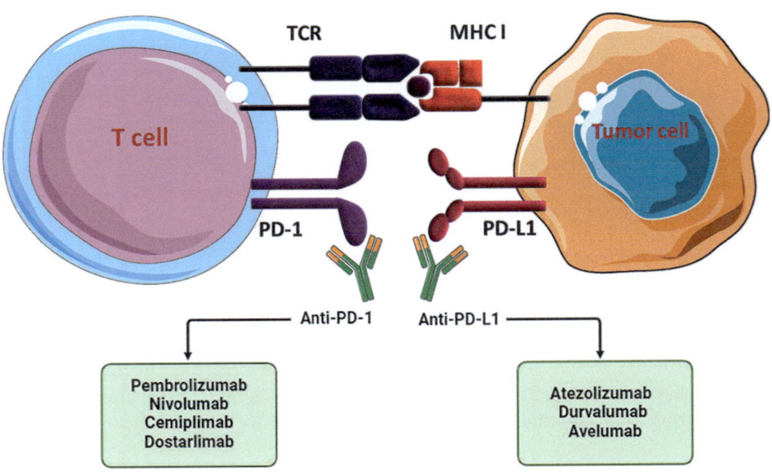

Fig. 5.2 Cancer immunotherapy using FDA-approved PD-1 and PD-L1 blocking antibodies. Created using elements from Servier Medical Art (https://smart.servier.com), licensed under CC BY 4.0 (https://creativecommons.org/licenses/by/4.0/)

5.3.1.3 PD-L1 Inhibitors

PD-L1 is widely expressed in tumor cells and limits the antitumor response of T cells by interaction with PD-1. Atezolizumab, durvalumab, and avelumab are FDA-approved PD-L1 inhibitors (Fig. 5.2).

Atezolizumab (Tecentriq) is a humanized IgG1 mAb against PD-L1. In 2016, atezolizumab received approval for the treatment of urothelial carcinoma. It also has been effective in the treatment of NSCLC, non-Hodgkin's lymphoma, acute myeloid leukemia, and other locally advanced or metastatic solid tumors [21]. Durvalumab is an IgG1 mAb targeting PD-L1. The FDA granted durvalumab accelerated approval in May 2017 for the treatment of locally advanced/metastatic urothelial carcinoma. In addition, It has been used in several solid tumors and hematological malignancies [22]. Avelumab (Imfinzi) is a fully human mAb IgG1 targeting PD-L1. In March 2017, avelumab received accelerated approval for the treatment of patients with metastatic Merkel cell carcinoma (mMCC). Then, it was also used in other malignancies such as NSCLC, cancer, diffuse large B cell lymphoma, glioblastoma, intestinal, gastric, breast, ovarian, and head and neck cancers [23].

5.3.1.4 LAG-3 Inhibitors

LAG-3 is an immune checkpoint that is expressed on variety of immune cells including Treg, NK, and activated T and B cells. The upregulation of LAG-3 expression has been observed on tumor-infiltrating $CD8^+$ T cells as well as tumor cells in multiple types of cancers. LAG-3 overexpression is associated with tumor progression and poor outcomes [29].

Anti-LAG-3 agents include anti-LAG-3 mAbs, LAG-3-immunoglobulin fusion proteins, and LAG-3 bispecific antibodies. Since blocking LAG-3 alone is not able to generate a strong antitumor response, a LAG-3 inhibitor is used in combination with another ICI. The combination therapy with anti-LAG-3 and anti-PD-1 potentiates the efficacy of immunotherapy. The expression of LAG-3 together with PD-1 on tumor-infiltrating lymphocytes (TILs) makes it a good target for these drugs. Relatlimab (an IgG4 anti-LAG-3 mAb) in combination with nivolumab (Opdualag) has been approved for the treatment of melanoma patients. Fianlimab mAbs is another LAG-3 inhibitory antibody.

Tebotelimab, RO7247669, and EMB-02 are examples of bispecific antibodies investigated in clinical trials that target LAG-3 and PD-1 simultaneously. XmAb841 is another bispecific antibody that binds CTLA-4 and LAG-3 [29, 30]. Eftilagimod alpha is a recombinant soluble LAG-3 Ig fusion protein that activates APCs by binding to MHC-II and boosts the antitumor T cell response. LAG-3 blockers along with other ICIs or chemotherapy can be useful in improving the response to cancer [31].

5.3.2 Emerging ICIs

In addition to the ICIs mentioned in the previous sections, dozens of other ICIs have been developed that have been effective in the treatment of cancers. TIM-3 is one of the promising targets in cancer immunotherapy. TIM-3 is expressed on a range of immune cells, including lymphocytes, dendritic cells (DCs), and macrophages. The increased expression of TIM-3 in various cancers has been associated with the disease progression. TIM-3 inhibitors such as MBG453 and TSR-022 have been used in several clinical trials [32].

TIGIT is one of the novel ICs that has been strongly noticed. TIGIT is mainly expressed on T cells and can inhibit adaptive immune responses. Tiragolumab, domvanalimab, vibostolimab, etigilimab, ociperlimab are among the TIGIT mAbs that have been tested in different cancers, which have been associated with acceptable toxicity and appropriate response in many cases. Administration of tiragolumab together with atezolizumab for the treatment of NSCLC patients is one of the clinical trials designed based on this IC [33].

B7-H3 and B7-H4 are members of the B7 family of receptors that are expressed on immune cells as well as tumor cells and play a key role in cancer progression. Various types of agents targeting the B7-H3 have been developed for cancer therapy, including blocking mAbs such as enoblituzumab, a bispecific antibody binding to CD3 and B7-H3 (obrindatamab), antibody-drug conjugates (ADCs) such as DS-7300 (an anti-B7-H3 antibody conjugated to a DNA topoisomerase I inhibitor) or ^{131}I-omburtamab (a radiolabeled anti-B7-H3 mAb) and B7-H3 chimeric antigen receptor (CAR)-T cell. For B7-H4 also, several inhibitory antibodies have been designed, including FPA150, 1H3 [34–36].

VISTA is an immune checkpoint structurally similar to the B7 family, which is overexpressed on tumor-infiltrating immune cells and can suppress the antitumor immune response. Anti-VISTA antibodies also have been evaluated in clinical studies. A clinical trial has been implemented to assess the effect of the combination of KVA12123 (a VISTA inhibitor) and pembrolizumab in solid tumors [37].

The CD47–SIRPα axis is a negative regulator of phagocytosis and the function of lymphocytes. CD47 is involved in suppressing the immune response against the tumor. Therefore, inhibitors of CD47–SIRPα pathway can be effective in inhibiting cancer growth. So far, various CD47–SIRPα inhibitors have been studied in cancer patients [38] (Table 5.4).

CD39/CD73 and CD38/CD203a/CD73 pathway are involved in the production of adenosine from ATP. A2AR and A2BR are the main receptors for adenosine. Adenosine is an immunosuppressive metabolite that inhibits inflammation and increasing the concentration of adenosine in the TME is one of the mechanisms of tumor escape from the immune system [39, 40].

CD38 is expressed on a range of immune cells such as T cells, NK cells, and DCs. Along with CD73, this molecule is also involved in the hydrolysis of ATP to adenosine. CD38 with its ectoenzyme activity hydrolyzes nicotinamide adenine dinucleotide (NAD) to adenosine diphosphate ribose (ADPR) and this metabolite is finally converted to adenosine by CD73. Overexpression of CD38 in hematological malignancies indicates the role of this immune checkpoint in the disease progression [41]. Isatuximab and daratumumab are two approved inhibitors of this CD38 molecule. Isatuximab is a CD38 targeting monoclonal antibody that in March 2020 was approved by the FDA for the treatment of multiple myeloma in combination with pomalidomide and dexamethasone. This drug has also been effective in non-Hodgkin's lymphoma and ALL [42]. Daratumumab is another CD38 inhibitor that first received approval in November 2015 for the treatment of MM patients [42]. Unlike other ICIs that are effective in cancer treatment mostly by intensifying the immune response in the tumor environment, induction of antibody-dependent cellular cytotoxicity (ADCC), complement-dependent cytotoxicity (CDC), and antibody-dependent cell-mediated phagocytosis (ADCP), which eliminates the $CD38^+$ tumor cells, are the major mechanisms of the effect of CD38 blockers in controlling multiple myeloma. However, these drugs have not been successful in solid tumors compared to hematological malignancies [41].

Targeting other immune checkpoints is an expanding field, and the list is growing. These ICIs are described in Table 5.4.

5.3.3 ICI Combination Therapy

Although ICIs have been beneficial for the treatment of cancers, ICI monotherapy alone is not enough to achieve favorable clinical outcomes due to tumor resistance. Consequently, mixtures of therapeutic methods have been used to improve the response. Combination therapy with different ICIs in one of these approaches to enhance the efficacy of the treatment, for example, anti-PD-1/PD-L1 with anti-CTLA-4 or newer checkpoint blockers including anti-LAG-3, anti-TIM-3, and anti-TIGIT. Recently, novel blockers such as bispecific antibodies against PD-L1 and LAG-3 have been developed. However, it should be noted that with additional ICIs, the possibility of severe adverse events increases [43].

In addition, combinations of ICIs and other anticancer agents including chemotherapy and radiotherapy are effective in improving OS, FPS, and improved objective response rate (ORR) in many cases. Increased response to vinorelbine, cyclophosphamide, and fluorouracil (5-FU) along with anti-PD-1 and anti-PD-L1 inhibitors are examples of this method. A study has evaluated the effect of the combination of PD-1 inhibitor with cyclophosphamide and radiation therapy (RT) in the treatment of HNSCC [44]. Another setting is the simultaneous use of ICIs and anti-angiogenic agents. Angiogenesis is a crucial mechanism for tumor growth. Active angiogenesis also has suppressive effects on immune cells in the TME. Vascular endothelial growth factor (VEGF) signaling is one of the most important pathways of tumor angiogenesis. The effects of angiogenesis inhibitors have been proven in harnessing the growth of solid tumors. It has been found that angiogenesis inhibitors such as bevacizumab, axitinib, and

Table 5.4 Different combination therapies with ICIs in cancer clinical trials

Therapeutic approach	Agents	Condition	References
ICI + ICI	Atezolizumab + durvalumab	Advanced SCLC	[47]
	Nivolumab + ipilimumab	Metastatic uveal melanoma	[48]
ICI + chemotherapy	Nivolumab + gemcitabine and cisplatin	Biliary tract cancer	[49]
	Anti-PD-1 + nanoparticle albumin-bound (nab)-paclitaxel	Refractory melanoma	[50]
	Pembrolizumab + doxorubicin	Soft tissue sarcomas	[51]
ICI + radiation therapy (RT)	Nivolumab and RT	Advanced NSCLC	[52]
	Anti-PD-1/PD-L1 and RT	NSCLC and HNSCC	[53]
ICI + angiogenesis inhibitors	Atezolizumab + bevacizumab (VEGF inhibitor)	HCC	[54]
	Sintilimab + IBI305 (VEGF inhibitor)	HBV-associated HCC	[55]
	Nivolumab + regorafenib (dual VEGFR2/TIE2 tyrosine kinase inhibitor)	Gastric and CRC	[56]
	Nivolumab and ipilimumab + cabozantinib (VEGFR2/c-Met inhibitor)	RCC	[57]
	Avelumab + axitinib (VEGFR inhibitor)	HCC	[58]
	Pembrolizumab + lenvatinib (multi-kinase VEGFR inhibitor)		[59]
ICI + HER2 inhibitors	Embrolizumab + trastuzumab (anti-HER2)	HER2-expressing metastatic esophagogastric cancer	[60]
	Pembrolizumab + margetuximab (anti-HER2)	HER2-positive gastroesophageal adenocarcinoma	[61]
ICI + poly(ADP-ribose) polymerase (PARP) inhibitors	Durvalumab + olaparib (PARP inhibitor)	High-risk HER2-negative stage II/III breast cancer	[62]
	Pembrolizumab + niraparib (PARP inhibitor)	Ovarian carcinoma	[63]
	Nivolumab + niraparib, ipilimumab + niraparib	Advanced pancreatic cancer	[64]

ICI + MAPK/ERK signaling pathway inhibitors	Atezolizumab + vemurafenib (BRAF inhibitor) and cobimetinib (MEK inhibitor)	Unresectable mutation positive melanoma	[65]
	Spartalizumab + dabrafenib (BRAF inhibitor) and trametinib (MEK inhibitor)	BRAF unresectable or metastatic melanoma	[66]
	Ipilimumab + vemurafenib	Metastatic melanoma	[67]
ICI + hormone receptor inhibitors	Pembrolizumab + aromatase inhibitor	Metastatic hormone receptor positive breast cancer	[68]
ICI + cancer vaccines	Ipilimumab + DCs-based mRNA vaccine	Stage III or IV melanoma	[46]
	Ipilimumab + GVAX (GMCSF cell-based vaccines)	PDA	[69]
	Nivolumab + ISA 101 (synthetic long-peptide human HPV vaccine)	HPV-16-positive tumors	[70]
ICI + adoptive cell therapy (ACT)	PD-1 inhibitor + mesothelin-specific CAR T cells	MPM	[71]
	Pembrolizumab + anti-CD19 CAR T cells	Leukemia	[72]
ICI + CXCR4 inhibitors	Cemiplimab + motixafortide (CXCR4 inhibitor)	Metastatic PDAC	[73]
	Nivolumab + mavorixafor (CXCR4 inhibitor)	Advanced RCC	[74]

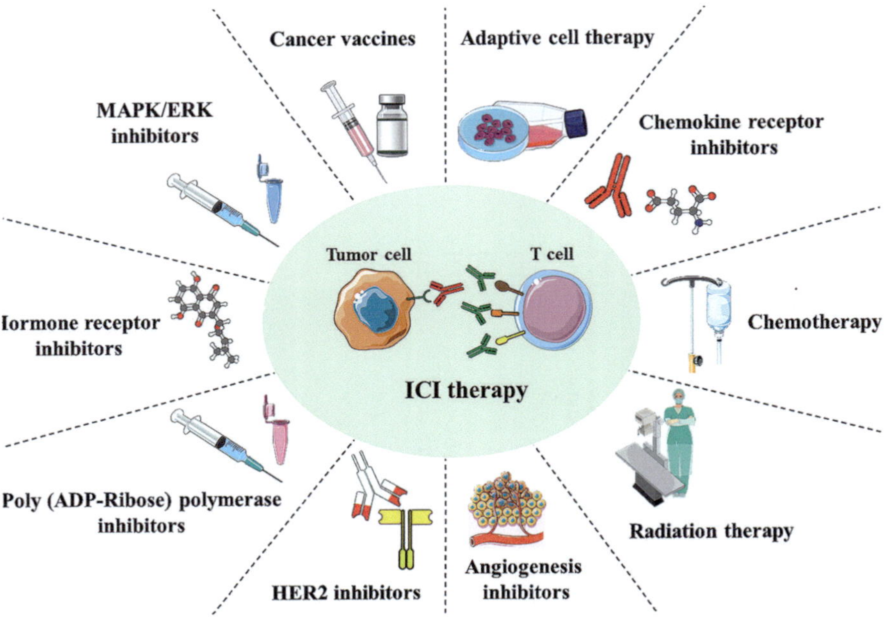

Fig. 5.3 Treatment of cancer using immune checkpoint inhibitors (ICIs) in combination with other methods. MAPK/ERK mitogen-activated protein kinases/extracellular signal-regulated kinases; HER2 human epidermal growth factor receptor 2. Created using elements from Servier Medical Art (https://smart.servier.com), licensed under CC BY 4.0 (https://creativecommons.org/licenses/by/4.0/), and from NIAID NIH BioArt Source (bioart.niaid.nih.gov)

regorafenib along with ICIs such as atezolizumab, pembrolizumab, and nivolumab increase the antitumor response in NSCLC, HCC, CRC, and gastric cancer [44]. The use of ICIs in combination with tyrosine kinase inhibitors and MAPK/ERK and PI3K/AKT/mTOR signaling pathways inhibitors or DNA repair systems inhibitors are other therapeutic strategies that recently have been studied in cancer patients.

Adoptive cell therapy (ACT) is a novel method in tumor therapy. Recently, the administration of tumor specific CAR-T cells and ICIs have been used in preclinical and clinical studies, for example the combination of anti-CD19 CAR-T cells with pembrolizumab for the treatment of leukemia.

Using cancer vaccines along with ICIs in animal models and clinical studies has also shown promising results [44, 45]. Based on a recent study, the combination of ipilimumab and DCs-based mRNA vaccination has been associated with a better clinical response in melanoma patients [46]. Different strategies for combinatorial treatment of cancer with ICIs and other anticancer agents are summarized in Table 5.4 and Fig. 5.3.

5.4 Predictive Biomarkers of Cancer Treatment with ICIs

Only about 30% of cancer patients receiving ICIs experience the clinical benefits of this therapeutic approach, other cases have no response or show resistance to the immunotherapy. Considering this, it is very important to use proper biomarkers to select patients for ICI treatment. Several types of biomarkers have been identified in this regard. Biomarkers are also helpful means to predict response (positive predictive biomarkers) or resistance (negative predictive biomarkers) to ICI cancer therapy. PD-L1, tumor mutational burden (TMB), and microsatellite instability (MSI) are FDA-approved biomarkers that are important for predicting the response to ICIs therapy in cancers [75].

5.4.1 FDA-Approved Predictive Biomarkers for Clinical Response to ICIs

5.4.1.1 PD-L1 Expression

The expression status of PD-L1 on tumor and immune cells is an important predictor of the response to ICI therapy. A study conducted by Topalian et al. on the effect of anti-PD-1 on various cancers provided valuable evidence regarding the correlation of anti-PD-L1 expression in tumor tissue with treatment outcome. Thirty-six percent of patients who were PD-L1 positive had an objective response [76]. So far, several studies have confirmed the correlation of PD-L1 expression with the response to ICIs treatment in various cancers. PD-L1 was the first predictive biomarker that received FDA-approval for NSCLC in 2015 [75]. Other cancers for which this biomarker is approved include gastric or gastroesophageal junction adenocarcinoma, cervical cancer, urothelial carcinoma, head and neck squamous cell carcinoma (HNSCC), esophageal squamous cell carcinoma (ESCC), and triple-negative breast carcinoma (TNBC([75]. PD-L1 expression can be used for the prediction of maintenance therapy with ICIs after chemotherapy [77]. PD-L1 expression evaluation by immunohistochemistry (IHC) is an approved method that can be considered before treatment with PD-1 or PD-L1 inhibitors. In this way, a tumor proportion score (TPS) is defined for each patient that represents the percentage of tumor cells that express PD-L1. The correlation between TPS and response to ICIs has been reported in several studies, for example, the longer progression-free survival (PFS) and OS in response to pembrolizumab in NSCLC patients with TPS ≥50% [26]. For other tumors such as gastric cancer, cervical carcinoma, bladder and renal cancer, combined positive score (CPS) has shown a better correlation with ICI therapy response. CPS considers the PD-L1 expression in both tumor and immune cells including lymphocytes and macrophages [78]. However, the standardization of this method is challenging due to several variables: different antibodies have been used to determine PD-L1 expression cutoffs, and different scoring systems have been defined, including TPS and CPS. Furthermore, the predictive value of PD-L1 expression varies based on ICIs type and patient conditions. PD-L1 expression can be altered during chemotherapy or radiotherapy. The tissue type and sample preparation process are also influential factors. Nevertheless, PD-L1 is still a valuable marker. The FDA has approved the administration of pembrolizumab in addition to chemotherapy for metastatic NSCLC patients with PD-L1 TPS $\geq$1% [78].

5.4.1.2 Tumor Mutational Burden

Tumor mutational burden (TMB) has been suggested as a predictive biomarker for ICI treatment outcome. TMB defines the number of mutations that occur in each megabase of DNA [26]. Accumulation of mutations can lead to the formation of neoantigens. These antigens are recognized by T cells and the specific immune response against the tumor is activated. Therefore, tumors with higher TMB are more vulnerable to ICI therapy [75]. In 2020, TMB was approved as a biomarker for administration of anti-PD-1 in unresectable or metastatic solid tumors. Defective damage response (DDR) genes mutations are intrinsic factors that affect TMB. Environmental factors such as smoking and radiation can also be involved in increasing TMB [75]. TMB is more common in lung cancer, melanoma, and bladder cancer. A study in 2014 showed that melanoma patients with high TMB (TMB-H) had better clinical outcome in response to anti-CTLA-4. Subsequent studies confirmed the association of TMB with response to ICI therapy, and TMB was suggested to be a potential predictor of ICI therapy response [77]. A study on NSCLC patients with TMB-H treated with pembrolizumab found ORR and PFS. Similar results have been reported in the treatment with nivolumab and ipilimumab. KEYNOTE-158 study in various solid tumors treated with pembrolizumab has shown a significant response in patients with TMB-H [26]. A retrospective study on 27 types of cancer revealed that the clinical outcome of treatment with PD-1/PD-L1 antibody was better in TMB-H cases. NSCLC patients receiving low-dose ipilimumab with TMB $\geq$10 had significantly longer PFS. In another study, using the combination of nivolumab and ipilimumab, the PFS was longer in patients with TMB $\geq$10 [79].

TMB can be evaluated by whole-genome sequencing (WGS) and next-generation sequencing (NGS) assays. Different thresholds have been reported to determine the TMB-H. Standardization of TMB assessment because of different cancer types, tissue preparation, and sequencing parameters is a challenging issue [75].

5.4.1.3 Defective DNA Mismatch Repair and Microsatellite Instability

Intrinsic errors that occur during DNA replication are corrected by the DNA mismatch repair (MMR) system. MLH1, MSH2, PMS2, and MSH6 are major proteins of the DNA MMR system and loss of function of these proteins can influence the MMR. Mutations mainly occur in MLH1 and MSH2 genes [77].

Deficient mismatch repair (dMMR) causes numerous mutations in the genome. These mutations mostly target microsatellite regions. Microsatellites are repeated sequences of a small DNA motif (1–6 nucleotides) in the genome, which may include 15–65 repetitions [79]. Microsatellites are spread throughout the genome, including regions near the coding genes. The dMMR leads to the accumulation of errors in microsatellites and microsatellite instability (MSI). Therefore, the MSI is a potential tumorigenesis factor. High MSI (MSI-H)/dMMR phenotype has been observed in 15% of colorectal cancers [80]. Furthermore, MSI/dMMR can cause the production of tumor neoantigens. The increase of these antigens is related to more infiltration of lymphocytes into the tumor and augmenting the antitumor immune response, as well as better immunotherapy outcomes [75, 79]. MSI-H/dMMR CRC patients have a significantly better response to PD-1 inhibitors [81]. Therefore, MSI/dMMR is considered as a biomarker for ICI therapy. In 2017, MSI/dMMR received the FDA approval as a predictive biomarker for the treatment of patients with unresectable or metastatic solid tumors by pembrolizumab. Defects in MMR can be determined by immunohistochemistry (IHC) for MLH1, MSH2, PMS2, and MSH6, as well as PCR and NGS for MSI-H [75].

5.4.2 *Other Predictive Biomarkers*

5.4.2.1 DNA Damage and Repair-Related Genes

DDR pathway plays an important role in maintaining DNA integrity by repairing DNA damages. With defective DDR, the genome becomes unstable and prone to tumorigenesis. DDR pathways consist of more than 450 proteins [82]. Loss of function mutations leading to dysfunctional DDR. Analysis of the DDR mutational landscape has shown that the most common mutated genes of DDR in different tumors (including NSCLC, bladder, CRC, and prostate cancers) are TP53, ARID1A, ATM, SMARCA4, MDM2, BRCA2, BRCA1, MUTYH, CHEK2, ATR, and MSH6 [28]. DDR defects lead to increased TMB. Altered DDR pathway in tumor is significantly associates with ICIs efficacy. For example, a study of urothelial carcinoma patients treated with atezolizumab or nivolumab showed that response and OS were better in patients with DDR pathway dysfunction [82, 83].

DNA polymerase epsilon is involved in DNA replication and repair. The POLE gene product is responsible for the catalytic activity of this polymerase. Mutations in the POLE gene lead to polymerase defects and the accumulation of mutations in the genome. These mutations in the tumor tissue lead to the production of neoantigens, the increase of TILs, and the enhancement of the antitumor immune response [75, 79]. Garmezy et al. found that cancer patients treated with PD-1 alone or with CTLA-4 containing pathogenic POLE mutations had improved clinical benefit rate, PFS, and OS [84].

5.4.2.2 Tumor Infiltrating Lymphocytes

TME is a complex of blood vessels, immune cells, and various factors present in the tumor environment. TILs play an important role in antitumor response. There is a lot of evidence about the effect of TILs on OS improvement and clinical outcomes in cancer. Lymphocytes are the major component of TIL. The increase of $CD8^+$ CTLs in the tumor is associated with a favorable prognosis. Tissue-resident effector memory (TEM) CTLs ($CD45RO^+$ $CCR7^-$ $CD62L^-$ cells) with their inflammatory activity are very protective in reinfection. The increase of these cells in the tumor tissue inhibits the tumor growth. The presence of TEM cells is related to the improvement of OS in some tumors [85]. $CD4^+$ helper cells are one of the most important antitumor cells. Recently, the role of T follicular helper (Tfh) has been highlighted in tumors. These cells play an essential role in the expansion and differentiation of B cells into plasma cells in lymph node follicles. Increased frequency of B cells in cancer is associated with better survival and prognosis. Plasma cells ($CD20^+$ $CD38^+$ $CD138^+$) are antibody producing cells that play a prominent role in antitumor immune response. A study has indicated that the presence of $CD20^+$ B cells and plasma cells along with $CD4^+$ and $CD8^+$ T cells in advanced ovarian cancer is associated with improved OS [85]. NK cells are a group of lymphocytes that do not have specific antigen receptors found in T and B cells. These cells are involved in inhibiting tumor growth with their cytotoxicity and the production of IFN-γ and TNF-α cytokines. The relationship between the reduction of these cells and the reduction of OS in cancer patients have been confirmed [85].

Pathological assessment is the traditional method of quantification of TILs. Digital immune scores and digital prognostic scores are new methods that have been used for the evaluation of TILs to predict the prognosis and estimate the risk of recurrence of tumors. Immune scores have become a standard method to monitor the progress of various tumors [85].

The association of TILs with the patient's response to ICIs has introduced it as a potential predictive factor. The systematic characterization of $CD8^+$ TILs is used as a marker to predict response to ICIs [26].

A systematic review and meta-analysis of cancer patients treated with ICIs showed that high $CD8^+$ TILs are associated with better OS, PFS, and ORR [86].

In an innovative study, Park et al. used artificial intelligence (AI)-assisted analysis of TILs as a biomarker for assessing response to ICIs in NSCLC. They used an AI-powered whole-slide images (WSI) analyzer to evaluate TILs in NSCLC. The presence of TILs in tumor tissue was defined in three immune phenotypes including inflamed (TILs distributed intratumorally), immune-excluded (TILs excluded, out of cancer stroma), and immune-desert (scant TILs in TME). The results showed that ICI-treated patients (anti-PD-1 or anti-PD-L1) who had inflamed immunophenotype experienced a better response to treatment and longer PFS [87].

5.4.2.3 Hematology Biomarkers

Absolute neutrophil counts (ANC), absolute lymphocyte counts (ALC), and derived neutrophil-to-lymphocyte ratio (dNLR) are useful parameters in evaluating response to ICI treatment. Increased ALC during ICI treatment is associated with better outcomes. In multiple myeloma (MM) patients treated with ipilimumab, increased ALC in the 12th week of ICI treatment was associated with improved OS. In another study in MM patients treated with ipilimumab, ALC was associated with longer PFS. Higher ANC and dNLR may be related to poor response to ICI therapy. A prospective study of metastatic MM patients treated with ipilimumab found a significant decrease in OS and PFS in the presence of increased ANC. In addition, decreased dNLR was associated with greater OS and PFS. An association between the increase of $CD4^+$ and $CD8^+$ T lymphocytes with good outcomes in ICI therapy has been reported [79].

5.4.3 Other Factors Affecting ICI Therapy Efficacy

5.4.3.1 Microbiota

Gut microbiome consisting of inhabitant microorganisms and related genes, proteins, and factors have important effects on the physiology of the body, including on the homeostasis of the immune system. The association of many inflammatory diseases such as IBD, celiac disease and cardiovascular disease with the reduced diversity of intestinal bacteria indicates the importance of gut microbiota [88]. Microbiota can influence the immune system function, for example, the activation of innate immunity, maturation of DCs, differentiation of T cells, and production of cytokines [89]. There is extensive evidence of the role of gut microbiota in the response to ICI therapy. Lack of enough microbial diversity affects the response to ICIs. The presence of some species such as *Bifidobacterium*, *Faecalibacterium*, *Lactobacillus*, and *Akkermansia* has been associated with a better response to ICI therapy [26]. A study showed that increased *Prevotella*/*Bacteroides* ratio augments the efficacy of anti-PD-1/PD-L1 treatment in gastrointestinal cancer [89]. A study of patients with lung and kidney cancer revealed that those who had a poor response to anti-PD-1 therapy lacked *Akkermansia muciniphila* in their gut microbiota and supplementation with *Akkermansia muciniphila* improved the response. In melanoma patients, it was found that the amount of *Bifdobacterium longum*, *Collinsella aerofaciens*, and *Enterococcus faecium* in the intestinal flora is positively correlated with an improved outcome [79].

Antibiotics can affect the OS of cancer patients receiving ICIs. The correlation of antibiotic administration with response to ICI treatment has been identified in NSCLC patients. In several studies, the effect of antibiotics in worse clinical outcomes for ICI therapy has been demonstrated. According to a study, patients who received antibiotics before treatment with anti-PD-1/PD-L1 and anti-CTLA-4 were associated with shorter OS and PFS [88]. Therefore, before treatment with ICIs, factors like antibiotics and diet that can change the composition of microbiota should be considered [26].

Modifying the gut microbiota can enhance the response to ICI therapy. Several studies have focused on the modulation of gut microbiota to potentiate the efficacy of immunotherapy. Fecal microbiota transplant (FMT) is a method that alters the composition of gut microbiota by transferring intestinal microbiota from one host to the target host [89]. FMT studies on animal models have been promising in improving the efficacy of treatment with ICIs [88]. Multiple clinical trials have also been conducted in this regard. In phase I of a clinical trial (NCT03353402), a 30% responsiveness rate to FMT is reported for refractory metastatic melanoma patients who received anti-PD-1 [89]. Microbial ecosystem therapy (MET) is a method similar to FMT in which distinct combinations of live bacterial strains are specifically selected from stool for transfer to the host. In a clinical trial (NCT03686202), MET has been used in combination with ICI therapy for various solid tumors [88]. Oral restorative microbiota therapy (RMT) capsules are another way to change the microbiota. The clinical trial number NCT04105270 was designed to evaluate the efficacy of ICI in NSCLC using RMT. In addition, in some studies, the administration of probiotics has been associated with better PFS and OS after ICI therapy [88].

5.4.3.2 Diet

Nutritional status can have important effects on the function of the immune system and consequently on the antitumor immune response. Based on this, several studies have investigated the effect of different diets on antitumor immunotherapy. Specifically in the field of ICI therapy, fasting, ketogenic diet, protein-restricted diet, high fiber diet, and various vitamins have been studied. The ketogenic diet (KD) consists of a high percentage of fat, adequate protein, and a small amount of carbohydrate so that about 90% of the calories is provided by fat. The effects of this regimen on tumor immunotherapy have been documented [90, 91]. A study of mice model of glioblastoma has shown that KD can increase the infiltration of T cells in the tumor. It also improves the antitumor response by reducing the expression of CTLA-4 and PD-1 on TILs and also reducing the expression of PD-L1 on tumor cells [92]. Therefore, it is potentially important in the efficacy of ICI therapy.

Protein-restricted diet can also be involved in increasing response to ICI therapy through antitumor effects. Induction of endoplasmic reticulum (ER) stress in tumor cells, suppression of tumor cells proliferation, reduction of Treg cells in TME, and boosting the activity of T cells are among the antitumor mechanisms of this diet. Studies on animal models of cancer have shown that a protein-restricted diet increases the effect of ICIs. In addition, improved response to ICI therapy following a fiber diet has been reported [91].

5.5 Conclusion

The field of cancer immunotherapy using immune checkpoint inhibitors has revolutionized oncology treatment in recent years. This chapter has highlighted the significant progress made in developing and implementing ICIs, from the first approval of ipilimumab for melanoma to the expanding array of approved agents targeting various immune checkpoints. The success of ICIs in multiple cancer types has demonstrated the power of harnessing the immune system to combat tumors. However, despite these advances, challenges remain. The limited response rates to ICI monotherapy and the emergence of resistance mechanisms highlight the need for continued research and innovation. Combination approaches, whether using multiple ICIs or combining ICIs with other treatment modalities, show promise in expanding the benefits of immunotherapy to a broader patient population.

The identification and validation of predictive biomarkers represent a critical area of ongoing research. While PD-L1 expression, TMB, and MSI have proven useful, they are imperfect predictors of response. The exploration of novel biomarkers, including immune cell phenotypes and gene signatures, may lead to more precise patient selection and treatment strategies. Furthermore, the growing understanding of how factors such as the gut microbiome and diet influence ICI efficacy opens new avenues for enhancing treatment outcomes. These insights may lead to innovative approaches to modulate the immune response and improve ICI effectiveness. As the field continues to grow, the focus will likely shift toward personalized immunotherapy strategies that are tailored to individual patients based on their tumor characteristics, immune profile, and other relevant factors. The ongoing research into novel immune checkpoints and combination approaches promises to further expand the reach and efficacy of cancer immunotherapy. In conclusion, while immune checkpoint blockade has already transformed cancer treatment, its full potential is yet to be realized. Continued research, clinical trials, and interdisciplinary collaboration will be necessary in overcoming current limitations and unlocking the full power of the immune system in the fight against cancer.

Acknowledgments The authors gratefully acknowledge the valuable assistance provided by Maryam Sadr.

References

1. Alturki NA. Review of the immune checkpoint inhibitors in the context of cancer treatment. J Clin Med. 2023;12(13)
2. Dutta S, Ganguly A, Chatterjee K, Spada S, Mukherjee S. Targets of immune escape mechanisms in cancer: basis for development and evolution of cancer immune checkpoint inhibitors. Biology. 2023;12(2)
3. Wahli MN, Hayoz S, Hoch D, Ryser CO, Hoffmann M, Scherz A, et al. The role of immune checkpoint inhibitors in clinical practice: an analysis of the treatment patterns, survival and toxicity rates by sex. J Cancer Res Clin Oncol. 2023;149(7):3847–58.

4. Sun Q, Hong Z, Zhang C, Wang L, Han Z, Ma D. Immune checkpoint therapy for solid tumours: clinical dilemmas and future trends. Signal Transduct Target Ther. 2023;8(1):320.
5. Couzin-Frankel J. Breakthrough of the year 2013. Cancer immunotherapy. Science (New York, NY). 2013;342(6165):1432–3.
6. Jin Y, Li H, Zhang P, Yu M, Zhang H, Li X. The regulatory approvals of immune checkpoint inhibitors in China and the United States: a cross-national comparison study. Int J Cancer. 2023;152(11):2351–61.
7. Cameron F, Whiteside G, Perry C. Ipilimumab: first global approval. Drugs. 2011;71(8):1093–104.
8. Keam SJ. Tremelimumab: first approval. Drugs. 2023;83(1):93–102.
9. Poole RM. Pembrolizumab: first global approval. Drugs. 2014;74(16):1973–81.
10. Markham A, Duggan S. Cemiplimab: first global approval. Drugs. 2018;78(17):1841–6.
11. Paik J. Nivolumab plus relatlimab: first approval. Drugs. 2022;82(8):925–31.
12. Markham A. Dostarlimab: first approval. Drugs. 2021;81(10):1213–9.
13. Keam SJ. Toripalimab: first global approval. Drugs. 2019;79(5):573–8.
14. Hoy SM. Sintilimab: first global approval. Drugs. 2019;79(3):341–6.
15. Markham A, Keam SJ. Camrelizumab: first global approval. Drugs. 2019;79(12):1355–61.
16. Lee A, Keam SJ. Tislelizumab: first approval. Drugs. 2020;80(6):617–24.
17. Dhillon S. Penpulimab: first approval. Drugs. 2021;81(18):2159–66.
18. Lee A. Serplulimab: first approval. Drugs. 2022;82(10):1137–41.
19. Markham A. Zimberelimab: first approval. Drugs. 2021;81(17):2063–8.
20. Keam SJ. Cadonilimab: first approval. Drugs. 2022;82(12):1333–9.
21. Markham A. Atezolizumab: first global approval. Drugs. 2016;76(12):1227–32.
22. Syed YY. Durvalumab: first global approval. Drugs. 2017;77(12):1369–76.
23. Kim ES. Avelumab: first global approval. Drugs. 2017;77(8):929–37.
24. Markham A. Envafolimab: first approval. Drugs. 2022;82(2):235–40.
25. Dhillon S, Duggan S. Sugemalimab: first approval. Drugs. 2022;82(5):593–9.
26. Basudan AM. The role of immune checkpoint inhibitors in cancer therapy. Clin Pract. 2022;13(1):22–40.
27. Rowshanravan B, Halliday N, Sansom DM. CTLA-4: a moving target in immunotherapy. Blood. 2018;131(1):58–67.
28. Tremelimumab. Drugs R D. 2010;10(2):123–32.
29. Ibrahim R, Saleh K, Chahine C, Khoury R, Khalife N, Cesne AL. LAG-3 inhibitors: novel immune checkpoint inhibitors changing the landscape of immunotherapy. Biomedicine. 2023;11(7)
30. Sauer N, Szlasa W, Jonderko L, Oślizło M, Kunachowicz D, Kulbacka J, et al. LAG-3 as a potent target for novel anticancer therapies of a wide range of tumors. Int J Mol Sci. 2022;23(17)
31. Li Y, Ju M, Miao Y, Zhao L, Xing L, Wei M. Advancement of anti-LAG-3 in cancer therapy. FASEB J. 2023;37(11):e23236.
32. He Y, Cao J, Zhao C, Li X, Zhou C, Hirsch FR. TIM-3, a promising target for cancer immunotherapy. Onco Targets Ther. 2018;11:7005–9.
33. Rousseau A, Parisi C, Barlesi F. Anti-TIGIT therapies for solid tumors: a systematic review. ESMO Open. 2023;8(2):101184.
34. Getu AA, Tigabu A, Zhou M, Lu J, Fodstad Ø, Tan M. New frontiers in immune checkpoint B7-H3 (CD276) research and drug development. Mol Cancer. 2023;22(1):43.
35. Kanchan RK, Doss D, Khan P, Nasser MW, Mahapatra S. To kill a cancer: targeting the immune inhibitory checkpoint molecule, B7-H3. Biochim Biophys Acta Rev Cancer. 2022;1877(5):188783.
36. Mortezaee K. B7x in cancer immunity and immunotherapy. Int Immunopharmacol. 2023;118:110133.
37. Noelle RJ, Lines JL, Lewis LD, Martell RE, Guillaudeux T, Lee SW, et al. Clinical and research updates on the VISTA immune checkpoint: immuno-oncology themes and highlights. Front Oncol. 2023;13:1225081.

38. Son J, Hsieh RC, Lin HY, Krause KJ, Yuan Y, Biter AB, et al. Inhibition of the CD47-SIRPα axis for cancer therapy: a systematic review and meta-analysis of emerging clinical data. Front Immunol. 2022;13:1027235.
39. Horenstein AL, Chillemi A, Zini R, Quarona V, Bianchi N, Manfredini R, et al. Cytokine-induced killer cells express CD39, CD38, CD203a, CD73 ectoenzymes and P1 adenosinergic receptors. Front Pharmacol. 2018;9:196.
40. Cekic C, Day YJ, Sag D, Linden J. Myeloid expression of adenosine A2A receptor suppresses T and NK cell responses in the solid tumor microenvironment. Cancer Res. 2014;74(24):7250–9.
41. van de Donk N, Usmani SZ. CD38 antibodies in multiple myeloma: mechanisms of action and modes of resistance. Front Immunol. 2018;9:2134.
42. Dhillon S. Isatuximab: first approval. Drugs. 2020;80(9):905–12.
43. Walsh RJ, Sundar R, Lim JSJ. Immune checkpoint inhibitor combinations-current and emerging strategies. Br J Cancer. 2023;128(8):1415–7.
44. Vafaei S, Zekiy AO, Khanamir RA, Zaman BA, Ghayourvahdat A, Azimizonuzi H, et al. Combination therapy with immune checkpoint inhibitors (ICIs); a new frontier. Cancer Cell Int. 2022;22(1):2.
45. Li B, Jin J, Guo D, Tao Z, Hu X. Immune checkpoint inhibitors combined with targeted therapy: the recent advances and future potentials. Cancer. 2023;15(10)
46. De Keersmaecker B, Claerhout S, Carrasco J, Bar I, Corthals J, Wilgenhof S, et al. TriMix and tumor antigen mRNA electroporated dendritic cell vaccination plus ipilimumab: link between T-cell activation and clinical responses in advanced melanoma. J Immunother Cancer. 2020;8(1)
47. Shi A, Li L, Yang D, Min Y, Jiang L, Dong X, et al. 98P First-line atezolizumab/durvalumab plus platinum-etoposide combined with radiotherapy in extensive-stage small cell lung cancer. Immuno-Oncol Technol. 2022;16:100202.
48. Pelster MS, Gruschkus SK, Bassett R, Gombos DS, Shephard M, Posada L, et al. Nivolumab and ipilimumab in metastatic uveal melanoma: results from a single-arm phase II study. J Clin Oncol. 2021;39(6):599–607.
49. Ueno M, Ikeda M, Morizane C, Kobayashi S, Ohno I, Kondo S, et al. Nivolumab alone or in combination with cisplatin plus gemcitabine in Japanese patients with unresectable or recurrent biliary tract cancer: a non-randomised, multicentre, open-label, phase 1 study. Lancet Gastroenterol Hepatol. 2019;4(8):611–21.
50. Li JJ, Wang JH, Dingv Y, Li DD, Wen XZ, Zhao JJ, et al. Efficacy and safety of anti-PD-1 inhibitor combined with nab-paclitaxel in Chinese patients with refractory melanoma. J Cancer Res Clin Oncol. 2022;148(5):1159–69.
51. Lee EK, Xiong N, Cheng SC, Barry WT, Penson RT, Konstantinopoulos PA, et al. Combined pembrolizumab and pegylated liposomal doxorubicin in platinum resistant ovarian cancer: a phase 2 clinical trial. Gynecol Oncol. 2020;159(1):72–8.
52. Ansari J, Farrag A, Ali A, Abdelgelil M, Murshid E, Alhamad A, et al. Concurrent use of nivolumab and radiotherapy for patients with metastatic non-small cell lung cancer and renal cell carcinoma with oligometastatic disease progression on nivolumab. Mol Clin Oncol. 2021;15(4):214.
53. Schubert P, Rutzner S, Eckstein M, Frey B, Schweizer C, Haderlein M, et al. Prospective evaluation of all-lesion versus single-lesion radiotherapy in combination with PD-1/PD-L1 immune checkpoint inhibitors. Front Oncol. 2020;10:576643.
54. Finn RS, Qin S, Ikeda M, Galle PR, Ducreux M, Kim TY, et al. Atezolizumab plus bevacizumab in unresectable hepatocellular carcinoma. N Engl J Med. 2020;382(20):1894–905.
55. Ren Z, Xu J, Bai Y, Xu A, Cang S, Du C, et al. Sintilimab plus a bevacizumab biosimilar (IBI305) versus sorafenib in unresectable hepatocellular carcinoma (ORIENT-32): a randomised, open-label, phase 2-3 study. Lancet Oncol. 2021;22(7):977–90.
56. Fukuoka S, Hara H, Takahashi N, Kojima T, Kawazoe A, Asayama M, et al. Regorafenib plus nivolumab in patients with advanced gastric or colorectal cancer: an open-label, dose-escalation, and dose-expansion phase Ib trial (REGONIVO, EPOC1603). J Clin Oncol. 2020;38(18):2053–61.

57. Choueiri TK, Powles T, Albiges L, Burotto M, Szczylik C, Zurawski B, et al. Cabozantinib plus nivolumab and ipilimumab in renal-cell carcinoma. N Engl J Med. 2023;388(19):1767–78.
58. Kudo M, Motomura K, Wada Y, Inaba Y, Sakamoto Y, Kurosaki M, et al. Avelumab in combination with axitinib as first-line treatment in patients with advanced hepatocellular carcinoma: results from the phase 1b VEGF liver 100 trial. Liver Cancer. 2021;10(3):249–59.
59. Kawazoe A, Fukuoka S, Nakamura Y, Kuboki Y, Wakabayashi M, Nomura S, et al. Lenvatinib plus pembrolizumab in patients with advanced gastric cancer in the first-line or second-line setting (EPOC1706): an open-label, single-arm, phase 2 trial. Lancet Oncol. 2020;21(8):1057–65.
60. Janjigian YY, Maron SB, Chatila WK, Millang B, Chavan SS, Alterman C, et al. First-line pembrolizumab and trastuzumab in HER2-positive oesophageal, gastric, or gastro-oesophageal junction cancer: an open-label, single-arm, phase 2 trial. Lancet Oncol. 2020;21(6):821–31.
61. Catenacci DVT, Kang YK, Park H, Uronis HE, Lee KW, Ng MCH, et al. Margetuximab plus pembrolizumab in patients with previously treated, HER2-positive gastro-oesophageal adenocarcinoma (CP-MGAH22-05): a single-arm, phase 1b-2 trial. Lancet Oncol. 2020;21(8):1066–76.
62. Pusztai L, Yau C, Wolf DM, Han HS, Du L, Wallace AM, et al. Durvalumab with olaparib and paclitaxel for high-risk HER2-negative stage II/III breast cancer: results from the adaptively randomized I-SPY2 trial. Cancer Cell. 2021;39(7):989–98.e5.
63. Konstantinopoulos PA, Waggoner S, Vidal GA, Mita M, Moroney JW, Holloway R, et al. Single-arm phases 1 and 2 trial of niraparib in combination with pembrolizumab in patients with recurrent platinum-resistant ovarian carcinoma. JAMA Oncol. 2019;5(8):1141–9.
64. Reiss KA, Mick R, Teitelbaum U, O'Hara M, Schneider C, Massa R, et al. Niraparib plus nivolumab or niraparib plus ipilimumab in patients with platinum-sensitive advanced pancreatic cancer: a randomised, phase 1b/2 trial. Lancet Oncol. 2022;23(8):1009–20.
65. Gutzmer R, Stroyakovskiy D, Gogas H, Robert C, Lewis K, Protsenko S, et al. Atezolizumab, vemurafenib, and cobimetinib as first-line treatment for unresectable advanced BRAF(V600) mutation-positive melanoma (IMspire150): primary analysis of the randomised, double-blind, placebo-controlled, phase 3 trial. Lancet (London, England). 2020;395(10240):1835–44.
66. Dummer R, Long GV, Robert C, Tawbi HA, Flaherty KT, Ascierto PA, et al. Randomized phase III trial evaluating spartalizumab plus dabrafenib and trametinib for BRAF V600-mutant unresectable or metastatic melanoma. J Clin Oncol. 2022;40(13):1428–38.
67. Amin A, Lawson DH, Salama AK, Koon HB, Guthrie T Jr, Thomas SS, et al. Phase II study of vemurafenib followed by ipilimumab in patients with previously untreated BRAF-mutated metastatic melanoma. J Immunother Cancer. 2016;4:44.
68. Ge X, Yost SE, Lee JS, Frankel PH, Ruel C, Cui Y, et al. Phase II study combining pembrolizumab with aromatase inhibitor in patients with metastatic hormone receptor positive breast cancer. Cancer. 2022;14(17)
69. Le DT, Lutz E, Uram JN, Sugar EA, Onners B, Solt S, et al. Evaluation of ipilimumab in combination with allogeneic pancreatic tumor cells transfected with a GM-CSF gene in previously treated pancreatic cancer. J Immunother. 2013;36(7):382–9.
70. Massarelli E, William W, Johnson F, Kies M, Ferrarotto R, Guo M, et al. Combining immune checkpoint blockade and tumor-specific vaccine for patients with incurable human papillomavirus 16-related cancer: a phase 2 clinical trial. JAMA Oncol. 2019;5(1):67–73.
71. Adusumilli PS, Zauderer MG, Rivière I, Solomon SB, Rusch VW, O'Cearbhaill RE, et al. A phase I trial of regional mesothelin-targeted CAR T-cell therapy in patients with malignant pleural disease, in combination with the anti-PD-1 agent pembrolizumab. Cancer Discov. 2021;11(11):2748–63.
72. Maude SL, Hucks GE, Seif AE, Talekar MK, Teachey DT, Baniewicz D, et al. The effect of pembrolizumab in combination with CD19-targeted chimeric antigen receptor (CAR) T cells in relapsed acute lymphoblastic leukemia (ALL). J Clin Oncol. 2017;35(15_suppl):103.
73. Manji GA, May MS, Pellicciotta I, Ana SS, Sender N, Pan SM, et al. CheMo4METPANC: a phase 2 study with combination chemotherapy (gemcitabine and nab-paclitaxel), chemokine (C-X-C) motif receptor 4 inhibitor (motixafortide), and immune checkpoint block-

ade (cemiplimab) in metastatic treatment-naïve pancreas adenocarcinoma. J Clin Oncol. 2023;41(16_suppl):TPS4200–TPS.

74. Choueiri TK, Atkins MB, Rose TL, Alter RS, Ju Y, Niland K, et al. A phase 1b trial of the CXCR4 inhibitor mavorixafor and nivolumab in advanced renal cell carcinoma patients with no prior response to nivolumab monotherapy. Investig New Drugs. 2021;39(4):1019–27.
75. Wang Y, Tong Z, Zhang W, Zhang W, Buzdin A, Mu X, et al. FDA-approved and emerging next generation predictive biomarkers for immune checkpoint inhibitors in cancer patients. Front Oncol. 2021;11:683419.
76. Topalian SL, Hodi FS, Brahmer JR, Gettinger SN, Smith DC, McDermott DF, et al. Safety, activity, and immune correlates of anti-PD-1 antibody in cancer. N Engl J Med. 2012;366(26):2443–54.
77. Bindal P, Gray JE, Boyle TA, Florou V, Puri S. Biomarkers of therapeutic response with immune checkpoint inhibitors. Ann Transl Med. 2021;9(12):1040.
78. De Marchi P, Leal LF, Duval da Silva V, da Silva ECA, Cordeiro de Lima VC, Reis RM. PD-L1 expression by tumor proportion score (TPS) and combined positive score (CPS) are similar in non-small cell lung cancer (NSCLC). J Clin Pathol. 2021;74(11):735–40.
79. Li N, Hou X, Huang S, Tai R, Lei L, Li S, et al. Biomarkers related to immune checkpoint inhibitors therapy. Biomed Pharmacother. 2022;147:112470.
80. Mulet-Margalef N, Linares J, Badia-Ramentol J, Jimeno M, Sanz Monte C, Manzano Mozo JL, et al. Challenges and therapeutic opportunities in the dMMR/MSI-H colorectal cancer landscape. Cancer. 2023;15(4)
81. Sahin IH, Akce M, Alese O, Shaib W, Lesinski GB, El-Rayes B, et al. Immune checkpoint inhibitors for the treatment of MSI-H/MMR-D colorectal cancer and a perspective on resistance mechanisms. Br J Cancer. 2019;121(10):809–18.
82. Sun W, Zhang Q, Wang R, Li Y, Sun Y, Yang L. Targeting DNA damage repair for immune checkpoint inhibition: mechanisms and potential clinical applications. Front Oncol. 2021;11:648687.
83. Shi C, Qin K, Lin A, Jiang A, Cheng Q, Liu Z, et al. The role of DNA damage repair (DDR) system in response to immune checkpoint inhibitor (ICI) therapy. J Exp Clin Cancer Res. 2022;41(1):268.
84. Garmezy B, Gheeya J, Lin HY, Huang Y, Kim T, Jiang X, et al. Clinical and molecular characterization of POLE mutations as predictive biomarkers of response to immune checkpoint inhibitors in advanced cancers. JCO Precis Oncol. 2022;6:e2100267.
85. Paijens ST, Vledder A, de Bruyn M, Nijman HW. Tumor-infiltrating lymphocytes in the immunotherapy era. Cell Mol Immunol. 2021;18(4):842–59.
86. Li F, Li C, Cai X, Xie Z, Zhou L, Cheng B, et al. The association between CD8+ tumor-infiltrating lymphocytes and the clinical outcome of cancer immunotherapy: a systematic review and meta-analysis. EClinicalMedicine. 2021;41:101134.
87. Park S, Ock CY, Kim H, Pereira S, Park S, Ma M, et al. Artificial intelligence-powered spatial analysis of tumor-infiltrating lymphocytes as complementary biomarker for immune checkpoint inhibition in non-small-cell lung cancer. J Clin Oncol. 2022;40(17):1916–28.
88. Duttagupta S, Hakozaki T, Routy B, Messaoudene M. The gut microbiome from a biomarker to a novel therapeutic strategy for immunotherapy response in patients with lung cancer. Curr Oncol. 2023;30(11):9406–27.
89. Zhang C, Zhang C, Wang H. Immune-checkpoint inhibitor resistance in cancer treatment: current progress and future directions. Cancer Lett. 2023;562:216182.
90. Zitvogel L, Kroemer G. Boosting the immunotherapy response by nutritional interventions. J Clin Invest. 2022;132(11)
91. Zhang X, Li H, Lv X, Hu L, Li W, Zi M, et al. Impact of diets on response to immune checkpoint inhibitors (ICIs) therapy against tumors. Life. 2022;12(3)
92. Lussier DM, Woolf EC, Johnson JL, Brooks KS, Blattman JN, Scheck AC. Enhanced immunity in a mouse model of malignant glioma is mediated by a therapeutic ketogenic diet. BMC Cancer. 2016;16:310.

Chapter 6
Cancer Immunotherapy Using Immune Checkpoint Inhibitors: Current Approaches and Future Directions

6.1 Introduction

Immune checkpoint inhibitors (ICIs) have emerged as a major therapeutic in cancer immunotherapy which are associated with good clinical outcomes in many patients. In recent years, these medications have been increasingly used to boost the antitumor immune responses in different cancers such as melanoma, lymphoma, lung, bladder, and renal cell cancers. Several monoclonal antibodies against inhibitory molecules such as CTLA-4 (ipilimumab), PD-1 (nivolumab, pembrolizumab, cemiplimab), and its ligand PD-L1 (atezolizumab, avelumab, durvalumab) have been approved by the United States Food and Drug Administration (FDA). Since immune checkpoints are regulators of immune responses, blocking these receptors can lead to uncontrolled immune responses and autoimmunity, which are known as immune-related adverse events (irAEs). irAEs can occur in all organs, but they are more probable in certain organs, mainly skin, gastrointestinal tract, and lung, or in organs that are more sensitive to autoimmune diseases such as the thyroid and joints (Fig. 6.1). irAEs mostly develop in the first 3 months of the ICI therapy, although they may appear several months after the treatment. These complications can be mild or severe and even cause death in some patients. Usually, acute irAEs symptoms are manageable by glucocorticoids and stopping the administration of ICIs [1, 2]. Here, the clinical features of the irAEs caused by ICIs in different organs during cancer treatment are discussed.

L. Tayebi, M. Abdolmaleki, *Immune System Regulation*,
https://doi.org/10.1007/978-981-95-8026-2_6

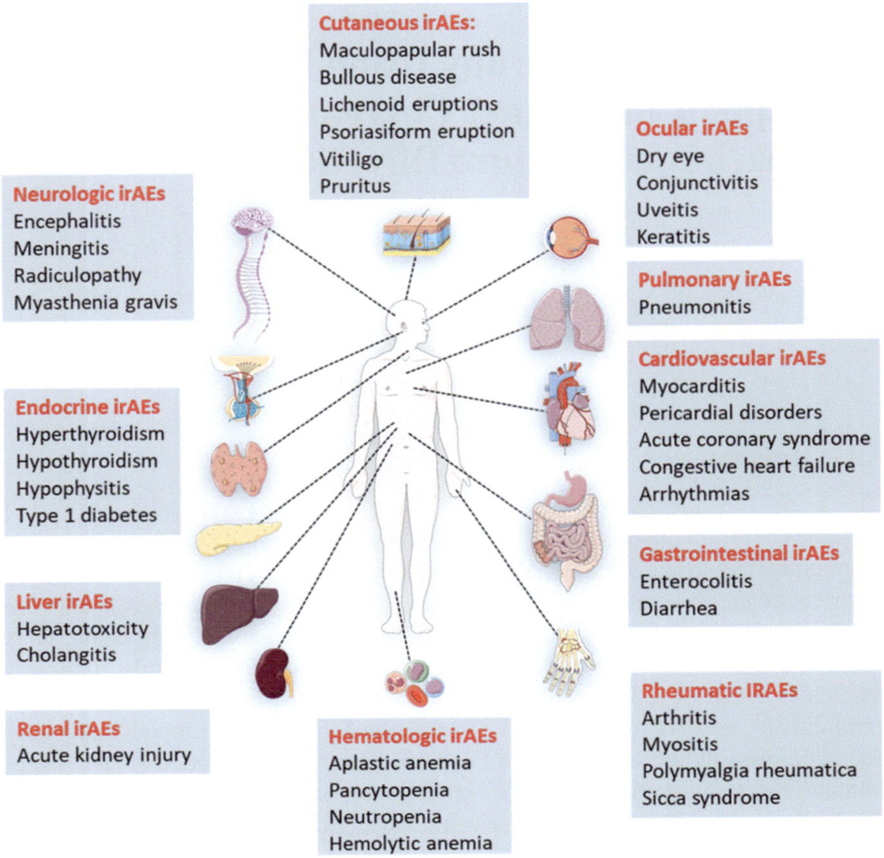

Fig. 6.1 Immune-related adverse events induced by immune checkpoint inhibitors in different organs. (The figure is adapted from Ref. (90) created using elements from Servier Medical Art (https://smart.servier.com), licensed under CC BY 4.0 (https://creativecommons.org/licenses/by/4.0/))

6.2 Cutaneous irAEs

Skin complications are among the most common irAEs related to ICI therapy. Cutaneous irAEs (cirAEs) usually appear within the first few weeks of treatment. The incidence of cirAEs in patients receiving ICIs is estimated between 30% and 60%. The incidence rate is 44–59% for anti-CTLA-4 and 34–42% for anti-PD-1 therapy. The combination of CTLA-4 and PD-1 inhibitors raises the risk of cirAEs (59–72% of treated patients). cirAEs consist of heterogeneous clinical manifestations including maculopapular rash (MPR), pruritus, eczema, lichenoid eruptions, psoriasiform dermatitis, vitiligo, bullous disorders, sarcoidosis, scleroderma, alopecia, Stevens-Johnson syndrome (SJS), toxic epidermal necrolysis (TEN), and drug-induced hypersensitivity syndrome (DIHS)/drug reaction with eosinophilia and systemic symptoms (DRESS). Most of the cirAEs are mild or moderate and usually self-limiting; however, in some cases, severe cutaneous adverse reactions (SCARs) may appear, including SJS/TEN, DIHS/DRESS, and acute generalized exanthematous pustulosis (AGEP). MPR, pruritus, psoriasiform rash, eczema, and lichenoid eruptions are the most frequent ICIs-induced cirAEs. Regarding the pathogenesis of cirAEs, various mechanisms have been suggested, including type IV hypersensitivity reactions, activation of autoreactive T cells and B cells, and proinflammatory cytokines [3–5]. The characteristics of cirAEs have been summarized in Table 6.1.

6.2.1 *Maculopapular (Morbilliform) Rush*

MPR is one of the most common cirAEs, which is more likely to develop with anti-CTLA-4 than with other inhibitors. It occurs in 49–68% of anti-CTLA-4 and 20% of anti-PD-1/PD-L1 therapy cases. The morbilliform rash is usually observed 3–6 weeks after immunotherapy, which typically appears as faint erythematous macules and papules in the trunk and the extensor side of the extremities. Most MPRs are mild and self-limiting; however, sometimes it turns into a severe cutaneous disease. To control the symptoms and prevent the development of more serious lesions such as blisters and epidermal detachment, the patient must be monitored [3, 5]. Type IV hypersensitivity reaction mediated by cytotoxic T cells is a notable pathophysiological mechanism in this situation. Topical corticosteroids are prescribed for MPR grade 1 and 2, and in severe cases (grade 3 and 4), systemic corticosteroids are recommended [3, 6].

6.2.2 *Pruritus*

Pruritus is also common in cirAEs, which can occur alone or with other skin involvement; 14–47% of patients undergoing ICI treatment experience pruritus. Anti-CTLA-4 monotherapy and anti-CTLA-4/PD-1 combination therapy account for 25–36% and 33–47% of this complication, respectively. It is usually developed after three treatment cycles. Recently, the incidence has been increasing with LAG-3/PD-1 therapy in melanoma patients. Symptoms present as macular rash and eczematous reactions [5, 7]. It is often mild and occurs mostly in the scalp and trunk. The severe form is observed in less than 1% of the patients. T cell cytokines, especially Th2 response and the related cytokines including IL-4, IL-13, and IL-31, play an important role in the pathogenesis of pruritus. This complication is managed with topical moisturizers, corticosteroids, and oral antihistamines [3, 6].

Table 6.1 Cutaneous irAEs induced by ICI immunotherapy

Type of irAE	Symptoms	Onset time	Frequency	Treatment	References
Maculopapular rush	Erythematous macules and papules of trunk and extremities	3–6 weeks	49–68% for anti-CTLA-4, 20% for anti-PD-1/PD-L1	Topical steroids, emollients, oral antihistamines, systemic steroids for higher grades	[3, 6]
Pruritus	Irritating sensation, trunk, and scalp itching	3–10 weeks	25–36% for anti-CTLA-4, 33–47% for combination therapy	Topical steroids, emollients, moisturizers, oral antihistamines	[3, 11]
Lichenoid eruptions	Classic lichen planus (flat-topped, violaceous plaques on the extremities and the trunk), hypertrophic lichen planus, oral lichen planus	6–12 weeks	0.5–6%	Topical steroids, systemic steroids for higher grades	[5, 8]
Psoriasiform eruptions	Scaly erythematous plaques of trunk and extremities	3–12 weeks	More frequent with anti-PD-1 therapy (3–12% of patients)	Topical steroids, vitamin D analogs, narrowband ultraviolet B phototherapy	[5, 12]
Vitiligo-like depigmentation	Macular or patchy depigmentation	Several weeks to months	2–9% for CTLA-4, 7–11% for anti-PD-1	No definitive treatment	[3, 9]
Bullous disease	Tense bullae, subepidermal blisters	Several weeks to months	1% for anti-PD-1/PD-L1	Topical or systemic steroids	[6, 13]
SJS/TEN	Flaccid bullae, targetoid patches, detachment of the epidermis, erosions, mucosal involvement	1–20 weeks	Rare	High-dose corticosteroids, ICI discontinuation, TNF inhibitors	[5, 14]
DIHS/DRESS	Fever, facial swelling, diffuse erythema, internal organ involvement	Several weeks to months	Rare	Systemic corticosteroids, ICI discontinuation, TNF inhibitors	[5, 14]

6.2.3 Lichenoid Eruptions

Lichenoid eruptions emerge about 6–12 weeks after immunotherapy and occur in 0.5–6% of patients. It is more common in patients receiving PD-1/PD-L1 inhibitors. Clinical manifestations include itchy rashes, pruritic, purple, flat-topped, and keratotic papules usually on the extensor surfaces of the extremities and trunk. Nails, oral, and genital mucosa are involved in some patients. In ICI-associated lichenoid eruptions, spongiosis, parakeratosis, necrosis, and eosinophils are observed, which is different from typical lichen planus (LP). Activation of cytotoxic T cells, increased production of IFN-γ and infiltration of $CD14^{+}$ $CD16^{+}$ monocytes with overexpression of TLR2 and TLR4 are involved in the pathogenesis of the disease. High-potency topical corticosteroids are effective in ameliorating the lesions. For higher grades, methotrexate and TNF-α inhibitors are helpful [3, 5, 6, 8].

6.2.4 Psoriasiform Eruptions

Psoriasiform eruptions are more prevalent during treatment with PD-1/PD-L1 inhibitors than CTLA-4 inhibitors. It affects about 3–12% of patients receiving PD-1 inhibitors. This complication can occur as newly onset psoriasis (de novo psoriasis), which includes 70% of patients, or develops as a result of the activation of preexisting psoriasis in patients who have a history of psoriasis (30%). Usually, the complication appears during the 3–12 weeks of the treatment. Plaque psoriasis is the most common variant of this eruption, which is erythematous scaly plaques localized on the extensor surfaces of extremities and the trunk. Other types include palmoplantar, pustular, guttate, and inverse psoriasis. Th17 cytokines such as IL-17, IL-22, TNF-α, and IL-23 play a critical key role in the development of these eruptions. Lesions can be treated with topical corticosteroids and narrowband ultraviolet B phototherapy. For steroid-resistant cases, other agents such as methotrexate are used [3, 5].

6.2.5 Vitiligo-Like Depigmentation (VLD)

Vitiligo is an autoimmune disorder that causes patchy depigmentation of the skin. It occurs following damage to melanocytes in the epidermis. ICI-induced VLD is a type of cirAEs that is similar to vitiligo. It seems that due to the antigenic similarity between melanocytes and melanoma tumor cells, such as melan-A proteins, tyrosinase-related proteins 1 and 2, and GP100, $CD8^{+}$ cytotoxic T cells become activated against these antigens that lead to melanocyte destruction. The incidence rate of VLD during anti-PD-1 therapy is about 7–11% and for anti-CTLA-4 therapy 2–9%. The median onset time of VLD is about 26 weeks. Clinical manifestations include multiple flecked macules that expand into larger patches, mostly in a symmetrical pattern [3, 6]. Regardless of the unpleasant appearance, VLD is considered a favorable prognosis in the treatment of melanoma, which is associated with prolonged survival rates in patients [9].

6.2.6 Bullous Disease

This type of cirAEs is less common and appears for a relatively long time from the start of treatment (13th–18th week) and is observed in about 1% of patients receiving anti-PD-1/PD-L1. Pemphigoid (BP) is the most dominant form of these lesions. Other types such as bullous lichenoid dermatitis and linear IgA bullous dermatosis are less common. Symptoms are similar to classic BP including pruritic prodromal non-bullous phase and tense bullae filled with serous fluid predominantly on the trunk and extremities. Autoantibodies against basement membrane proteins BP180 and BP230, which are common between melanoma tumor cells and normal skin, play a pivotal role pathogenesis of the disease. Low-grade BP is managed with topical corticosteroids and for higher grades, systemic corticosteroids and rituximab (a B cell-depleting anti-CD20 antibody) are recommended [3, 6].

6.2.7 Severe Cutaneous Adverse Reactions (SCARs)

SCARs are rare ICI-related cirAEs, but are important because they may be life-threatening. The onset time is ranging from the first to the 20th week of immunotherapy. Few cases of SJS/TEN have been observed following the administration of pembrolizumab, nivolumab, and atezolizumab. Mortality rates for SJS, SJS-TEN overlap syndrome, and TEN have been reported at 10%, 30%, and 50%, respectively. Symptoms similar to classical SJS/TEN appear in the forms of fever, malaise, diffuse erythema, flaccid bullae, and epidermal detachment. Furthermore, lesions can spread to mucosal tissues including the oral cavity, conjunctivae, genitalia, gastrointestinal and respiratory tracts. Patients with ICI-induced morbilliform eruption are more susceptible to ICI-induced SJS/TEN. Thereby these patients should be monitored for related signs on their skin, such as blister formation or a positive Nikolsky sign [3, 5, 8]. DRESS is another SCARs presented with fever, facial edema, exanthema, pustular, purpuric, urticarial, or lichen planus (LP)-like skin lesions, morbilliform eruption in the trunk and extremities, hematologic problems, and multi-organ involvement [10]. Administration of high-dose corticosteroids, intravenous immunoglobulin (IVIg), TNF inhibitors, and discontinuation of ICI therapy are required for patient management [5, 8].

6.3 Endocrine irAEs

Endocrine disorders are among the most frequent ICI-induced irAEs, which can affect up to 40% of patients. Various organs regulating the endocrine system are affected, including the thyroid, parathyroid pituitary, adrenal glands, and pancreatic beta cells (Table 6.2). The endocrine dysfunction leads to the development of hypo- and hyperthyroidism, hypophysitis, hypoparathyroidism, insulin-deficient diabetes mellitus, and primary adrenal insufficiency. In addition, in some cases, hypogonadism, hypoparathyroidism, and autoimmune polyglandular syndrome have been reported. Thyroid and pituitary disorders are the most common immune-related endocrine events. Most of these endocrinopathies can be managed with hormone replacement treatment [15, 16].

6.3.1 Thyroid

Thyroid dysfunction varies depending on the type of ICI therapy. The median onset time is 6–10 weeks after the treatment and sometimes it occurs several months later. It is more likely to develop after anti-PD-1. Thyroid irAEs have been reported in about 5% of patients treated with anti-CTLA-4, 10% of anti-PD-1/PD-L1 therapy cases, and 15–20% of anti-PD-1/CTLA-4 combination therapy. In addition, based on recent data, the incidence of thyroiditis or hypothyroidism in patients receiving anti-LAG-3 and anti-PD-1 is estimated to be up to 18%. Acute inflammation and activation of $CD4^+$ T and $CD8^+$ T cells are involved in thyroid damage. In addition, antithyroid peroxidase (TPOAb) and anti-thyroglobulin (TgAb) antibodies have also been detected. Patients with baseline TPOAb and TgAb are more prone to thyroid disorders. Therefore, evaluating the presence of thyroid autoantibodies or their early increase during ICI therapy can be helpful criteria for the prediction of thyroid dysfunction occurrence [16, 17].

6.3.1.1 Hyperthyroidism

Increased production and secretion of thyroid hormones is considered as hyperthyroidism, and thyrotoxicosis is defined as a clinical syndrome of elevated thyroid hormones. In this condition, thyrotropin (TSH) decreases and free thyroxine (FT4) and free triiodothyronine (FT3) increase. ICI-induced thyrotoxicosis can occur in the form of destructive thyroiditis or autoimmune hyperthyroidism (Graves' disease) [18]. The incidence rate of hyperthyroidism for the administration of anti-PD-1 (3.2%) is higher than that of anti-CTLA-4 (1.7%) and anti-PD-L1 (0.6%), and anti-PD-1/anti-CTLA-4 combination therapy reaches 8% [19]. The median time of onset for hyperthyroidism is between 6 and 7 weeks. The thyrotoxic phase is usually transient and asymptomatic. The symptoms include weight loss, anxiety,

Table 6.2 Endocrine irAEs induced by ICI immunotherapy

Type of irAE	Symptoms	Onset time	Frequency	Treatment	References
Hyperthyroidism	Anxiety, tremors, fatigue, weakness, tachycardia, palpitation, disturbed sleep, increased perspiration, poor concentration, dyspnea	6–7 weeks	3.2% for anti-PD-1 1.7% for anti-CTLA-4 0.6% for anti-PD-L1 8% for anti-PD-1/CTLA-4	Monitoring of thyroid function, beta-blockers for alleviation of symptoms	[19, 28, 29]
Hypothyroidism	Fatigue, weight gain bradycardia, mood impairment, cold intolerance, impaired memory, dry skin, visual disturbances, constipation	6–12 weeks	3.9–8.5% for anti-PD-1/PD-L1 2.5–5.2% for anti-CTLA-4 10.2–16.4% for anti-PD-1/CTLA-4	Monitoring of TSH, levothyroxine	[19, 20, 29, 30]
Hypophysitis	Fatigue, nausea, headache, dizziness, visual disturbances, loss of appetite, insomnia, labile mood, vision disturbances, nausea	9–28 weeks	5% for anti-CTLA-4 1% for anti-PD-1/PD-L1 Up to 10% for anti-PD-1/CTLA-4	Methylprednisolone, hydrocortisone	[23, 29, 31]
Type 1 diabetes mellitus	Elevated blood glucose, polydipsia, polyuria, weight loss, dry mouth, dizziness	3–103 weeks (with median onset time of 25 weeks)	0.2–1.4% for ICI monotherapy 1.5% for anti-PD-1/CTLA-4	Insulin therapy, endocrine follow-up	[26, 29, 32]

palpitations, and tremors. Thyrotoxicosis is usually mild and may not be diagnosed [16, 18].

6.3.1.2 Hypothyroidism

Another form of thyroid abnormality is hypothyroidism, which is characterized by increased TSH and reduced FT4 and FT3. Hypothyroidism appears approximately 6–12 weeks after administration of ICIs [18]. The incidence of hypothyroidism during treatment with anti-PD-1/PD-L1 (3.9–8.5%) is higher than anti-CTLA-4 (2.5–5.2%) and combination therapy affects 10.2–16.4% of the patients [19, 20]. In many cases, thyroiditis leads to hypothyroidism. However, sometimes thyroiditis turns to transient thyrotoxicosis in the first weeks of treatment. More than half of the cases of thyrotoxicosis can end in hypothyroidism. Asymptomatic hypothyroidism may be revealed during the evaluation of thyroid hormones, or it can be a typical hypothyroidism with fatigue, depression, constipation, and weight gain symptoms [16].

6.3.1.3 Diagnosis and Treatment

All patients undergoing ICI therapy should be monitored for thyroid function every 4–8 weeks. If the TSH level is more than 10 mIU/mL in two separate evaluations, or if a slight increase in TSH is observed along with a decrease in free T4, the diagnosis is primary hypothyroidism. In subclinical hypothyroidism, the TSH level is less than 10 mIU/mL and the free T4 level is normal. If TSH level is decreased and free T4 and/or T3 are elevated, it should be considered as thyrotoxicosis [16, 17]. The treatment choice for ICI-related hypothyroidism is levothyroxine as hormone replacement. In thyrotoxicosis, the thyrotoxic phase—which is caused by destructive thyroiditis—is temporary and the treatment is mainly supportive, including beta blockers to reduce the symptoms. If Graves' disease is confirmed, antithyroidal agents such as methimazole or surgery are options depending on the patient's condition. According to various studies, high-dose glucocorticoid administration is not effective in thyroid irAEs [16, 21].

6.3.2 Pituitary Gland

6.3.2.1 Hypophysitis

Hypophysitis is the inflammation of the pituitary gland and can be induced by ICIs. The frequency of hypophysitis is different based on the type of ICI. The incidence of ICI-induced hypophysitis in patients treated with CTLA-4 inhibitor and PD-1/PD-L1 is 5% and 1%, respectively, and the incidence is reported up to 10% in combination treatment [22]. Even though some studies indicate a higher incidence rate, Jessel et al. reported that hypophysitis incidence in patients treated with ipilimumab plus nivolumab is 19% [23]. Hypophysitis is more common in combination therapy with anti-LAG-3/PD-1 compared to anti-PD-1 monotherapy. The median onset time of the complication following CTLA-4 inhibitor therapy is 9 weeks; for PD-1/PD-L1 inhibitor, it takes longer and is about 28 weeks, while in combination therapy with CTLA-4 inhibitor and PD-1/PD-L1 inhibitor, it is 4 weeks. Symptoms may be nonspecific, including headache, nausea, hypotension, loss of appetite, fatigue, and pituitary gland enlargement. Severe hypophysitis is associated with low blood pressure, hyponatremia, and coma [22–24]. Depending on the type of hormonal dysfunction, several disorders can appear in the hypophysitis, including central hypothyroidism, secondary adrenal insufficiency, hypogonadotropic hypogonadism, and central diabetes insipidus (CDI). CDI is a rare event and occurs as a result of antidiuretic hormone (ADH) insufficiency [16].

6.3.2.2 Diagnosis and Treatment

Diagnosis of the disease is based on clinical presentation, imaging especially MRI, and laboratory tests including assessment of hypothalamic–pituitary–thyroid axis (TSH, FT3, and FT4), hypothalamic–pituitary–adrenal axis (ACTH and cortisol), and hypothalamic–pituitary–gonad axis (FSH, LH, and T/E2) [22]. A decrease in morning cortisol level <3 mg/dL along with low to inappropriately normal ACTH level indicates secondary adrenal insufficiency. Hypogonadotropic hypogonadism is diagnosed with decreased morning testosterone or estrogen and low or inappropriately normal LH and FSH. Manifestations of polydipsia, polyuria, nocturia, and extreme thirst can be indicative of central diabetes insipidus, which must be differentiated from primary polydipsia and nephrogenic diabetes insipidus [16, 25]. Treatment of adrenal insufficiency is based on glucocorticoid replacement by hydrocortisone and prednisone. In the case of concomitant central hypothyroidism, the patient must first undergo glucocorticoid replacement to resolve the adrenal crisis and then be treated with thyroid hormones. In ICI-associated hypophysitis and thyroid disorders, there is no need to stop ICI administration as long as hormone replacement is undergoing. The treatment choice of men with hypogonadotropic hypogonadism is testosterone replacement. Desmopressin can be prescribed to control severe thirst and polyuria in central diabetes insipidus patients [16, 24].

6.3.3 Diabetes

The incidence of type 1 diabetes mellitus (T1DM) is estimated to be about 0.2–1.4% of patients treated with ICI and mostly (71%) occur during anti-PD-1/L1 therapy. The T1DM incidence rate after combination therapy with CTLA-4 inhibitors and PD-1/PD-L1 inhibitors is higher than monotherapy and is estimated up to 1.5%.

Typically, other irAEs such as pancreatitis and thyroiditis can also occur in ICI-dependent DM cases [21, 26]. Despite the low frequency, ICI-induced T1DM can be life-threatening due to its rapid onset. The disease presents with various symptoms, including asymptomatic hyperglycemia, polyuria, polydipsia, and diabetic ketoacidosis (DKA) [26].

It seems that ICI-induced DM develops because of the autoimmune destruction of insulin-producing pancreatic beta cells. The expression of PD-L1 in these cells is a protective mechanism against the cytotoxic T cells responses. Therefore, blocking this pathway can trigger the activation of T cells and damage to the beta cells. Screening of ICI-induced DM is made by random blood glucose assessment. When the diagnosis is confirmed, other markers such as the c-peptide, hemoglobin A1c, urinary and serum ketones should be checked. In these patients, the blood glucose is highly elevated (marked hyperglycemia) and C peptide is low or undetectable. Hemoglobin A1c (HbA1c) can increase depending on different stages between diagnosis and follow-up. Ketoacidosis has also been observed in many cases. Diabetic ketoacidosis is present in a large percentage of ICI-induced DM patients, which requires immediate follow-up and treatment. According to common terminology criteria for adverse events (CTCAE) grading, this disease is divided into four grades. In regards to the severity of the disease, the treatment includes insulin administration and, if necessary, suspension of ICI therapy should be considered. Unlike other irAEs, glucocorticoids are not recommended in this condition because of their effects on increasing the blood glucose level [21, 26, 27].

6.4 Ocular irAEs

ICI-related ocular toxicities are rare and about 1% of patients experience these complications but they may cause serious damage to the eyes in some cases. Most of ocular irAEs are observed during treatment with ipilimumab, followed by nivolumab and pembrolizumab. The low rate may be related to the immune-privileged status of the eye [33]. Various types of ocular irAEs have been reported, including blepharitis, dry eye, conjunctivitis, uveitis, keratitis, scleritis, and choroidal retinitis, Vogt–Koyanagi–Harada (VKH)-like syndrome, inflammatory orbital disease, optical neuropathy, and Graves' syndrome-like oculopathy. Dry eye and uveitis are the most common reported forms. Ocular adverse events have been reported in several clinical trials with different ICIs [34–36]. Martens et al. reviewed 290 case reports of cancer patients (61.7% melanoma, 19.3% lung cancer, 19% other cancers) treated with ICIs who experienced ocular irAEs and revealed that uveitis was the most common complication. Of note, since dry eye disease is common, it is probably underestimated and is considered to be about 1–24%. Another reason is that dry eye is not a serious complication and can be easily resolved [37]. Alba-Linero et al., by reviewing 35 clinical trials of ICIs (including CTLA-4, PD-1, and PD-L1 inhibitors) applied in different cancers, showed that uveitis, orbital inflammatory disease, and alterations of the ocular surface are the most commonly reported ocular irAEs [38].

Overall, the findings of retrospective studies show that ocular irAEs are not very common in cancer patients treated with ICIs, and among them, dry eye is the most observed condition. Uveitis, conjunctivitis, and keratitis have also been reported in the next ranks of complications. Administration of topical corticosteroids and artificial tears have been the most common treatments to improve the symptoms [36, 39–42].

6.4.1 Dry Eye

Dry eye is usually ignored due to its prevalence in healthy people; however, it can occur during ICI administration. Dry eye affects the ocular surface and tear secretion. Dry eye can be categorized as hyperevaporative (evaporation of the tear film) form or it may be associated with a decrease in tear secretion. It is characterized by dryness of cornea and conjunctiva, redness, pain, photophobia, and blurred vision. Patients may experience meibomian glands and lid inflammation. In some cases, dry eye is caused by a more serious systemic complication such as Sjögren's syndrome. Artificial tears, anti-inflammatory agents, and warm compress are useful in improving the symptoms [34, 43].

6.4.2 Blepharitis and Conjunctivitis

These side effects may occur after ICI therapy, which are manifested by various symptoms including itching, chronic eyelid redness, eye irritation, burning sensation, photophobia, and increased lacrimation and mucoid discharge. To manage the condition, warm compress, antihistamine eye drops, anti-inflammatory ointment, and artificial tears and topical corticosteroids are helpful. With proper care, symptoms usually resolve quickly [34, 43].

6.4.3 Uveitis and Keratitis

Uveitis is one of the common ocular irAEs that can occur with CTLA-4 and PD-1 inhibitors. The uveal tract includes iris, ciliary body, and choroid and inflammation in these parts leads to uveitis. Four types of uveitis can be detected in ICI-treated patients including anterior uveitis (involving the anterior chamber of the eye), intermediate uveitis (inflammation of the vitreous body), posterior uveitis (choroiditis), and panuveitis (inflammation of all uveal components of the eye). A wide range of clinical symptoms are present such as ocular pain, photophobia, tearing, blurred vision, conjunctival congestion, corneal edema, and floaters. Keratitis, which is usually associated with corneal epithelial erosion and corneal ulcer, is characterized by pain, photophobia, tearing, eye redness, and impaired vision. Topical or systemic corticosteroid administration is effective in treating the complications [34, 44].

6.5 Rheumatic irAEs

Rheumatic irAEs include several disorders such as arthritis, polymyalgia rheumatic, myositis, and Sicca syndrome (Table 6.3). Because of challenging diagnosis, long time occurrence after immunotherapy (up to 2 years), and lack of precise epidemiological information, the estimated incidences of rheumatic irAEs are variable and probably are underestimated. The frequency of these complications varies according to the type and dose of ICIs. The incidence in patients receiving anti-CTLA-4 is higher compared to PD-1/PD-L1 antibody. NSAIDs, disease-modifying antirheumatic drugs (DMARDs), and corticosteroids along with ICI immunotherapy withholding are effective in controlling the patient's symptoms [45, 46]. Table 6.3 shows the clinical features of ICI-induced rheumatic irAEs.

Table 6.3 Rheumatic irAEs induced by ICI immunotherapy

Type of irAE	Symptoms	Onset time	Frequency	Treatment	References
Inflammatory arthritis	Arthralgia, joint pain, and swelling.	1.3–12 months	1–7%, anti-CTLA-4 (3–9%), anti-PD-1/PD-L1 (7–11%)	NSAID, analgesics, glucocorticoids, DMARDs	[48, 52]
Myositis	Muscle inflammation, muscle weakness, diplopia	1 month	1%	Glucocorticoid, biological agents, IVIg	[47, 53]
Polymyalgia rheumatica (PMR)	Acute joint pain, morning stiffness of neck, shoulders, and hips	3 months	2%	Glucocorticoids	[47, 51]
Sicca syndrome	Dry mouth and dry eyes	3 months	1.2–24.2%	Saliva substitutes, sialogogues, artificial tears, glucocorticoids	[47, 48, 54]

6.5.1 Arthritis

Arthritis is the most common feature of ICI-induced rheumatoid complications, with an incidence of 1.5–22%. Moreover, an incidence rate of 3–9% for anti-CTLA-4, 7–11% for anti-PD-1/PD-L1, and 11% for combination therapy is reported. Symptoms may appear several months (average time of 1.3–12 months) after the initiation of ICI therapy. Different types of ICI-associated arthritis are similar to rheumatoid arthritis, psoriatic arthritis, or reactive arthritis. The pattern of the arthritis can be different according to the type of ICI. For example, during treatment with anti-PD-1/PD-L1, small joints inflammation is more common, but with anti-CTLA-4 or combination therapy, knee involvement and reactive-arthritis-like symptoms are more likely [47–49]. Mild to moderate arthritis with symptoms of morning stiffness and joint pain can be managed with nonsteroidal anti-inflammatory drugs, analgesics, and glucocorticoids. For persistent symptoms, systemic glucocorticoids are the next choice. In cases of refractory arthritis to glucocorticoids, DMARDs are prescribed [48].

6.5.2 Myositis

ICI-induced myositis affects about 1% of patients. Myositis is not a common complication, but it is a serious irAE. It can occur less than 1 month from the start of immunotherapy. The characteristics of ICI-induced myositis are identical to classical inflammatory myositis including weakness of the proximal limbs; however, it has distinct symptoms, including ptosis and ocular motility disorders. Respiratory muscle involvement has also been reported in this irAE. Usually, myositis-specific/-associated antibodies are undetectable in ICI-induced myositis; instead, anti-striated muscle antibodies such as anti-titin and anti-Kv1.4 antibodies are present. In muscle biopsy, myofiber necrosis and infiltration of $CD4^+$ T cells, $CD8^+$ T cells, and B cells have been observed [48, 50]. In ICI-induced myositis, similar to polymyositis, muscle damage markers including creatine kinase and myoglobin are elevated. Patients are treated with corticosteroids, and in severe cases, intravenous immunoglobulin, plasma exchange, and immunosuppressive agents can be considered [47, 48].

6.5.3 Polymyalgia Rheumatica (PMR)

About 2% of ICI-induced rheumatic cases are accompanied by a PMR-like syndrome. Similar to the classic form of the disease, patients over 50 years of age are more involved, and giant cell arteritis may also be observed in the pathological assessment. Shoulder and pelvic girdle pain are the main symptoms of PMR. The incidence rate of this irAE is higher for treatment with anti-PD-1/PD-L1 antibodies compared to anti-CTLA-4 antibodies. PMR usually responds to glucocorticoids. In addition, DMARDs can be used in certain cases [47, 48, 51].

6.5.4 Sicca Syndrome

ICI-induced Sicca syndrome presents with symptoms like Sjögren's syndrome, with dry eyes and mouth. It usually occurs after 3 months of immunotherapy. Treatment with anti-PD-1/PD-L1 antibodies has a higher risk of developing Sicca syndrome. Most patients lack anti-Ro and anti-La autoantibodies. Management is based on low-dose glucocorticoids along with symptomatic treatment [47, 48].

6.6 Neurologic irAEs

Neurologic irAEs involve both central and peripheral nervous systems, but the central nervous system irAEs are more frequent (Table 6.4). Neurologic irAEs occur in 1–5% of patients treated with anti-CTLA-4, anti-PD-1, or PD-L1 monotherapy. The incidence for combination therapy is about 12%. ICI-induced neurological abnormalities are important because they might be life-threatening; therefore, rapid diagnosis is crucial. These complications are more likely to occur in melanoma and non-small cell lung cancer [55].

6.6.1 Central Nervous System Complications

6.6.1.1 Encephalitis

ICI-induced encephalitis is a relatively rare irAE that has been reported in 0.86% of patients. Altered mental status is a common symptom and seizure has been observed in 30% of the patients. There are two clinical subtypes of encephalitis: diffuse meningoencephalitic type with fever, headache, and altered level of consciousness and focal encephalitic type presents with neuropsychiatric changes, cranial nerve abnormalities, extrapyramidal signs, and brainstem or cerebellum involvement symptoms. MRI findings are normal in half of the cases, but abnormal neuroimaging is more frequent in focal encephalitis patients. About 90% of affected patients have abnormal cerebrospinal fluid (CSF) analysis including lymphocytic pleocytosis and elevated protein [56, 57]. Autoantibodies have been found in about 50% of the patients, which include intracellular onconeural anti-Ma2 and anti-Hu, anti-glutamic acid decarboxylase 65 (GAD65), and anti-N-methyl-D-aspartate (NMDA)

Table 6.4 Neurologic irAEs induced by ICI immunotherapy

Type of irAE	Symptoms	Onset time	Frequency	Treatment	References
Encephalitis	Fever, headache, seizure, altered level of consciousness. Confusion	4–630 days (with median onset time of 65 days)	0.8%	Corticosteroids, intravenous immunoglobulin	[56, 60]
Meningitis	Altered mental status, headache, fever, nausea, vomiting, photophobia	Median of 2 cycles of immunotherapy	0.4%	Corticosteroids	[56, 58]
Radiculopathies and neuropathies	Ataxia, bilateral proximal weakness, areflexia, sensory and autonomic disturbances	26–167 days	1.2%	Corticosteroids, intravenous immunoglobulin	[55, 56, 61]
Myasthenia gravis	Limb weakness, bulbar dysfunction, diplopia, ptosis, dysphonia, dysphagia	2–11 weeks (with median onset time of 6 weeks)	Rare	High-dose steroids, pyridostigmine, intravenous immunoglobulin	[59, 62, 63]

antibodies. This complication is managed with corticosteroids, and in severe cases, intravenous immunoglobulin (IVIg) or plasmapheresis is suggested. The mortality rate is reported up to 20% [55].

6.6.1.2 Meningitis

Meningitis can occur in isolation or along with encephalitis in a very small percentage (0.38%) of patients receiving ICI. However, considering the symptom of headache in patients, there may be additional cases in the form of low-grade aseptic meningitis. The risk of developing meningitis is higher with anti-CTLA-4 therapy. Like classical meningitis, the characteristics of irAEs meningitis include altered mental status, headache, fever, nausea, vomiting, and photophobia. Symptoms appear after a median of 2 cycles of immunotherapy (up to 14 cycles in some cases). In CSF analysis, nonspecific lymphocytic pleocytosis and moderately elevated protein are observed. The prognosis of meningitis is better than encephalitis and can be managed with steroids [55, 56, 58].

6.6.2 Peripheral Nervous System Complications

6.6.2.1 Radiculopathies and Neuropathies

A study of 920 patients receiving ICI has revealed that the frequency of peripheral neuropathy is about 1.2%. This neuropathy can occur in different phenotypes. The most common form is acute polyradiculoneuropathy. The symptoms include ataxia, bilateral proximal weakness, areflexia, and sensory and autonomic disturbances. Increased protein levels and the presence of leukocytes are among the CSF findings. Neural autoantibodies are usually not present. Corticosteroids are effective in the treatment of symptoms, and in severe cases, IVIg is recommended [55, 56].

6.6.2.2 Myasthenia Gravis

ICI-induced myasthenia gravis (MG) usually occurs without a previous history of MG. The median onset time was about 6 weeks after starting immunotherapy in one study. Clinical symptoms include fluctuating weakness induced by exercise, bulbar dysfunction, and vision problems. More than half of the patients have bulbar or respiratory muscle weakness. Myasthenia gravis occurs more often in patients treated with anti-CTLA-4. Anti-acetylcholine receptor antibodies are found in about 60% of the patients. This disease is managed with high-dose steroids and pyridostigmine, which are effective in the majority of patients. For severe disease, IVIg and plasma exchange are useful. The mortality rate due to respiratory failure is high (up to 30%) and ICIs withdrawal should be considered. Concomitant occurrence of MG with myositis or myocarditis increases the mortality rate [55, 56, 59].

6.7 Gastrointestinal irAEs

ICI-induced enterocolitis is the most common irAE of the gastrointestinal tract that can affect 40% of patients. Clinical manifestations include diarrhea, abdominal pain, vomiting, pyrexia, blood or mucus in stool. Bowel perforation is one of the severe consequences that can be life-threatening. The prominent feature of ICI colitis is diarrhea. The onset time of diarrhea and colitis is around the 6th–8th weeks of ICI administration. Approximately 8–22% of patients receiving anti-CTLA-4 develop colitis, and for diarrhea, it is about 30–40%. GI-irAEs are less frequent following PD-1/PD-L1 inhibitor therapy (about 1%). Other disorders of the GI tract are rare, including esophagitis, gastritis, duodenitis, and ileitis [64–66]. The presence of $CD4^+$ and $CD8^+$ T cells in the intestine plays an important role in the pathology of ICI-induced colitis. The increase of inflammatory cytokines such as TNF-α, IFN-γ, IL-17, and IL-6 has been proven in this disease. Acute or chronic inflammation and increased intraepithelial lymphocytes are among the histopathological features of this type of colitis [67]. The diagnosis is made by biochemical and endoscopic evaluations and examination of stool microscopy with culture to rule out infectious colitis. Treatment is based on the severity of the symptoms. Patients with grade 1 diarrhea/colitis should receive supportive care including hydration and a low-fiber diet. Management of higher grades colitis consists of systemic corticosteroid administration, fluid replacement, electrolyte balance, and discontinuation of ICI therapy [65, 67, 68].

6.8 Pulmonary irAEs

ICI-induced pneumonitis or checkpoint inhibitor pneumonitis (CIP) is a serious irAE, especially in non-small cell lung cancer (NSCLC) patients. NSCLC is the most prevalent lung malignancy in recent years. ICI therapy has increased the survival rate of these patients. Because of the destruction of lung tissue, CIP is more likely to occur in NSCLC. According to epidemiological studies, CIP affects 7–19% of NSCLC patients [69]. However, the frequency of CIP in NSCLC patients has been reported to be 3–6.3% in different clinical trials. The incidence of CIP is higher in patients receiving ICI combination therapy and can be fatal in severe cases [70]. CIP is defined with dyspnea, cough, fever, hypoxia, and pulmonary infiltrates on chest imaging. Chest computed tomography (CT), bronchoalveolar lavage (BAL), or lung biopsy and blood tests are helpful in diagnosis. CIP should be differentiated from infection or chemotherapy/radiotherapy-induced pneumonitis. Steroids are recommended for these patients and according to the CTCAE guideline, for grade 3, stopping immunotherapy should be considered. Smokers, patients of $\geq$65 years old, and those with previous lung disease are more likely to develop CIP [69–71].

Various immunological factors are involved in CIP, including the increase of $CD8^+$ T cells and Th1 and Th17 cells in the lung environment. In a systematic study, expansion of T cell clones into IFN-γ^+ IL-17^- $CD8^+$ T cells and $CXCR3^+$ $CCR6^+$ Th17/Th1 cells and their correlation with the development of CIP was found [72]. Decreased expression of CTLA-4 and PD-1 in BAL fluid Tregs during ICI therapy can reduce the suppressive function of these cells and facilitate the development of CIP. Furthermore, elevated inflammatory factors such as IL-6, IL-17, IL-35, and CRP and their effects in the development of CIP have been shown in several studies. In CIP, like some other irAEs, the possibility of antigenic cross-reaction is assumed. Destruction of tumor cells caused by ICI therapy can lead to epitope spreading and damage to lung tissue [69].

Immunological markers are useful in CIP prediction and diagnosis. The presence of anti-CD74 autoantibodies is a potential predictive biomarker. Other criteria that are relevant to the disease severity and prognosis include increasing neutrophil-to-lymphocyte ratio (NLR), platelet-to-lymphocyte ratio (PLR), and decrease in eosinophils. It should be noted that the percentage of eosinophils to the percentage of eosinophils at the early stages is very helpful in differentiating CIP from infection or tumor-associated pneumonitis [69, 73].

6.9 Cardiovascular irAEs

A range of cardiovascular toxicity has been reported following ICI therapy, including myocarditis, pericardial disorders, acute coronary syndromes, congestive heart failure, arrhythmias, atrioventricular block, Takotsubo-like syndrome, vasculitis, and venous thromboembolism [74]. Due to the challenging diagnosis, the incidence of cardiovascular toxicity is not exactly known; however, it is more likely to occur with combination therapy. A meta-analysis of cardiovascular irAEs in patients treated with anti-CTLA-4 and anti-PD-1/PD-L1 has reported an incidence rate of 3.1% for monotherapy and 5.8% for combination therapy [75]. Furthermore, it is assumed that 4.2% of patients undergoing ICI therapy are affected by cardiovascular complications [76]. Cardiovascular irAEs can be associated with nonspecific symptoms of fatigue, weakness, muscle pain, and more specific symptoms such as palpitations, shortness of breath, chest pain, pulmonary or lower extremity edema, and irregular heartbeat [74]. Cardiovascular irAEs are suspected in patients with cardiovascular symptoms, abnormal electrocardiogram, and increased troponin. Since immune checkpoints are important regulatory elements in maintaining cardiac cell self-tolerance, ICIs can change this condition in favor of inflammation [77].

6.9.1 ICI-Associated Myocarditis

Myocarditis is the most prevalent cardiovascular irAEs with a frequency of 0.5–1.7%. ICI-induced myocarditis is associated with a poor prognosis and a significant mortality rate. Combination therapy, mainly with nivolumab and ipilimumab, increases the risk of myocarditis. In addition, combination therapy causes more severe myocarditis compared to monotherapy. The median onset time of myocarditis is 1–2 months after initiation of ICI therapy. Myocardial infiltration of $CD4^+$ T cells, $CD8^+$ T cells, and macrophages and cardiomyocytes necrosis are pathological findings of ICI-related myocarditis [74]. Furthermore, elevated levels of cytokines including IL-2, IFN-γ, TNF-α, IL-1, and IL-6 have been detected in myocarditis, which are involved in inflammation and tissue damage [78]. Clinical symptoms include chest pain, shortness of breath, and fatigue or more serious consequences such as hemodynamic instability, sever arrhythmias, multi-organ failure, and sudden death. The mortality rate of ICI-associated myocarditis is estimated at 26% [79, 80]. Diagnosis of myocarditis is performed using assessment of cardiac biomarkers, electrocardiogram, and cardiovascular imaging. Patient management is based on glucocorticoid administration and rapid discontinuation of ICI therapy. In case of steroid resistance, second-line immunosuppressive agents including mycophenolate mofetil, anti-CD3 antibody, anti-CD52 antibody, and CTLA-4 agonist can be considered [79]. Pericardial disease related to ICI is a rare complication that can occur separately or together with myocarditis. It can lead to pericardial effusion and cardiac tamponade. Symptoms of the disease include chest pain, difficulty breathing, and respiratory failure [78].

6.10 Liver irAEs

The incidence of ICI-induced liver damage or immune-mediated liver injury caused by checkpoint inhibitors (ILICI) is estimated between 2% and 25% (based on the type and dose of treatment). The highest rate is related to combination therapy. The onset time ranges between 1 and 3 months from the start of immunotherapy. Liver damage is mostly mild. About 20% of affected patients may progress to grade 3 and 4. Only a few cases of death have been reported. The pathological pattern of damage is more hepatocellular rather than cholestatic/mixed. Hepatic imaging and pathological evaluation are helpful in diagnosing. In liver imaging, nonspecific symptoms such as hepatomegaly, periportal edema, and lymphadenopathy may be seen. Usually, autoantibodies are not present. Histological evidence include hepatitis with a panlobular distribution, presence of hepatocellular necrosis, and lymphocyte infiltration, especially $CD8^+$ T cells and plasma cells [81, 82]. Cholangitis is another form that has been reported in patients treated with anti-PD-1/PD-L1 and can occur as bile duct thickening or diffuse intrahepatic and extrahepatic biliary strictures. An increase in the levels of liver enzymes including aspartate transaminase (AST) and alanine transaminase (ALT) is a common and nonspecific finding in ILICI, which also increases in other conditions such as cancer progression, biliary disease, infections such as hepatitis viruses, and the use of certain drugs. Although ICI hepatotoxicity and autoimmune hepatitis (AIH) have similarities and are caused by immune response, they differ in some characteristics. AIH autoantibodies have not been found in ILICI. No increase in IgG levels has been observed in ILICI. AIH responds better to steroid therapy compared to ILICI. Treatment of the patient includes the administration of corticosteroids. For higher grades, increasing the corticosteroid dose and in cases of corticosteroid resistance, the use of other immunosuppressants such as mycophenolate mofetil is recommended [83].

6.11 Renal irAEs

Acute kidney injury (AKI) is another type of adverse event related to cancer ICI therapy. The characteristics of AKI are acute tubular necrosis, acute tubulointerstitial nephritis, and glomerular lesions [84]. Based on different meta-analyses, the incidence rate of AKI in patients undergoing ICI therapy varies from less than 1% to 5%. ICI-associated AKI usually manifests 3–4 months after initiation of treatment. The most common type of ICI-related renal toxicity is acute tubulointerstitial nephritis (ATIN). The clinical findings are elevated serum creatinine levels, mild proteinuria, and occasionally pyuria and microhematuria. Other renal irAEs are less common including pauci-immune vasculitis, C3 glomerulonephritis, thrombotic microangiopathy, and immune complex glomerulonephritis [84–86]. According to the American Society of Clinical Oncology (ASCO) guideline, serum creatinine monitoring is required before each dose of ICI. Management of AKI includes discontinuation of ICI, corticosteroid administration, and withholding other ATIN-related medications such as proton pump inhibitors (PPIs) and nonsteroidal anti-inflammatory drugs (NSAIDs). ICI-AKI usually responds well to corticosteroids [87].

6.12 Hematologic irAEs

There are different data about the frequency of ICI-associated hematological toxicities. A study of 5923 patients from 19 clinical trials focusing on ICI therapy revealed an incidence rate of 3.6% for hematological irAEs, 1% immune thrombocytopenia [ITP], 0.6% aplastic anemia or pancytopenia, 0.6% neutropenia, 0.6% hemolytic anemia, 0.4% hemophagocytic lymphohistiocytosis (HLH), and 0.3% bicytopenia or pure red cell aplasia. Hematological irAEs induced by ICI are usually serious complications. The mortality rate is approximately 14% and the incidence of high-grade irAEs is estimated at 0.7%. Hematological irAEs in patients undergoing ICI therapy can occur in any time of the treatment; however, they are more common in the first 10 weeks of the immunotherapy [88]. Since hematological irAEs are rare in different types, their mechanisms and clinical manifestations are not very clear. Among the factors involved in the pathological mechanism, autoantibodies (thrombocytopenia and neutropenia), $CD8^+$ T cells (bone marrow failure), and cytokines (HLH and thromboses) can be mentioned [89].

6.13 Conclusion

The emergence of ICIs has revolutionized cancer treatment and offered new hope for patients with various malignancies. However, as this chapter has extensively detailed, the use of the immune system against tumors comes with a significant risk of irAEs affecting multiple organ systems. The wide spectrum of irAEs, ranging from mild and manageable to severe and potentially life-threatening, highlights the need for vigilant monitoring and prompt intervention in patients undergoing ICI therapy. The variability in onset timing, clinical presentation, and severity of irAEs adds complexity to their management, requiring a multidisciplinary approach involving oncologists, organ specialists, and immunologists. While some irAEs, such as skin reactions and endocrinopathies, are relatively common and well-characterized, others, such as neurological and cardiac complications, are rarer but can have profound impacts on patient outcomes. The underlying mechanisms of irAEs, often involving the activation of autoreactive T cells or the production of autoantibodies, highlight the delicate balance between enhancing antitumor immunity and maintaining self-tolerance. The management of irAEs typically involves immunosuppression, primarily with corticosteroids, which presents a challenge in balancing the control of adverse events with maintaining the antitumor efficacy of ICI therapy. The development of more targeted approaches to manage irAEs without compromising cancer treatment remains an important area of ongoing research.

As the use of ICIs expands to more cancer types and combination therapies become more common, understanding and managing irAEs will become increasingly important. Future directions in this field may include the development of more precise biomarkers to predict irAE risk, personalized monitoring strategies, and novel therapeutic approaches to prevent or mitigate these adverse events while preserving the benefits of cancer immunotherapy. In conclusion, while irAEs present significant challenges in the use of ICIs, their effective management is key to maximizing the potential of these groundbreaking therapies in cancer treatment. Continued research and clinical experience will be essential in refining approaches to irAE prevention, early detection, and management, ultimately improving patient outcomes in the era of cancer immunotherapy.

Acknowledgments The authors gratefully acknowledge the valuable assistance provided by Maryam Sadr.

References

1. Poto R, Troiani T, Criscuolo G, Marone G, Ciardiello F, Tocchetti CG, et al. Holistic approach to immune checkpoint inhibitor-related adverse events. Front Immunol. 2022;13:804597.
2. Johnson DB, Nebhan CA, Moslehi JJ, Balko JM. Immune-checkpoint inhibitors: long-term implications of toxicity. Nat Rev Clin Oncol. 2022;19(4):254–67.
3. Teng YS, Yu S. Molecular mechanisms of cutaneous immune-related adverse events (irAEs) induced by immune checkpoint inhibitors. Curr Oncol. 2023;30(7):6805–19.
4. Cao T, Zhou X, Wu X, Zou Y. Cutaneous immune-related adverse events to immune checkpoint inhibitors: from underlying immunological mechanisms to multi-omics prediction. Front Immunol. 2023;14:1207544.
5. Watanabe T, Yamaguchi Y. Cutaneous manifestations associated with immune checkpoint inhibitors. Front Immunol. 2023;14:1071983.
6. Geisler AN, Phillips GS, Barrios DM, Wu J, Leung DYM, Moy AP, et al. Immune checkpoint inhibitor-related dermatologic adverse events. J Am Acad Dermatol. 2020;83(5):1255–68.
7. Nikolaou V, Tsimpidakis A, Stratigos A. Cutaneous adverse reactions of immunotherapy in patients with advanced melanoma. Cancer. 2023;15(7)
8. Muhaj F, Karri PV, Moody W, Brown A, Patel AB. Mucocutaneous adverse events to immune checkpoint inhibitors. Front Allergy. 2023;4:1147513.
9. Coelho JQ, Romão R, Sousa MJ, Azevedo SX, Fidalgo P, Araújo A. Vitiligo-like lesions as a predictor of response to immunotherapy in non-small cell lung cancer: comprehensive review and case series from a university center. Curr Oncol. 2024;31(2):1113–28.
10. Wei BM, Fox LP, Kaffenberger BH, Korman AM, Micheletti RG, Mostaghimi A, et al. Drug-induced hypersensitivity syndrome/drug reaction with eosinophilia and systemic symptoms. Part I. Epidemiology, pathogenesis, clinicopathological features, and prognosis. J Am Acad Dermatol. 2024;90(5):885–908.

11. Apalla Z, Rapoport B, Sibaud V. Dermatologic immune-related adverse events: the toxicity spectrum and recommendations for management. Int J Womens Dermatol. 2021;7(5, Part A):625–35.
12. Cutroneo P, Ingrasciotta Y, Isgrò V, Rullo EV, Berretta M, Fiorica F, et al. Psoriasis and psoriasiform reactions secondary to immune checkpoint inhibitors. Dermatol Ther. 2021;34(2):e14830.
13. Niebel D, Wilsmann-Theis D, Bieber T, Berneburg M, Wenzel J, Braegelmann C. Bullous pemphigoid in patients receiving immune-checkpoint inhibitors and psoriatic patients-focus on clinical and histopathological variation. Dermatopathology. 2022;9(1):60–81.
14. Satoh TK, Neulinger MM, Stadler P-C, Aoki R, French LE. Immune checkpoint inhibitor-induced epidermal necrolysis: a narrative review evaluating demographics, clinical features, and culprit medications. J Dermatol. 2024;51(1):3–11.
15. Wright JJ, Powers AC, Johnson DB. Endocrine toxicities of immune checkpoint inhibitors. Nat Rev Endocrinol. 2021;17(7):389–99.
16. Cardona Z, Sosman JA, Chandra S, Huang W. Endocrine side effects of immune checkpoint inhibitors. Front Endocrinol. 2023;14
17. Karaviti D, Kani E-R, Karaviti E, Gerontiti E, Michalopoulou O, Stefanaki K, et al. Thyroid disorders induced by immune checkpoint inhibitors. Endocrine. 2024;85:67.
18. Profili NI, Castelli R, Gidaro A, Merella A, Manetti R, Palmieri G, et al. Endocrine side effects in patients treated with immune checkpoint inhibitors: a narrative review. J Clin Med. 2023;12(15)
19. Barroso-Sousa R, Barry WT, Garrido-Castro AC, Hodi FS, Min L, Krop IE, et al. Incidence of endocrine dysfunction following the use of different immune checkpoint inhibitor regimens: a systematic review and meta-analysis. JAMA Oncol. 2018;4(2):173–82.
20. Chera A, Stancu AL, Bucur O. Thyroid-related adverse events induced by immune checkpoint inhibitors. Front Endocrinol. 2022;13
21. Hattersley R, Nana M, Lansdown AJ. Endocrine complications of immunotherapies: a review. Clin Med (Lond). 2021;21(2):e212–e22.
22. Chen P, Li J, Tan H. Progress and challenges of immune checkpoint inhibitor-induced hypophysitis. J Clin Med. 2023;12(10)
23. Jessel S, Weiss SA, Austin M, Mahajan A, Etts K, Zhang L, et al. Immune checkpoint inhibitor-induced hypophysitis and patterns of loss of pituitary function. Front Oncol. 2022;12
24. Castillero F, Castillo-Fernández O, Jiménez-Jiménez G, Fallas-Ramírez J, Peralta-Álvarez MP, Arrieta O. Cancer immunotherapy-associated hypophysitis. Future Oncol. 2019;15(27):3159–69.
25. Di Dalmazi G, Ippolito S, Lupi I, Caturegli P. Hypophysitis induced by immune checkpoint inhibitors: a 10-year assessment. Exp Rev Endocrinol Metab. 2019;14(6):381–98.
26. Liao D, Liu C, Chen S, Liu F, Li W, Shangguan D, et al. Recent advances in immune checkpoint inhibitor-induced type 1 diabetes mellitus. Int Immunopharmacol. 2023;122:110414.
27. Quandt Z, Young A, Anderson M. Immune checkpoint inhibitor diabetes mellitus: a novel form of autoimmune diabetes. Clin Exp Immunol. 2020;200(2):131–40.
28. De Leo S, Lee SY, Braverman LE. Hyperthyroidism. Lancet. 2016;388(10047):906–18.
29. Goyal I, Pandey MR, Sharma R, Chaudhuri A, Dandona P. The side effects of immune checkpoint inhibitor therapy on the endocrine system. Indian J Med Res. 2021;154(4):559–70.
30. Chaker L, Bianco AC, Jonklaas J, Peeters RP. Hypothyroidism. Lancet. 2017;390(10101):1550–62.
31. Faje A. Hypophysitis: evaluation and management. Clin Diabet Endocrinol. 2016;2(1):15.
32. DiMeglio LA, Evans-Molina C, Oram RA. Type 1 diabetes. Lancet. 2018;391(10138):2449–62.
33. Zhou YW, Xu Q, Wang Y, Xia RL, Liu JY, Ma XL. Immune checkpoint inhibitor-associated ophthalmic adverse events: current understanding of its mechanisms, diagnosis, and management. Int J Ophthalmol. 2022;15(4):646–56.
34. Liu X, Wang Z, Zhao C, Wang H, Guo X, Zhou J, et al. Clinical diagnosis and treatment recommendations for ocular toxicities of targeted therapy and immune checkpoint inhibitor therapy. Thorac Cancer. 2020;11(3):810–8.

35. Antoun J, Titah C, Cochereau I. Ocular and orbital side-effects of checkpoint inhibitors: a review article. Curr Opin Oncol. 2016;28(4):288–94.
36. Park RB, Jain S, Han H, Park J. Ocular surface disease associated with immune checkpoint inhibitor therapy. Ocul Surf. 2021;20:115–29.
37. Martens A, Schauwvlieghe PP, Madoe A, Casteels I, Aspeslagh S. Ocular adverse events associated with immune checkpoint inhibitors, a scoping review. J Ophthalmic Inflamm Infect. 2023;13(1):5.
38. Alba-Linero C, Alba E. Ocular side effects of checkpoint inhibitors. Surv Ophthalmol. 2021;66(6):951–9.
39. Voskens CJ, Goldinger SM, Loquai C, Robert C, Kaehler KC, Berking C, et al. The price of tumor control: an analysis of rare side effects of anti-CTLA-4 therapy in metastatic melanoma from the ipilimumab network. PLoS One. 2013;8(1):e53745.
40. Zimmer L, Goldinger SM, Hofmann L, Loquai C, Ugurel S, Thomas I, et al. Neurological, respiratory, musculoskeletal, cardiac and ocular side-effects of anti-PD-1 therapy. Eur J Cancer. 2016;60:210–25.
41. Fortes BH, Liou H, Dalvin LA. Ophthalmic adverse effects of immune checkpoint inhibitors: the Mayo Clinic experience. Br J Ophthalmol. 2021;105(9):1263–71.
42. Voskens C, Cavallaro A, Erdmann M, Dippel O, Kaempgen E, Schuler G, et al. Anti-cytotoxic T-cell lymphocyte antigen-4-induced regression of spinal cord metastases in association with renal failure, atypical pneumonia, vision loss, and hearing loss. J Clin Oncol. 2012;30(33):e356–7.
43. Zhou L, Wei X. Ocular immune-related adverse events associated with immune checkpoint inhibitors in lung cancer. Front Immunol. 2021;12:701951.
44. Zhang H, Houadj L, Wu KY, Tran SD. Diagnosing and managing uveitis associated with immune checkpoint inhibitors: a review. Diagnostics. 2024;14(3)
45. Chatzidionysiou K, Liapi M, Tsakonas G, Gunnarsson I, Catrina A. Treatment of rheumatic immune-related adverse events due to cancer immunotherapy with immune checkpoint inhibitors-is it time for a paradigm shift? Clin Rheumatol. 2021;40(5):1687–95.
46. Cappelli LC, Bingham CO 3rd. Expert perspective: immune checkpoint inhibitors and rheumatologic complications. Arthritis Rheumatol. 2021;73(4):553–65.
47. Pacholczak-Madej R, Kosałka-Węgiel J, Kuszmiersz P, Mituś JW, Püsküllüoğlu M, Grela-Wojewoda A, et al. Immune checkpoint inhibitor related rheumatological complications: cooperation between rheumatologists and oncologists. Int J Environ Res Public Health. 2023;20(6)
48. Dang QM, Watanabe R, Shiomi M, Fukumoto K, Nobashi TW, Okano T, et al. Rheumatic immune-related adverse events due to immune checkpoint inhibitors-a 2023 update. Int J Mol Sci. 2023;24(6)
49. Shen P, Deng X, Hu Z, Chen Z, Huang Y, Wang K, et al. Rheumatic manifestations and diseases from immune checkpoint inhibitors in cancer immunotherapy. Front Med. 2021;8:762247.
50. Zhong H, Zhou J, Xu D, Zeng X. Rheumatic immune-related adverse events induced by immune checkpoint inhibitors. Asia Pac J Clin Oncol. 2021;17(3):178–85.
51. Reid P, Cappelli LC. Treatment of rheumatic adverse events of cancer immunotherapy. Best Pract Res Clin Rheumatol. 2022;36(4):101805.
52. Jeurling S, Cappelli LC. Treatment of immune checkpoint inhibitor-induced inflammatory arthritis. Curr Opin Rheumatol. 2020;32(3):315–20.
53. Solimando AG, Crudele L, Leone P, Argentiero A, Guarascio M, Silvestris N, et al. Immune checkpoint inhibitor-related myositis: from biology to bedside. Int J Mol Sci. 2020;21(9)
54. Warner BM, Baer AN, Lipson EJ, Allen C, Hinrichs C, Rajan A, et al. Sicca syndrome associated with immune checkpoint inhibitor therapy. Oncologist. 2019;24(9):1259–69.
55. Wang N. Neurologic complications of cancer immunotherapy. Continuum. 2023;29(6):1827–43.
56. Alsalem AN, Scarffe LA, Briemberg HR, Aaroe AE, Harrison RA. Neurologic complications of cancer immunotherapy. Curr Oncol. 2023;30(6):5876–97.

57. Zhao Z, Zhang C, Zhou L, Dong P, Shi L. Immune checkpoint inhibitors and neurotoxicity. Curr Neuropharmacol. 2021;19(8):1246–63.
58. Nannini S, Koshenkova L, Baloglu S, Chaussemy D, Noël G, Schott R. Immune-related aseptic meningitis and strategies to manage immune checkpoint inhibitor therapy: a systematic review. J Neuro-Oncol. 2022;157(3):533–50.
59. Hundsberger T, Schreiner B, Roth P. Immune checkpoint inhibitors induced side effects of the peripheral nervous system. Curr Opin Neurol. 2023;36(5):427–31.
60. Stuby J, Herren T, Schwegler Naumburger G, Papet C, Rudiger A. Immune checkpoint inhibitor therapy-associated encephalitis: a case series and review of the literature. Swiss Med Wkly. 2020;150:w20377.
61. Plaçais L, Michot JM, Champiat S, Romano-Martin P, Baldini C, Joao MS, et al. Neurological complications induced by immune checkpoint inhibitors: a comprehensive descriptive case-series unravelling high risk of long-term sequelae. Brain Commun. 2021;3(4):fcab220.
62. Marco C, Simó M, Alemany M, Casasnovas C, Domínguez R, Vilariño N, et al. Myasthenia gravis induced by immune checkpoint inhibitors: an emerging neurotoxicity in neuro-oncology practice: case series. J Clin Med. 2022;12(1)
63. Zubair AS, Roy B, Baehring JM, Nowak RJ. Myasthenia gravis in the setting of immune checkpoint inhibitor therapy: practical considerations and opinion-based approach to acute management. Cureus. 2022;14(10):e30638.
64. Cappello G, Molea F, Campanella D, Galioto F, Russo F, Regge D. Gastrointestinal adverse events of immunotherapy. BJR Open. 2021;3(1):20210027.
65. Nicolaides S, Boussioutas A. Immune-related adverse events of the gastrointestinal system. Cancer. 2023;15(3)
66. Cheng Y, Ling F, Li J, Chen Y, Xu M, Li S, et al. An updated review of gastrointestinal toxicity induced by PD-1 inhibitors: from mechanisms to management. Front Immunol. 2023;14:1190850.
67. Terrin M, Migliorisi G, Dal Buono A, Gabbiadini R, Mastrorocco E, Quadarella A, et al. Checkpoint inhibitor-induced colitis: from pathogenesis to management. Int J Mol Sci. 2023;24(14)
68. Kelly-Goss MR, Badran YR, Dougan M. Update on immune checkpoint inhibitor enterocolitis. Curr Gastroenterol Rep. 2022;24(12):171–81.
69. Guo X, Chen S, Wang X, Liu X. Immune-related pulmonary toxicities of checkpoint inhibitors in non-small cell lung cancer: diagnosis, mechanism, and treatment strategies. Front Immunol. 2023;14:1138483.
70. Hao Y, Zhang X, Yu L. Immune checkpoint inhibitor-related pneumonitis in non-small cell lung cancer: a review. Front Oncol. 2022;12:911906.
71. Chuzi S, Tavora F, Cruz M, Costa R, Chae YK, Carneiro BA, et al. Clinical features, diagnostic challenges, and management strategies in checkpoint inhibitor-related pneumonitis. Cancer Manag Res. 2017;9:207–13.
72. Kim ST, Sheshadri A, Shannon V, Kontoyiannis DP, Kantarjian H, Garcia-Manero G, et al. Distinct immunophenotypes of T cells in bronchoalveolar lavage fluid from leukemia patients with immune checkpoint inhibitors-related pulmonary complications. Front Immunol. 2020;11:590494.
73. Shibata Y, Murakami S, Kato T. Overview of checkpoint inhibitor pneumonitis: incidence and associated risk factors. Expert Opin Drug Saf. 2021;20(5):537–47.
74. Raschi E, Rossi S, De Giglio A, Fusaroli M, Burgazzi F, Rinaldi R, et al. Cardiovascular toxicity of immune checkpoint inhibitors: a guide for clinicians. Drug Saf. 2023;46(9):819–33.
75. Rubio-Infante N, Ramírez-Flores YA, Castillo EC, Lozano O, García-Rivas G, Torre-Amione G. Cardiotoxicity associated with immune checkpoint inhibitor therapy: a meta-analysis. Eur J Heart Fail. 2021;23(10):1739–47.
76. Drobni ZD, Alvi RM, Taron J, Zafar A, Murphy SP, Rambarat PK, et al. Association between immune checkpoint inhibitors with cardiovascular events and atherosclerotic plaque. Circulation. 2020;142(24):2299–311.

77. Thuny F, Naidoo J, Neilan TG. Cardiovascular complications of immune checkpoint inhibitors for cancer. Eur Heart J. 2022;43(42):4458–68.
78. Lessomo FYN, Mandizadza OO, Mukuka C, Wang ZQ. A comprehensive review on immune checkpoint inhibitors induced cardiotoxicity characteristics and associated factors. Eur J Med Res. 2023;28(1):495.
79. Wang D, Bauersachs J, Berliner D. Immune checkpoint inhibitor associated myocarditis and cardiomyopathy: a translational review. Biology. 2023;12(3)
80. Zotova L. Immune checkpoint inhibitors-related myocarditis: a review of reported clinical cases. Diagnostics. 2023;13(7)
81. Bessone F, Björnsson ES. Drug-induced liver injury due to biologics and immune check point inhibitors. Med Clin North Am. 2023;107(3):623–40.
82. Hercun J, Vincent C, Bilodeau M, Lapierre P. Immune-mediated hepatitis during immune checkpoint inhibitor cancer immunotherapy: lessons from autoimmune hepatitis and liver immunology. Front Immunol. 2022;13:907591.
83. Cunningham M, Gupta R, Butler M. Checkpoint inhibitor hepatotoxicity: pathogenesis and management. Hepatology. 2024;79(1):198–212.
84. Tonooka A, Ohashi R. Current trends in anti-cancer molecular targeted therapies: renal complications and their histological features. J Nippon Med Sch. 2022;89(2):128–38.
85. Catalano M, Roviello G, Galli IC, Santi R, Nesi G. Immune checkpoint inhibitor induced nephrotoxicity: an ongoing challenge. Front Med. 2022;9:1014257.
86. Mamlouk O, Danesh FR. Immune checkpoint inhibitor-associated nephrotoxicity. Nephron. 2023;148(1):11–5.
87. Rao Ullur A, Côté G, Pelletier K, Kitchlu A. Immunotherapy in oncology and the kidneys: a clinical review of the evaluation and management of kidney immune-related adverse events. Clin Kidney J. 2023;16(6):939–51.
88. Michot JM, Lazarovici J, Tieu A, Champiat S, Voisin AL, Ebbo M, et al. Haematological immune-related adverse events with immune checkpoint inhibitors, how to manage? Eur J Cancer. 2019;122:72–90.
89. Kroll MH, Rojas-Hernandez C, Yee C. Hematologic complications of immune checkpoint inhibitors. Blood. 2022;139(25):3594–604.
90. Servier Medical Art. https://smart.servier.com. Licensed under Creative Commons Attribution 4.0 (https://creativecommons.org/licenses/by/4.0/).

Chapter 7
Immune Checkpoint Dysregulation in Autoimmune Diseases: Mechanisms and Clinical Implications

7.1 Introduction

Autoimmune diseases have been increasing in recent decades, and the prevalence is estimated to be 3–5%. Multiple genetic and environmental factors are involved in susceptibility to autoimmune diseases. Some of the autoimmune disorders are monogenic. A clear example is autoimmune polyendocrinopathy syndrome type 1 (APS1), which is caused by a mutation in the autoimmune regulator (AIRE) gene. In this disease, the negative selection of T cells in the thymus is disrupted; as a result, self-reactive T cells enter the peripheral tissues. However, most autoimmune diseases are polygenic. HLAs, immune checkpoints (ICs), cytokines, and cytokine receptors (such as TGF-β, TNF, IL-2, IL-12, IL-7Ra, and IL-2RA) and several signaling molecules (e.g., STAT3, PTPN22, STAT4, SOCS1) are among the important genes involved in autoimmune diseases [1]. Central and peripheral tolerances are critical in preventing the development of inflammatory and autoimmune diseases. By the central tolerance, autoreactive lymphocytes are deleted. In the thymus, negative selection, T cells that recognize self-peptides with high affinity are eliminated. However, some autoreactive lymphocytes may be present in the peripheral tissues. Peripheral tolerance includes precise regulatory mechanisms that modulate the function of the immune system. It maintains immune homeostasis and limits the activation of autoreactive T cells. Regulatory cells, such as Treg, Breg, tolerogenic DC, as well as ICs, on the immune cell surface are important components of peripheral tolerance. Regulation of T cell activation is coordinated by co-activation and co-inhibitory receptors. Inhibitory receptors prevent overactivation of immune cells [2]. The role of immune checkpoints in peripheral tolerance is well established. IC-deficient animal models have highlighted the role of these molecules in the maintenance of immune tolerance. CTLA-4 knockout mice suffer from severe lymphoproliferative disease. Genetic ablation of PD-1 in mice causes lupus-like symptoms, while mice deficient for PD-1/LAG-3 develops multiple organ autoimmunity.

L. Tayebi, M. Abdolmaleki, *Immune System Regulation*,
https://doi.org/10.1007/978-981-95-8026-2_7

In addition, administration of anti-PD1 or anti-LAG-3 to nonobese diabetic (NOD) mice accelerates the development of autoimmune diabetes, and deletion of PD-1, TIM-3, and TIGIT genes in experimental autoimmune encephalomyelitis (EAE) worsens the disease in mice. As described in Chap. 6, cancer patients treated with immune checkpoint inhibitors, such as anti-CTLA-4, anti-PD-1, or anti-PD-L1, are predisposed to autoimmune diseases. Genome-wide association studies (GWAS) have revealed the association of several single-nucleotide polymorphisms (SNPs) within IC genes with autoimmune diseases. CTLA-4 has been widely studied in many autoimmune disorders, including Graves' disease, systemic lupus erythematosus (SLE), and type 1 diabetes (T1D). PD-1 is another immune checkpoint that is strongly implicated in autoimmunity [3]. In this chapter, the relationship of important immune checkpoints, mainly CTLA-4, PD-1, and TIM-3, with various autoimmune diseases, such as rheumatoid diseases, autoimmune thyroid disease, MS, and T1D, is discussed.

7.2 Rheumatic Diseases

7.2.1 Rheumatoid Arthritis

Rheumatoid arthritis (RA) is a chronic inflammatory autoimmune disease characterized by joint destruction and deformity. In systemic RA, other tissues may also be damaged, including the lung, kidneys, skin, nervous system, digestive system, heart, and eye. The prevalence of RA worldwide is about 0.5–2% and is more common in women. The presence of rheumatoid factor (RF) autoantibodies and anti-citrullinated protein antibodies (ACPAs) is the main immunological marker of the disease, which is found in 50–80% of cases. In ACPA-positive patients, the most important genetic factors related to RA risk are HLA-DR alleles, tyrosine phosphatase non-receptor type 22 (PTPN22) alleles, and TNF-receptor associated factor 1/complement component 5 (TRAF1/C5) related genes. Synovial macrophages are involved in joint inflammation by producing TNF-α, IL-1, and IL-6. The increase of these cytokines is associated with the stimulation of osteoclast and fibroblast-like synoviocytes (FLS) activity. FLS cells are the main source of matrix metalloproteinases (MMPs), prostaglandins, and leukotrienes in the synovium. This inflammatory process leads to cartilage degradation and bone erosion. Th1 and Th17 cells play an important role in the development of RA. IL-17 and IL-22 produced from T cells are involved in joint tissue destruction. The most common treatments for RA patients are nonsteroidal anti-inflammatory drugs (NSAIDs), glucocorticoids, and disease-modifying antirheumatic drugs (DMARDs). In recent years, several cytokine inhibitors have been developed to alleviate RA disease, such as TNF-α, IL-1, IL-6, IL-17, and RANKL inhibitors [4–6].

The involvement of CTLA-4 in RA has been demonstrated in many studies [7]. A meta-analysis evaluating the relationship between CTLA-4 gene polymorphisms and RA revealed that there is a significant association between the rs3087243 and rs231775 polymorphisms of CTLA-4 with the risk of RA [8]. A study indicated that increased serum level of soluble CTLA-4 was related to the severity of RA. They found that leflunomide (an immunosuppressive agent) downregulates the sCTLA-4 expression [9]. Chagollán et al. showed that the levels of soluble CTLA-4 (sCTL-A) 4 in RA patients were lower than those of healthy controls. In addition, the concentration of sCTLA-4 in early RA patients was lower compared to that of untreated RA patients, which might be related to the treatment of the patients. No membrane CTLA-4 expression was detected on $CD4^+$ and $CD8^+$ T cells in RA patients [10]. In contrast, according to another study, sCTLA-4 level in RA patients was higher than in healthy individuals. Furthermore, plasma sCTLA-4 was significantly higher in *methotrexate responders* than in nonresponders [11]. Decreased expression of CTLA-4 on Treg cells can disrupt their function and is associated with RA severity [12]. Abatacept is a fusion protein consisting of the IgG1 Fc region fused to the extracellular domain of CTLA-4. It can inhibit T cell activation by blocking CD28-CD80/CD86 interaction. Abatacept is effective in reducing the severity of RA. Abatacept administration is associated with lower inflammation and improved clinical symptoms, and it can reduce the risk of RA development in high-risk individuals [13, 14].

Some PD-1 gene polymorphisms are related to RA susceptibility. For example, the rs11568821 polymorphism is associated with an increased risk of RA [15]. Elevated concentration of sPD-1 in serum and synovial fluid of RA patients has been reported in several studies. sPD-1 is increased in early RA and chronic RA compared to healthy subjects. The increase in sPD-1 level is related to positivity for IgM-RF and anti-CCP, IL-21 production, and more disease activity. It is assumed that sPD-1 can block the inhibitory effect of membrane PD-1 in suppressor T cells [16, 17]. The expression of PD-1 on T cells in RA patients and its correlation of PD-1 with disease progression have been reported in different studies. It has been shown that the percentages of $PD\text{-}1^+$ $CD4^+$ and $PD\text{-}1^+$ $CD8^+$ T cells in RA patients are higher than in healthy controls. Overexpression of PD-1 is associated with increased *erythrocyte sedimentation rate* (ESR), C-reactive protein (CRP), and more severe disease [18, 19]. On the contrary, the expression pattern of PD-1 and PD-L1 in the synovium of 51 RA patients showed that PD-1 was upregulated on the infiltrating lymphocytes in more than half of the patients. In addition, PD-L1 was detected in synovial lining cells in about 70% of patients, and its expression level was directly related to disease activity, RF-positive state, and the number of infiltrating T cells [20]. T follicular helper cells (*Tfh*) are localized in the B cell follicle of the lymph node and play a pivotal role in regulating the B cell response. Increased frequency of Tfh cells can lead to the uncontrolled expansion of B cells and the production of autoantibodies. The number of $CD4^+$ $PD\text{-}1^+$ $CXCR5^+$ Tfh increases in the peripheral blood of RA patients. There is a strong correlation between increased Tfh and anti-CCP in RA. These cells are involved in the activation of B cells producing autoreactive antibodies, such as RF and ACPAs, in RA [21, 22]. In addition, the assessment of cell populations in RA has shown that, besides the Tfh, the percentage of $PD1^+ICOS^+$ effector memory T *cells* (*Tem*) and $PD1^+$ $ICOS^+$ central memory T cells (Tcm) was increased. The frequency of these cells was positively related to the disease activity score 28 (DAS28). Moreover, the levels of IL-1β, IL-6, and MCP-1 in these patients were higher than healthy controls [23]. Zhao et al. showed that the population of PD-1^{hi} FoxP3$^-$ CXCR5$^-$ CXCR3$^+$ CD4$^+$ T cells was increased in RA. This cell subset was related to higher DAS28 and disease severity. Interestingly, the percentage of these cells decreased significantly after treatment [24].

Increased expression of TIM-3 on CD4$^+$ and CD8$^+$ T cells in peripheral blood and synovial fluid of RA patients is negatively correlated with disease activity. TIM-3 expression in the synovial tissue of RA patients has a significant increase compared to healthy individuals. TIM-3 and galectin-9 (*TIM-3 ligand*) upregulation on peripheral blood mononuclear cells (PBMCs) of patients is negatively associated with DAS28. Gal-9 mRNA expression of PBMCs is increased in patients with lower disease activity. This increased expression is positively related to FoxP3 mRNA expression in Tregs [25–27]. A study showed that sTIM-3 in the serum of RA patients was significantly increased compared to healthy controls. Elevated sTIM-3 was associated with inflammatory markers, such as ESR, ACPA titers, and *matrix metalloproteinase-3* (*MMP-3*). The increased level of sTIM-3 in the serum of RA patients was associated with severe joint damage. Therefore, sTIM-3 can be considered a marker of disease activity [28].

The association of −574T>G and 4259G>T polymorphism of the TIM-3 with RA susceptibility has been reported in several studies [29, 30].

7.2.2 Systemic Lupus Erythematosus

SLE is a severe multi-organ autoimmune disease. Its prevalence varies according to geographical area and genetic or environmental factors, but it has been increasing in recent decades. The prevalence of SLE in the United States is about 73 per 100,000 people. Fever, fatigue, brain fog, inflammatory arthropathy, and mucocutaneous lesions are common symptoms in patients. Butterfly rash, oral ulcers, synovitis, non-scarring alopecia, leukopenia, thrombocytopenia, and renal and neurological dysfunctions are other complications that are observed in SLE patients. SLE occurs because of loss of self-tolerance and dysregulation of the adaptive and innate immune response, activation of autoreactive T and B cells, and production of autoantibodies. Important immunological markers in this disease include elevated antinuclear, phospholipid, dsDNA, β2 glycoprotein I, and cardiolipin antibodies and low levels of C3 and C4 complement. Glucocorticoids and immunosuppressants, such as immunosuppressants and azathioprine, are effective in ameliorating the symptoms [31, 32].

A significant association between −1722TC and +49AG polymorphisms of the CTLA-4 gene with susceptibility to SLE has been proven [33–37]. Plasma sCTLA-4 is elevated in SLE. According to a study, CTLA4 expression in PBMCs of SLE patients was significantly increased compared to healthy controls [38]. Increased sCTLA-4 correlates with a higher SLE disease activity index (SLEDAI) [39].

Increased level of sCTLA-4 in SLE patients is associated with serum levels of IFN-α [40]. Jury et al. showed that CTLA-4 was increased on T cells of SLE patients, but no correlation was found between the expression of CTLA-4 and lupus disease activity status. Notably, CTLA-4 expression was limited to $FoxP3^-$ T cells and was not observed in $FoxP3^+$ $CD4^+$ T cells [41].

PD-1/PD-L1 axis is involved in the pathogenesis of SLE by affecting innate and adaptive immune responses [31]. PD1.5 polymorphism is associated with SLE risk, and PD1.3 polymorphism relates to susceptibility to lupus nephritis [31]. The percentage of $PD\text{-}1^+$ $CD4^+$ T cells is increased in SLE patients, and PD-1 upregulation is associated with higher INF-γ production [42].

The $CD19^+$ $PD\text{-}L1^+$ B cell population also increases in SLE, which is related to more disease activity [43]. Increased levels of sPD-1 and sPD-L1 have also been demonstrated in SLE patients. Elevated sPD-1 and sPD-L1 levels have been associated with the severity and activity (SLEDAI >8) of the disease. It seems that sPD-1 and sPD-L1 play a role in the activation of T lymphocytes by blocking the membrane-bound PD-1/PD-L1 signaling pathway [44]. Dysfunction of NK cells has been observed in SLE. The frequency of peripheral blood $TIM\text{-}3^+$ NK, $PD\text{-}1^+$ NK, and $TIM\text{-}3^+$ $PD\text{-}1^+$ NK cell subsets rises in SLE patients. Higher $TIM\text{-}3^+$ $PD\text{-}1^+$ NK cells are correlated with the presence of anti-dsDNA autoantibodies, increased inflammatory markers, such as CRP, as well as a higher disease activity and severity [45]. PD-L1-expressing neutrophils are also an important cell population in SLE. The increase of these cells has been observed in anti-nRNP/Sm-positive patients, patients with high antinuclear antibody (ANA) titer, and patients with high SLEDAI score. It has been reported that the number of $PD\text{-}L1^+$ neutrophils decreases after treatment. Presumably, the presence of these cells is a negative feedback mechanism against excessive autoimmune response to prevent tissue destruction [46].

TIM-3 expression is increased in PBMCs of SLE patients. It has been demonstrated that $CD3^+$ $CD4^+$ $TIM\text{-}3^+$ and $CD3^+$ $CD4^+$ $TIM\text{-}3^+$ Fas^+ T cells in the peripheral blood of SLE patients are more frequent than in healthy controls, which are related to the severity of the disease [47]. The presence of $CD14^+$ phagocyte cells expressing TIM-3 in SLE patients is accompanied by decreased peripheral apoptotic cells clearance and elevated levels of dsDNA [48]. Studies have shown that the levels of sTIM-3 are increased in the serum of SLE patients. The sTIM-3 levels are higher in patients with organ damage compared to patients without organ damage. There is a positive correlation between elevated sTIM-3 levels and anti-dsDNA and SLEDAI score. Overall, increased sTIM-3 is associated with disease activity [49, 50].

7.2.3 Ankylosing Spondylitis

Ankylosing spondylitis (AS) is an autoinflammatory disease involving axial bone and sacroiliac joints. Chronic inflammation leads to ankylosis. Clinical manifestations include spinal ankylosis and inflammation in the back, hips, knees, ankles, shoulders, and peripheral joints. Several genes are involved in susceptibility to AS, but the most important gene related to the risk of this disease is HLA-B27. Eighty to ninety-five percent of patients are HLA-B27 positive. In addition, some other HLA genotypes such as HLA-A3/A11 are associated with susceptibility to AS. The IL-23/17 axis plays a pivotal role in the progression of AS. NSAIDs, DMARDs, TNF blockers, and IL17-A antagonists are useful in reducing inflammation and pain [51, 52].

There is limited data regarding the correlation between CTLA-4 and AS disease, but based on the available evidence, CTLA-4 dysregulation can affect AS outcome. For example, it has been reported that increased serum sCTLA-4 is associated with higher BASDAI in spondyloarthritis [53, 54]. Among CTLA-4 gene polymorphisms, +49 A/G is more related to AS susceptibility. This correlation has been reported in European, Iranian, and Taiwanese populations [55–57].

Decreased expression of PD-1 and TIM-3 on lymphocytes of AS patients can be involved in the progression of the disease [58]. Some polymorphisms of these genes have been identified in AS patients. PD 1.9 C/T polymorphism is associated with AS risk in Asian populations [59]. In the case of TIM-3, the -574GT genotype is related to the decreased expression of this immune checkpoint on T cells and monocytes of AS patients [60]. Zhou et al. observed no difference in PD-1 expression levels on T cells from AS patients and healthy controls. They found that the expression of PD-1 on T cells, especially $CD4^+$ $CD25^+$ T cells of AS patients after in vitro stimulation, was significantly lower than that of the control group [61]. Evaluation of PD-1 expression on PBMCs of AS patients has revealed that the percentage of $PD\text{-}1^+$ $CD4^+$ T cells increases in these patients. Interestingly, the presence of this cell population was associated with lower modified Stokes ankylosing spondylitis spinal scores (mSASSS). The negative relationship between PD-1 gene expression and AS disease activity indicates the regulatory role of PD-1 in this disease [62, 63].

7.2.4 Sjogren's Syndrome (SS)

Sjogren's syndrome is another subset of rheumatological diseases and is defined as chronic inflammation of the tear and salivary glands. Sicca symptoms are the most common feature of this disease, which occurs in 98% of cases, and it has several types, including keratoconjunctivitis sicca, stomatitis sicca, rhinitis sicca, and tracheobronchitis sicca. Eye involvement is manifested as xerophthalmia, a burning sensation or soreness of the eyes, and sensitivity to light. Oral involvement presents with xerostomia, parotid gland enlargement, and difficulties when talking for long periods or chewing dry foods. Sjogren's syndrome can be divided into two forms, including the typical primary Sjögren's syndrome (pSS) and secondary Sjögren's syndrome (sSS), which occurs with other rheumatoid diseases, such as SLE, RA, and sclerosis. The prevalence of pSS is estimated at 61 per 100,000 population. The disease rate in women is much higher than that of men. Anti-Ro/SSA and anti-La/SSB are the most common autoantibodies in SS patients [64].

Gottenberg et al. indicated that there is no correlation between CTLA-4 CT60 and +49A/G with primary SS [65]. However, according to some studies, +49A;CT60A and +49A;CT60G haplotypes are related to susceptibility to primary SS. The +49A;CT60G haplotype is associated with Ro/La-positive autoantibody in pSS, while the +49A;CT60A haplotype has a protective role against Raynaud's phenomenon in pSS [66, 67]. Upregulation of CTLA-4, PD-1, Fas, and FasL has been identified in the salivary glands of primary SS patients, which indicates local immune regulatory mechanisms in this tissue [68].

Overexpression of PD-1, B7-H3, and B7-H1 in serum and salivary glands has been demonstrated in pSS [69].

$CXCR5^+$ $PD\text{-}1^+$ Tfh $CD8^+$ T cells are a subset of CD8 T cells that interact with B cells in the germinal center of lymphoid follicles. These cells have gene signatures similar to $CD4^+$ Tfh and are involved in regulating B cell autoimmune responses and controlling autoantibody production. Increased $CXCR5^+$ $PD\text{-}1^+$ $CD8^+$ T cell subset and $CXCR5^+$ $PD1^+$ $CD4^+$ Tfh have been reported in the peripheral blood of primary SS patients [22, 70, 71]. It has also been found that the frequency of peripheral $PD\text{-}1^+$ $CXCR5^-$ $CD4^+$ T helper cells (Tph) increases in the peripheral blood and labial glands of pSS patients, which is related to the activity and severity of the disease [71].

7.2.5 Systemic Sclerosis

Systemic sclerosis (SSc) or scleroderma is a rare but severe and complex disease characterized by fibrosis and thickness of the skin at the extremities, which can end in digital ulcerations. Severe pruritus and telangiectasias also occurred in the patients. Involvement of other organs is common, including pulmonary, renal, gastrointestinal tract, and musculoskeletal diseases. SSc has the highest mortality rate in rheumatic diseases. The main pathological findings in SSc are vasculopathy and endothelial damage. The increased levels of cell adhesion molecules, infiltration of immune cells such as T cells and macrophages, and production of proinflammatory cytokines, especially IL-6, are related to disease progression. IL-4, IL-13, and TGFβ are elevated in this disease, which are associated with tissue fibrosis. TGFβ, as a fibrotic mediator, stimulates fibroblast proliferation and differentiation and extracellular matrix (ECM) production. Raynaud phenomenon, SSc-specific autoimmune antibodies, and sclerodermatous changes on nail fold capillaroscopy are helpful criteria for early diagnosis of the disease [72, 73].

Numerous researches have been conducted on the correlation between CTLA-4 polymorphisms and SSc. This correlation is different between ethnicities. For example, in Japanese or African-American patients, the +49A allele is associated with susceptibility to SSc. Some studies have indicated the association of promoter polymorphism -318C/T with SSc in Iranian and Italian populations. In conclusion, among CTLA-4 polymorphisms, -318C/T shows a stronger association with SSc risk in different populations [74].

A study has demonstrated that the level of sCTLA-4 increases in the serum of SSc patients. The increase of this immune checkpoint in the serum of patients is associated with extensive skin fibrosis, higher pulmonary fibrosis rate, and more active disease [75].

Investigating the immune checkpoint expression on PBMCs of SSc patients revealed that PD-1 and TIGIT are co-expressed on different subsets of T cells. In addition, overexpression of TIM-3 has been identified on $CD16^+$ $CD56^{med}$ NK cells [76]. sPD-1, sPD-L1, and sPD-L2 are increased in the serum of SSc patients. The elevation of sPD-1 levels is correlated with the severity of SSc disease and with skin sclerosis in the case of diffuse cutaneous SSc. Furthermore, membrane PD-1 and PD-L2 on T cells, B cells, and peripheral blood macrophages are upregulated in SSc. PD-$L2^{hi}$ B cells produce more IL-10 compared to PD-$L2^{low}$ B cells, which seems to be involved in the regulation of T cell response [77–79]. High-throughput mass cytometry analysis showed the presence of PD-1^{hi} $CXCR5^-$ HLA-DR^+ $ICOS^-$ $CD4^+$ T cells in SSc patients. These T cell subsets show cytotoxic activity and are related to interstitial lung disease in the patients [80].

7.3 Central Nervous System Autoimmune Disease: Multiple Sclerosis

Multiple sclerosis (MS) is a demyelinating disease of the central nervous system (CNS) that affects motor (numbness or weakness of limbs), sensory (paresthesias), visual (blurred or doubled vision), and autonomic (bladder, bowel, and sexual dysfunction) systems. Fatigue, pain, depression, cognitive impairment, and anxiety are common complications in MS patients. More than 80% of MS cases manifest as clinically isolated syndrome (CIS). CIS is the first clinical onset of potential MS that is associated with inflammatory demyelination and destruction of one or more CNS sites. Another common form of the disease is relapsing-remitting MS (RRMS). RRMS is a progressive neurological disability that occurs periodically and is associated with a complete or partial recovery. In some RRMS patients, neurological damage develops without proper recovery. This form of MS is defined as a secondary progressive course (SPMS). Primary progressive MS (PPMS) is another type of disease in which symptoms are progressive from the onset. In general, the infiltration of adaptive and innate immune cells into the CNS causes demyelinating disease. The presence of $CD8^+$ T cells and Th1 and Th17 cells plays an important role in the disease development. B cells are also significant in the pathogenesis of MS. Antibody oligoclonal bands (OCB) are found in the cerebrospinal fluid (CSF) of more than 90% of MS patients. Various genetic factors are involved in MS. Correlation of HLA-DR and HLA-DQ variants with susceptibility to MS has been proven. HLA-DRB1∗15:01 is one of the most important genes associated with MS risk [81–84].

Immune checkpoints play an important role in the outcome of MS. Study of different inhibitory molecule expression profiles, including CTLA-4, PD-1, TIM-3,

TIGIT, and LAG-3, indicated that TIGIT and LAG-3 mRNA expression in MS patients were significantly lower than in healthy controls. Lower levels of TIGIT and LAG-3 were associated with disease progression and worse outcomes. In contrast, higher levels of TIGIT and LAG-3 were associated with a good prognosis. TIGIT was higher in OCB-positive CSF patients than in OCB-negative patients [85].

In the majority of related studies, no correlation between CTLA-4 polymorphisms and MS has been observed [86, 87]. However, the association of certain CTLA-4 polymorphisms with the risk of MS has been demonstrated in some studies. Wagner et al. reported that in HLA-DRB1*15:01 negative cases, the presence of the G allele in rs231775A NG is associated with MS susceptibility [88]. It has been shown that Jo31G and CT60G alleles are associated with susceptibility to MS and decreased CTLA-4 gene expression in RRMS and SPMS [89]. Mohammadzadeh et al. have evaluated the expression of some important immune checkpoints in MS patients. They found that the expressions of CTLA-4, PD-1, and TIM-3 were increased in PBMCs of patients compared to healthy controls [90]. Contrary to these findings, another study demonstrated that PD-1 expression is decreased on $CD4^+$ T cells and $CD8^+$ T cells in the peripheral blood of RRMS patients, and PD-1 downregulation is associated with increased levels of IFN-γ, IL-12, IL-17, and TGFβ [91]. Analysis of CTLA-4 and PD-L1 expressions on PBMCs of MS patients revealed that these markers were mainly expressed on Treg, naïve T, and activated $CD8^+$ T cells. CTLA-4 and PD-L1 mRNA expression levels in healthy subjects were higher than in untreated patients. The expression of both CTLA-4 and PD-L1 molecules in patients treated with fingolimod, IFNβ-1α, and dimethyl fumarate (DMF) was significantly higher than that of untreated RRMS patients. Therefore, the treatment of MS patients, especially with fingolimod, by inducing the expression of immune checkpoints can lead to a decrease in the autoreactive T cell response and attenuate the autoimmune reactions [92]. Abatacept (CTLA4-Ig) prevents T cell activation by inhibiting the CD28–B7 costimulatory pathway and can play a protective role in autoimmunity. Although in vivo studies of CTLA4-Ig administration in animal models of EAE have shown that this agent is effective in reducing the symptoms and severity of the disease, the results of clinical trials using CTLA4-Ig for the treatment of MS patients are controversial [93]. A phase 1 open-label study conducted by Viglietta et al. to evaluate the effect of CTLA4-Ig in RRMS patients showed that CTLA4-Ig is safe and effective in MS patients [94]. In contrast, the results of a phase II randomized trial indicated that CTLA4-Ig fusion protein was not successful in reducing disease activity in RRMS [95].

Saresella et al. have explored the TIM-3/GAL pathway in MS. PBMCs were isolated and stimulated with myelin basic protein (MBP) peptide. They found that the population of MBP-specific $TIM\text{-}3^+$ $CD4^+$, $Gal\text{-}9^+$ $CD4^+$ T cells, as well as apoptotic ($TIM\text{-}3^+$/annexin V^+) T cells, was elevated in benign MS. Blocking the TIM-3/Gal-9 pathway led to a decrease in the apoptosis of T cells from RRMS and benign MS patients and an increase in the production of IFN-γ and IL-17 compared to PPMS. They proposed that TIM-3/Gal-9 interaction is involved in the apoptosis of MBP-specific T cells in MS [96].

7.4 Autoimmune Thyroid Disease

Autoimmune thyroid disease (AITD) includes Graves' disease (GD) and Hashimoto's thyroiditis (HT). AITD is associated with the presence of T and B cells in the thyroid gland and the production of autoantibodies against thyroid antigens. The relationship of several immune-regulatory genes, such as CTLA-4, PD-1, CD40, FoxP3, CD25, and HLA family, especially HLA-DR3 allele, with susceptibility to AITD have been discovered [97]. In GD, binding of thyroid receptor autoantibodies (TRAbs) to thyroid-stimulating hormone (TSH) receptor (TSHR) expressed in the thyroid gland stimulates the production of excessive amounts of thyroid hormone, which leads to hyperthyroidism. Symptoms include goiter, sweating, tremors, palpitations, behavioral changes, irritability, and poor concentration. In some patients, abnormal manifestations of the eye (Graves' ophthalmopathy) and skin are observed. Laboratory findings include suppressed TSH, along with increased free triiodothyronine (FT3) and FT4. Elevated TRAb titer is one of the main immunological characteristics of GD [98]. HT is a chronic inflammation of the thyroid gland, which is associated with gradual thyroid destruction. HT leads to thyroid hormone deficiency and is the most common cause of hypothyroidism. HT is determined by decreasing FT3 and T4, increasing TSH levels, and autoantibodies against thyroid peroxidase (TPO-Ab) and thyroglobulin (Tg-Ab) [99, 100].

The association of polymorphisms of the CTLA-4 gene with autoimmune thyroiditis has been identified. +49A>G is strongly associated with a genetic predisposition to GD disease [101]. According to a meta-analysis, the +49A>G polymorphism in the CTLA-4 gene is associated with susceptibility to GD in Asian children [102]. CT60 has also been found to be associated with GD [103]. C55A polymorphism in exon 1 of CTLA-4 is also associated with HT risk [100]. In the case of PD-1, the correlation of rs36084323 and rs2227982 polymorphisms with HT has been indicated [104].

Evaluation of PD-1 expression on PBMCs of GD patients has revealed that PD-1^+ $CD8^+$ T cells, PD-1^+ $CD4^+$ T cells, and PD-1^+ $CD19^+$ B cells subsets are increased compared to healthy individuals [105–107]. Ortega-Rodríguez and coworkers showed that the PD-1^+ NK subset was increased in AITD. PD-1^- $CD56^{bright}$ NK cells from GD and HT patients had a high potency to produce IL-10, while PD-1^+ NK cells showed more cytotoxic activity. They found that there is a strong correlation between the proportion of PD-1^+ NK cells and autoantibodies or free T4 levels. An increased PD-1^+ $CD56^{bright}$ NK cell population was associated with anti-TPO antibody levels in HT patients. In addition, in GD patients, the percentage of PD-1^+ $CD56^{dim}$ NK cells had a positive correlation with anti-TPO levels. These findings indicate the possible role of NK cells expressing PD-1 in the pathogenesis of AITD [108].

The association of PD-1 expression and the function of Treg cells in AITD has been highlighted in AITD. Zhong et al. indicated that the expression of PD-1 and

PD-L1 on Tregs ($CD4^+CD25^+$) was significantly lower in GD patients. Serum FT3 concentration of patients was negatively correlated with PD-1 and PD-L1 expressions on Tregs. In addition, the effect of thyroid hormone on Treg cells was measured. The results of the PBMC culture in the presence of different concentrations of thyroid hormone showed that the high levels of T3 reduce the expression of PD-1 on Tregs and also dampen their suppressive activity. T3 injection to mice led to a decrease in PD-1 expression on Tregs. Tregs of these mice had a lower expression of IL-10 than control mice, which indicates the impaired suppressive function of these cells. Therefore, the pathological increase of thyroid hormones can affect the immune regulation in GD through the dysfunction of Tregs [107]. A study group showed that $PD\text{-}1^+$ $CD4^+$ T cells are highly infiltrated in the GD thyroid gland. Interestingly, PD-L1 is also expressed on thyroid follicular cells (TFCs), which indicates the role of the PD-1/PD-L1 axis in the AITD, and it may be involved in slowing down the disease progression [106]. In line with these findings, another study showed that $PD\text{-}1^+$ $CD4^+$ and $PD\text{-}1^+$ $CD8^+$ T cells in co-culture with mouse TFCs inhibited the apoptosis of these cells and stimulated thyroid hormone production in culture. The production of inflammatory cytokines, such as IFN-γ and IL-17, was also higher in the presence of $PD\text{-}1^+$ $CD4^+$ and $PD\text{-}1^+$ $CD8^+$ T cells than in PD-1-negative lymphocytes [109].

7.5 Psoriasis

Psoriasis is a chronic inflammatory disease involving the skin, which has a global prevalence of about 2%. Clinical symptoms appear as erythematous and pruritic plaques with silvery scales, usually on the trunk and extensor surfaces of the limbs. Inflammatory cell infiltration, epidermal basal layer keratinocyte hyperproliferation, and capillary dilatation are among the pathological characteristics of psoriasis. Chronic inflammation leads to dysregulation of keratinocyte proliferation and differentiation. The role of TNFα–IL23–Th17 axis in the plaque psoriasis development and the progression of the disease has been demonstrated. Psoriasis susceptibility 1(PSORS1) locus, located within MHC on chromosome 6p21, is one of the most important susceptibility factors to psoriasis [110–112]. The relationship between PD-1 and psoriasis has been extensively studied, while less information is available on the role of CTLA-4 in this disease. The expression of CTLA-4 in the skin lesions of patients with mild psoriasis is more than that of moderate and severe psoriasis patients, which means that the expression of this marker is inversely related to the severity of the disease. CTLA-4 Ig injection in the mouse model of psoriasis induced by (IMQ) imiquimod reduces epidermal hyperplasia and inflammation, while the CTLA-4 blocking antibody worsens the disease [113]. Lee et al. generated a recombinant CTLA-4 consisting of the CTLA-4 intracellular signaling domain and a cell-penetrating peptide (dNP2-ctCTLA-4) and assessed its effect on psoriasis. Administering dNP2-ctCTLA-4 to the IMQ-induced psoriasis mouse model improved the psoriasis area and severity index (PASI) score and inhibited the progression of psoriasis lesions. They demonstrated that dNP2-ctCTLA-4 exerts its effect by inducing the production of FoxP3^{+} Treg cells and reducing skin inflammation through these cells [114].

High expression of PD-1 on circulating T cells or high levels of PD-1^{+} T cells in psoriasis patients have been observed in many studies [115]. In contrast, Bartosińska et al. found that the percentage of CD4^{+} PD-1^{+} as well as CD8^{+} PD-1^{+} T cells was lower in psoriatic patients with and without arthritis compared to the control group. There was no correlation between PD-1 expression on T cells and disease severity [116]. Similarly, Adamczyk et al. showed that the percentage of PD-1^{+} T cells and PD-1^{+} B cells, as well as PD-L1^{+} B and T cells, in PBMCs of psoriasis patients was decreased compared to healthy individuals [117]. However, Peled and colleagues showed that PD-1 expression on circulating T cells of psoriatic arthritis (PsA) patients was significantly increased [118]. Some researchers have focused on the expression profile of PD-1 and PD-L1 in psoriasis skin lesions. A study has shown that PD-1 and PD-L1 expression on the immune cells of tissue biopsies of psoriasis patients is much higher than that of healthy controls. They argued that there is a negative correlation between PD-L1 expression levels and disease severity [119]. Jung et al., by examining chronic plaque psoriasis (CPP) skin biopsies, demonstrated that in the high PD-1 expression group, the psoriasis area and severity index (PASI) was significantly higher than the epidermal PD-1^{low} group. They concluded that the expression of PD-1 in the epidermis is related to the severity and longer duration of the disease [120].

7.6 Type 1 Diabetes

T1D is a heterogeneous disease characterized by insulin deficiency. The disease manifests as classic diabetes with polyuria, polydipsia, and weight loss. T1D mainly occurs in young people, so that ≥85% of all T1D cases are under 20 years old. The incidence of T1D is higher in children than in adults. The disease is the result of progressive autoimmune-mediated destruction of beta (β) cells of pancreatic islets. According to the proposed models, the progression of T1D consists of three stages: (1) normoglycemia (asymptomatic phase) and the presence of two or more islet-directed autoantibodies; (2) dysglycemia (early glucose metabolism alteration) along with autoantibody positivity, which indicates insufficient insulin secretion; (3) hypoglycemia, the clinical presentation of diabetes and the need for insulin therapy. Recent-onset T1D pathological features include patchy and variable insulitis (immune cells infiltration to the pancreatic islets), some insulin-negative and pseudo-atrophic islets, and some normal-appearing β cells in the islets. Autoantibodies associated with T1D include antibodies to insulin, glutamic acid decarboxylase (GAD), insulinoma-associated antigen-2 (IA-2), zinc transporter 8 (ZnT8), and islet cell antibodies (ICA), which can be detected in >90% of typical T1D cases. The role of HLA II alleles (especially DR and DQ) has been highlighted in T1D pathogenesis. DR4-DQ8 haplotype (HLA-DRB1∗04 with DQA1∗03:01-DQB1∗03:02) is associated with an increased risk of T1D development [121–123].

CTLA-4 + 49A/G (rs231775) polymorphism is an important genetic marker in T1D. The association of this SNP with increased risk of T1D has been identified in different populations, especially in Caucasians and Asians [124–126]. The GG genotype or the G allele of +49 G/A is associated with a high rate of IA-2A positivity in T1D patients. In addition, it has been demonstrated that +49G/A affects the expression of CTLA-4 on Treg cells in these patients, and the GG genotype of +49 G/A is associated with lower CTLA-4 expression [127]. By evaluating the checkpoint immune profile of 57 islet autoantibody-positive (AAb+) children, Bruzzaniti et al. showed that in these children, sCTLA-4, sPD-1, sPDL-2, and sBTLA levels were higher compared to those of recent-onset T1D and healthy children. Further investigations also revealed that the levels of sPD-1 and sBTLA were higher in AAb+ children who progressed to T1D (AAb-P) than those who did not progress to T1D (AAb-NP). Therefore, the expression of immune checkpoints is dysregulated in the early preclinical stages of T1D, and increased serum levels of sPD-1 are associated with a higher risk of T1D development in AAb+ children. sPD-1 as a decoy molecule can disrupt the PD-1/PDL-1 signaling pathway [128].

According to a study in the Japanese population, PD-1 mRNA levels and the percentage of $CD4^+$ $PD\text{-}1^+$ T cells in T1D patients were significantly lower than those of healthy controls. In addition, the 7785C/T genotype in PDCD1 was associated with PD-1 expression. This study suggests that the lower expression of PD-1 on T cells may be involved in T1AD development [129]. Another study showed that T cells derived from newly diagnosed T1D children fail to upregulate PD-1 during stimulation with anti-CD3/CD28 antibodies [130]. A study of PD-L1 expression in pancreatic biopsies of T1D patients has shown that this marker is upregulated in β cells, while its expression was not observed in insulin-deficient islets. Notably, the level of PD-L1 mRNA expression in recent-onset T1D patients was several times higher than in long-lasting T1D subjects. These findings highlight the possible role of PD-L1 in mitigating the autoimmune responses in T1D [131] (Table 7.1).

Table 7.1 The association between SNPs within the immune checkpoint genes and autoimmune diseases

Disease	Gene	SNP	Position	Papulation	Comment	Ref.
Rheumatoid arthritis (RA)	PD-1	rs36084323	chr2:241859444	Asian	G/G genotype	[132]
		rs11568821	chr2:241851760	Caucasian	significantly associated with RA risk may be used as a biomarker for early diagnosis of RA	[133]
	CTLA-4	rs231775 rs3087243	chr2:203867991 ch2:203874196	Asians and Caucasians and Mongolian	Based on 66 case-control studies including 21,681 cases and 23,457 controls, both SNPs were associated with the risk of RA	[134, 135]
	TIM-3	rs1036199	chr5:157104725	East-Asians	Switching T to G, replacement of neutral amino acid (arginine) by a hydrophobic one (leucine), alteration of TIM-3 structure	[136, 137]
	BTLA	rs76844316	chr3:112469762	Japanese	rs76844316:A/C and C/C, Asparagine to threonine, rs9288952: C to T, leucine to proline. A significant association between these SNPs in the BTLA gene that affects the expression and function of BTLA in lymphocytes	[138, 139]
		rs9288952	chr3:112466178	Taiwanese		
Systemic lupus erythematosus (SLE)	PD-1	rs11568821 rs10204525	chr2:241851760 chr2:241850169	Caucasians and Mexicans LN in European Latin-American	SLE risk in males, but no association was observed in the females. In Latin-American, PD1.3A (rs11568821) showed decreased SLE risk	[140, 141]
	CTLA-4	rs231775 rs17268364	chr2:203867991 chr2:203913095	Thai, Caucasians, Mongolians	No association with SLE	[135, 142, 143]
				Chinese		
	TIM-3	rs9313439 rs10515746	chr5:157086171 chr5:157109557	Chinese	No association with SLE	[144]

Behcet's disease (BD)	PD1	rs2227981 rs10204525	chr2:241851121 chr2:241850169	Chinese Han	Lack of association with BD	[145]
	CTLA-4	rs231775 rs5742909 rs231775	chr2:203867991 chr2:203867624 chr2:203867991	Turkey, China, Korea, Tunisia, UK, Middle East	No association find between +49 A/G, −318 C/T or CT60 A/G with BD	[146]
				Iranian Azari	Patients with A allele and AA genotype were more susceptible to BD	[147]
	TIM-3	rs9313439 rs10515746	chr5:157086171 chr5:157109557	Iranian	There were no significant differences in allele and genotype frequencies with BD	[148]
	BTLA	rs184489 rs9288952	chr8:26448265 chr3:112466178	Turkish	rs1844089 (T), rs9288952(C) increase the risk of BD. CT haplotype might have a potential function in the susceptibility to BD	[149]
Multiple sclerosis (MS)	PD-1	146G/A		German	There was a significant association	[150]
	CTLA-4	rs231775 rs5742909 rs3087243	chr2:203867991 chr2:203867624 chr2:203874196	Caucasians, Asians, Arabs Americas, Europe	There was no significant association between these SNPs with MS	[86, 151]
	TIM-3	rs10053538 rs10515746	chr5:157110499 chr5:157109557	Iranian	There were significant differences in genotype and allele distributions between MS patients and controls	[152]
	LAG3	rs1922452	chr12:6787028	Arab Jordanian	There was an association with MS	[153]
Systemic sclerosis (SSc)	PD-1	rs2227981	chr2:241851121	Italy	No association with SS	[154]
	CTLA-4	rs231775	chr2:203867991	Thai	No association with SS	[143]
Sjogren's syndrome (SS)	CTLA-4	rs231775 rs3087243	chr2:203867991 chr2:203874196	Caucasians	There was a lack of association between CTLA-4 CT60 or + 49A/G polymorphisms and pSS	[155]

(continued)

Table 7.1 (continued)

Disease	Gene	SNP	Position	Papulation	Comment	Ref.
Ankylosing spondylitis (AS)	PD-1	rs2227982	chr2:241851281	China	Five studies showed the association of this polymorphism with the risk of AS	[156]
	CTLA-4	rs231775	chr2:203867991	Caucasian, Mongolian	No association with AS	[135]
	TIM-3	rs10515746 (−574G/T) rs1036199 (+4259T/G)	chr5:157109557 chr5:157104725	China	Significant association with AS (−574G/T) No association with AS (+4259T/G)	[60]
Graves' disease (GD)	PD-L1	rs822339 rs2282055 rs1411262	chr9:5453172 chr9:5455732 chr9:5459419	Japanese, Northern European, United Kingdom	Associated with GD	[157]
	CTLA-4	rs231775 rs3087243	chr2:203867991 chr2:203874196	South-Indian Chinese (children & adolescents) Polish, Iranian, Caucasian, Asians	Associated with GD	[158, 159]
	TIM-3	rs10053538 rs1036199 rs10515746	chr5:157110499 chr5:157104725 chr5:157109557	Chinese Han Han Chinese population of North China	There was association between these SNPs with GD, but there was a significant correlation between rs10515746 and MG in Han Chinese population of North China.	[160, 161]
Hashimoto's disease (HD)	PD-1	rs36084323 rs2227982	chr2:241859444 chr2:241851281	Japan	rs36084323 AA and rs2227982 TT genotypes were lower in mild HD than in patients with severe HD	[104]
	CTLA-4	rs231775 rs3087243	chr2:203867991 chr2:203874196	South-Indian Asians, Iranian, Caucasian	CTLA-4 + 49A/G (rs231775) can be considered as a biomarker for HT	[158, 159, 162]

Psoriasis	PD-1	rs10204525	chr2:241850169	Chinese	The G allele of PD1.6 increases the risk of psoriasis	[163]
	CTLA-4	rs231775	chr2:203867991	Asian and Caucasian	CTLA-4 + 49A/G (rs231775) showed a protective effect for psoriasis in some subgroup	[164]
Type 1 diabetes (T1D)	PDL-1	rs2297137	chr9:5465732	Egyptian pediatric	Significantly associated with T1D	[165]
	CTLA-4	rs231775	chr2:203867991	Polish (children & adolescents) Caucasians and South Asians	Threonine to alanine substitution decrease CTLA-4 on T-cell, increase T activation, increases the risk of T1D development	[158, 166]
	TIM-3	rs10515746 rs1036199 rs10053538	chr5:157109557 chr5:157104725 chr5:157110499	German	No association with T1D	[167]
	BTLA	rs2705534 rs9288953 rs2171513	chr3:112489538 chr3:112484405 chr3:112466080	Japanese	No association with T1D	[168]

7.7 Conclusion

The exploration of immune checkpoints in autoimmune diseases presented in this chapter highlights the intricate balance between immune activation and regulation in maintaining self-tolerance. The detailed examination of various checkpoint molecules, particularly CTLA-4, PD-1, and TIM-3, reveals their crucial roles in modulating immune responses and their potential involvement in the pathogenesis of autoimmune disorders.

The chapter focuses on the complexity of immune checkpoint interactions in different autoimmune conditions, with many molecules exhibiting context-dependent functions and often being co-expressed with other regulatory receptors. The association of checkpoint gene polymorphisms with disease susceptibility and the altered expression patterns of these molecules in various autoimmune diseases provides valuable insights into the genetic and molecular basis of autoimmunity.

While the success of checkpoint inhibitors in cancer therapy has demonstrated the power of manipulating these pathways, their potential application in autoimmune diseases presents both opportunities and challenges. The dual nature of immune checkpoints in both restraining and potentially exacerbating autoimmune responses necessitates a suitable approach to their therapeutic targeting.

As research in this field progresses, integrating genomic, epigenomic, and functional data will be crucial for developing a more comprehensive understanding of immune checkpoint regulation in autoimmune contexts. This knowledge may pave the way for more targeted and personalized therapeutic strategies, potentially allowing for fine-tuning of immune responses in autoimmune diseases.

The future of autoimmune disease treatment may lie in harnessing the complex network of immune checkpoints to restore immune balance. However, this approach will require careful consideration of the potential risks, including the possibility of triggering or exacerbating other autoimmune conditions. Continued research into the tissue-specific and disease-specific roles of immune checkpoints will be essential for translating these findings into effective clinical applications.

In conclusion, while our understanding of immune checkpoints in autoimmune diseases has grown significantly, many questions remain. The ongoing exploration of these pathways promises to yield new insights into the fundamental mechanisms of autoimmunity and may lead to innovative therapeutic approaches for managing these complex disorders.

Acknowledgments The authors gratefully acknowledge the valuable assistance provided by Maryam Sadr.

References

1. Wang L, Wang FS, Gershwin ME. Human autoimmune diseases: a comprehensive update. J Intern Med. 2015;278(4):369–95.
2. Huang C, Zhu HX, Yao Y, Bian ZH, Zheng YJ, Li L, et al. Immune checkpoint molecules. Possible future therapeutic implications in autoimmune diseases. J Autoimmun. 2019;104:102333.
3. Grebinoski S, Vignali DA. Inhibitory receptor agonists: the future of autoimmune disease therapeutics? Curr Opin Immunol. 2020;67:1–9.
4. Radu AF, Bungau SG. Management of rheumatoid arthritis: an overview. Cells. 2021;10(11).
5. Wu D, Luo Y, Li T, Zhao X, Lv T, Fang G, et al. Systemic complications of rheumatoid arthritis: focus on pathogenesis and treatment. Front Immunol. 2022;13:1051082.
6. Jang S, Kwon EJ, Lee JJ. Rheumatoid arthritis: pathogenic roles of diverse immune cells. Int J Mol Sci. 2022;23(2).
7. Ceeraz S, Nowak EC, Burns CM, Noelle RJ. Immune checkpoint receptors in regulating immune reactivity in rheumatic disease. Arthritis Res Ther. 2014;16(5):469.
8. Zhou C, Gao S, Yuan X, Shu Z, Li S, Sun X, et al. Association between CTLA-4 gene polymorphism and risk of rheumatoid arthritis: a meta-analysis. Aging. 2021;13(15):19397–414.
9. Cao J, Zou L, Luo P, Chen P, Zhang L. Increased production of circulating soluble co-stimulatory molecules CTLA-4, CD28 and CD80 in patients with rheumatoid arthritis. Int Immunopharmacol. 2012;14(4):585–92.
10. García-Chagollán M, Ledezma-Lozano IY, Hernández-Bello J, Sánchez-Hernández PE, Gutiérrez-Ureña SR, Muñoz-Valle JF. Expression patterns of CD28 and CTLA-4 in early, chronic, and untreated rheumatoid arthritis. J Clin Lab Anal. 2020;34(5):e23188.
11. Malik AE, Slauenwhite D, McAlpine SM, Hanly JG, Marshall JS, Issekutz TB. Differences in IDO1(+) dendritic cells and soluble CTLA-4 are associated with differential clinical responses to methotrexate treatment in rheumatoid arthritis. Front Immunol. 2024;15:1352251.
12. Flores-Borja F, Jury EC, Mauri C, Ehrenstein MR. Defects in CTLA-4 are associated with abnormal regulatory T cell function in rheumatoid arthritis. Proc Natl Acad Sci USA. 2008;105(49):19396–401.
13. Rech J, Tascilar K, Hagen M, Kleyer A, Manger B, Schoenau V, et al. Abatacept inhibits inflammation and onset of rheumatoid arthritis in individuals at high risk (ARIAA): a randomised, international, multicentre, double-blind, placebo-controlled trial. Lancet. 2024;403(10429):850–9.
14. Pombo-Suarez M, Gomez-Reino JJ. Abatacept for the treatment of rheumatoid arthritis. Expert Rev Clin Immunol. 2019;15(4):319–26.
15. Zou Y, Zhang Z, Liu Y, Liu D, Xu W. Are programmed cell death 1 gene polymorphisms correlated with susceptibility to rheumatoid arthritis?: A meta-analysis. Medicine. 2017;96(35):e7805.
16. Greisen SR, Rasmussen TK, Stengaard-Pedersen K, Hetland ML, Hørslev-Petersen K, Hvid M, et al. Increased soluble programmed death-1 (sPD-1) is associated with disease activity and radiographic progression in early rheumatoid arthritis. Scand J Rheumatol. 2014;43(2):101–8.
17. Liu C, Jiang J, Gao L, Wang X, Hu X, Wu M, et al. Soluble PD-1 aggravates progression of collagen-induced arthritis through Th1 and Th17 pathways. Arthritis Res Ther. 2015;17:340.
18. Bartosińska J, Zakrzewska E, Król A, Raczkiewicz D, Purkot J, Majdan M, et al. Differential expression of programmed death 1 (PD-1) on CD4+ and CD8+ T cells in rheumatoid arthritis and psoriatic arthritis. Pol Arch Intern Med. 2017;127(12):815–22.
19. Luo Q, Ye J, Zeng L, Luo Z, Deng Z, Li X, et al. Elevated expression of PD-1 on T cells correlates with disease activity in rheumatoid arthritis. Mol Med Rep. 2018;17(2):3297–305.
20. Matsuda K, Miyoshi H, Hiraoka K, Hamada T, Yoshida S, Ishibashi Y, et al. Clinicopathological value of programmed cell death 1 (PD-1) and programmed cell death ligand 1 (PD-L1) expression in synovium of patients with rheumatoid arthritis. Clin Exp Med. 2018;18(4):487–94.

21. Cao G, Chi S, Wang X, Sun J, Zhang Y. CD4+CXCR5+PD-1+ T follicular helper cells play a pivotal role in the development of rheumatoid arthritis. Med Sci Monit. 2019;25:3032–40.
22. Chen Y, Yu M, Zheng Y, Fu G, Xin G, Zhu W, et al. CXCR5(+)PD-1(+) follicular helper CD8 T cells control B cell tolerance. Nat Commun. 2019;10(1):4415.
23. Zhou H, Hu B, Zhaopeng Z, Liu J, Zhong Q, Fan Y, et al. Elevated circulating T cell subsets and cytokines expression in patients with rheumatoid arthritis. Clin Rheumatol. 2019;38(7):1831–9.
24. Zhao L, Li Z, Zeng X, Xia C, Xu L, Xu Q, et al. Circulating CD4(+) FoxP3(−) CXCR5(−) CXCR3(+) PD-1(hi) cells are elevated in active rheumatoid arthritis and reflect the severity of the disease. Int J Rheum Dis. 2021;24(8):1032–9.
25. Lee J, Oh JM, Hwang JW, Ahn JK, Bae EK, Won J, et al. Expression of human TIM-3 and its correlation with disease activity in rheumatoid arthritis. Scand J Rheumatol. 2011;40(5):334–40.
26. Li S, Peng D, He Y, Zhang H, Sun H, Shan S, et al. Expression of TIM-3 on CD4+ and CD8+ T cells in the peripheral blood and synovial fluid of rheumatoid arthritis. APMIS. 2014;122(10):899–904.
27. Liu Y, Shu Q, Gao L, Hou N, Zhao D, Liu X, et al. Increased Tim-3 expression on peripheral lymphocytes from patients with rheumatoid arthritis negatively correlates with disease activity. Clini Immunol. 2010;137(2):288–95.
28. Matsumoto H, Fujita Y, Asano T, Matsuoka N, Temmoku J, Sato S, et al. T cell immunoglobulin and mucin domain-3 is associated with disease activity and progressive joint damage in rheumatoid arthritis patients. Medicine. 2020;99(44):e22892.
29. Chae SC, Park YR, Shim SC, Yoon KS, Chung HT. The polymorphisms of Th1 cell surface gene Tim-3 are associated in a Korean population with rheumatoid arthritis. Immunol Lett. 2004;95(1):91–5.
30. Xu J, Yang Y, Liu X, Wang Y. The −1541 C>T and +4259 G>T of TIM-3 polymorphisms are associated with rheumatoid arthritis susceptibility in a Chinese Hui population. Int J Immunogenet. 2011;38(6):513–8.
31. Curran CS, Gupta S, Sanz I, Sharon E. PD-1 immunobiology in systemic lupus erythematosus. J Autoimmun. 2019;97:1–9.
32. Morand EF, Fernandez-Ruiz R, Blazer A, Niewold TB. Advances in the management of systemic lupus erythematosus. BMJ. 2023;383:e073980.
33. Shojaa M, Aghaie M, Qorbani M, Khashayar P, Amoli M, Keshtkar AA, et al. Association of the CTLA-4 1722TC polymorphism and systemic lupus erythematosus: a systematic review and meta analysis. Med J Islam Repub Iran. 2014;28:132.
34. Zhu JM, Li BK, Chen GM, Feng CC, Cen H, Fan YG, et al. CTLA-4 -1722T/C polymorphism and systemic lupus erythematosus susceptibility: a meta-analysis involving ten separate studies. Immunol Investig. 2013;42(2):91–105.
35. Lee YH, Harley JB, Nath SK. CTLA-4 polymorphisms and systemic lupus erythematosus (SLE): a meta-analysis. Hum Genet. 2005;116(5):361–7.
36. Kishk RM, Abdellatif MA, Eldesouki RE, Fawzy M, Abdelhady SA, Fouad MM. Cytotoxic T lymphocyte antigen 4 gene +49 A/G (rs231775) polymorphism and susceptibility to systemic lupus erythematosus. Curr Rheumatol Rev. 2021;17(2):247–51.
37. Liu J, Zhang H. 1722T/C polymorphism (rs733618) of CTLA-4 significantly associated with systemic lupus erythematosus (SLE): a comprehensive meta-analysis. Hum Immunol. 2013;74(3):341–7.
38. Zahiri L, Malekmakan L, Masjedi F, Habibagahi Z, Habibagahi M. Association between IL-17A, FOXP3, and CTLA4 genes expression and severity of lupus nephritis. Iran J Kidney Dis. 2022;1(1):13–23.
39. Wong CK, Lit LC, Tam LS, Li EK, Lam CW. Aberrant production of soluble costimulatory molecules CTLA-4, CD28, CD80 and CD86 in patients with systemic lupus erythematosus. Rheumatology (Oxford). 2005;44(8):989–94.

40. Dahal LN, Barker RN, Ward FJ. The soluble isoform of CTLA-4 correlates with interferon-α activity in systemic lupus erythematosus. J Rheumatol. 2020;47(2):302–4.
41. Jury EC, Flores-Borja F, Kalsi HS, Lazarus M, Isenberg DA, Mauri C, et al. Abnormal CTLA-4 function in T cells from patients with systemic lupus erythematosus. Eur J Immunol. 2010;40(2):569–78.
42. Dolff S, Quandt D, Feldkamp T, Jun C, Mitchell A, Hua F, et al. Increased percentages of PD-1 on CD4+ T cells is associated with higher INF-γ production and altered IL-17 production in patients with systemic lupus erythematosus. Scand J Rheumatol. 2014;43(4):307–13.
43. Jia XY, Zhu QQ, Wang YY, Lu Y, Li ZJ, Li BQ, et al. The role and clinical significance of programmed cell death- ligand 1 expressed on CD19(+)B-cells and subsets in systemic lupus erythematosus. Clin Immunol. 2019;198:89–99.
44. Du Y, Nie L, Xu L, Wu X, Zhang S, Xue J. Serum levels of soluble programmed death-1 (sPD-1) and soluble programmed death ligand 1(sPD-L1) in systemic lupus erythematosus: association with activity and severity. Scand J Immunol. 2020;92(1):e12884.
45. Luo Q, Kong Y, Fu B, Li X, Huang Q, Huang Z, et al. Increased TIM-3(+)PD-1(+) NK cells are associated with the disease activity and severity of systemic lupus erythematosus. Clin Exp Med. 2022;22(1):47–56.
46. Luo Q, Huang Z, Ye J, Deng Y, Fang L, Li X, et al. PD-L1-expressing neutrophils as a novel indicator to assess disease activity and severity of systemic lupus erythematosus. Arthritis Res Ther. 2016;18:47.
47. Song LJ, Wang X, Wang XP, Li D, Ding F, Liu HX, et al. Increased Tim-3 expression on peripheral T lymphocyte subsets and association with higher disease activity in systemic lupus erythematosus. Diagn Pathol. 2015;10:71.
48. Zhao D, Guo M, Liu B, Lin Q, Xie T, Zhang Q, et al. Frontline Science: Tim-3-mediated dysfunctional engulfment of apoptotic cells in SLE. J Leukoc Biol. 2017;102(6):1313–22.
49. Zheng H, Guo X, Tian Q, Li H, Zhu Y. Distinct role of Tim-3 in systemic lupus erythematosus and clear cell renal cell carcinoma. Int J Clin Exp Med. 2015;8(5):7029–38.
50. Asano T, Matsuoka N, Fujita Y, Matsumoto H, Temmoku J, Yashiro-Furuya M, et al. Serum levels of T cell immunoglobulin and mucin-domain containing molecule 3 in patients with systemic lupus erythematosus. J Clin Med. 2020;9(11):3563.
51. Agrawal P, Tote S, Sapkale B. Diagnosis and Treatment of Ankylosing Spondylitis. Cureus. 2024;16(1):e52559.
52. Kim SH, Lee SH. Updates on ankylosing spondylitis: pathogenesis and therapeutic agents. J Rheum Dis. 2023;30(4):220–33.
53. Schütz C, Baraliakos X. What do we know about co-stimulatory and co-inhibitory immune checkpoint signals in ankylosing spondylitis? Clin Exp Immunol. 2023;213(3):288–300.
54. Toussirot E, Saas P, Deschamps M, Pouthier F, Perrot L, Perruche S, et al. Increased production of soluble CTLA-4 in patients with spondylarthropathies correlates with disease activity. Arthritis Res Ther. 2009;11(4):R101.
55. Wu J, Zhang L, Zhou Y. The association between CTLA-4 (+49 A/G) polymorphism and susceptibility to ankylosing spondylitis: a meta-analysis. Int J Rheum Dis. 2016;19(12):1237–43.
56. Azizi E, Massoud A, Amirzargar AA, Mahmoudi M, Soleimanifar N, Rezaei N, et al. Association of CTLA4 gene polymorphism in Iranian patients with ankylosing spondylitis. J Clin Immunol. 2010;30(2):268–71.
57. Huang CH, Wei JC, Chen CC, Chuang CS, Chou CH, Lin YJ, et al. Associations of the PTPN22 and CTLA-4 genetic polymorphisms with Taiwanese ankylosing spondylitis. Rheumatol Int. 2014;34(5):683–91.
58. Duan Z, Gui Y, Li C, Lin J, Gober HJ, Qin J, et al. The immune dysfunction in ankylosing spondylitis patients. Biosci Trends. 2017;11(1):69–76.
59. Yang M, Zou Y, Bai Y, Li M. The programmed cell death 1 gene polymorphisms (PD 1.3 G/A, PD 1.5 C/T and PD 1.9 C/T) and susceptibility to ankylosing spondylitis: a meta-analysis. J Orthop Sci. 2015;20(1):55–63.

60. Wang M, Ji B, Wang J, Cheng X, Zhou Q, Zhou J, et al. Tim-3 polymorphism downregulates gene expression and is involved in the susceptibility to ankylosing spondylitis. DNA Cell Biol. 2014;33(10):723–8.
61. Zhou L, Zhang Y, Xu H, Hu L, Zhang C, Sun L, et al. Decreased programmed death-1 expression on the T cells of patients with ankylosing spondylitis. Am J Med Sci. 2015;349(6):488–92.
62. Chen MH, Chen WS, Lee HT, Tsai CY, Chou CT. Inverse correlation of programmed death 1 (PD-1) expression in T cells to the spinal radiologic changes in Taiwanese patients with ankylosing spondylitis. Clin Rheumatol. 2011;30(9):1181–7.
63. Soleimanifar N, Assadiasl S, Al-Shammari MS, Rostamian A, Sadr M, Shahkarami S, et al. Evaluation of PD-1 gene expression profile and methylation of the regulatory regions in patients with ankylosing spondylitis. Iran J Immunol. 2024;21(2):166–75.
64. Stefanski AL, Tomiak C, Pleyer U, Dietrich T, Burmester GR, Dörner T. The diagnosis and treatment of Sjögren's syndrome. Dtsch Arztebl Int. 2017;114(20):354–61.
65. Gottenberg JE, Loiseau P, Azarian M, Chen C, Cagnard N, Hachulla E, et al. CTLA-4 +49A/G and CT60 gene polymorphisms in primary Sjögren syndrome. Arthritis Res Ther. 2007;9(2):R24.
66. Downie-Doyle S, Bayat N, Rischmueller M, Lester S. Influence of CTLA4 haplotypes on susceptibility and some extraglandular manifestations in primary Sjögren's syndrome. Arthritis Rheum. 2006;54(8):2434–40.
67. Lester S, Downie-Doyle S, Rischmueller M. CTLA4 polymorphism and primary Sjögren's syndrome. Arthritis Res Ther. 2007;9(3):401:author reply 2.
68. Bolstad AI, Eiken HG, Rosenlund B, Alarcón-Riquelme ME, Jonsson R. Increased salivary gland tissue expression of Fas, Fas ligand, cytotoxic T lymphocyte-associated antigen 4, and programmed cell death 1 in primary Sjögren's syndrome. Arthritis Rheum. 2003;48(1):174–85.
69. Li P, Yang Y, Jin Y, Zhao R, Dong C, Zheng W, et al. B7-H3 participates in human salivary gland epithelial cells apoptosis through NF-κB pathway in primary Sjögren's syndrome. J Transl Med. 2019;17(1):268.
70. Zhai X, Wang Y, Guo H, Liang Z, Feng M, Wu Y, et al. Altered levels of circulating CD8(+)CXCR5(+)PD-1(+)T follicular cytotoxic cells in primary Sjögren's syndrome. Clin Rheumatol. 2022;41(6):1697–708.
71. Chen W, Yang F, Lin J. Tph cells expanded in primary Sjögren's syndrome. Front Med. 2022;9:900349.
72. Rosendahl AH, Schönborn K, Krieg T. Pathophysiology of systemic sclerosis (scleroderma). Kaohsiung J Med Sci. 2022;38(3):187–95.
73. Volkmann ER, Andréasson K, Smith V. Systemic sclerosis. Lancet. 2023;401(10373):304–18.
74. Song GG, Lee YH. The CTLA-4 and MCP-1 polymorphisms and susceptibility to systemic sclerosis: a meta-analysis. Immunol Investig. 2013;42(6):481–92.
75. Sato S, Fujimoto M, Hasegawa M, Komura K, Yanaba K, Hayakawa I, et al. Serum soluble CTLA-4 levels are increased in diffuse cutaneous systemic sclerosis. Rheumatology (Oxford). 2004;43(10):1261–6.
76. Fleury M, Belkina AC, Proctor EA, Zammitti C, Simms RW, Lauffenburger DA, et al. Increased expression and modulated regulatory activity of coinhibitory receptors PD-1, TIGIT, and TIM-3 in lymphocytes from patients with systemic sclerosis. Arthritis Rheumatol. 2018;70(4):566–77.
77. Hirahara S, Katsumata Y, Kawasumi H, Kawaguchi Y, Harigai M. Serum levels of soluble programmed cell death protein 1 and soluble programmed cell death protein ligand 2 are increased in systemic lupus erythematosus and associated with the disease activity. Lupus. 2020;29(7):686–96.
78. Yanaba K, Hayashi M, Yoshihara Y, Nakagawa H. Serum levels of soluble programmed death-1 and programmed death ligand-1 in systemic sclerosis: association with extent of skin sclerosis. J Dermatol. 2016;43(8):954–7.

79. Fukasawa T, Yoshizaki A, Ebata S, Nakamura K, Saigusa R, Miura S, et al. Contribution of soluble forms of programmed death 1 and programmed death ligand 2 to disease severity and progression in systemic sclerosis. Arthritis Rheumatol. 2017;69(9):1879–90.
80. Elahee M, Mueller AA, Wang R, Marks KE, Sasaki T, Cao Y, et al. A PD-1(high)CD4(+) T cell population with a cytotoxic phenotype is associated with interstitial lung disease in systemic sclerosis. ACR Open Rheumatol. 2024.
81. Doshi A, Chataway J. Multiple sclerosis, a treatable disease. Clin Med (Lond). 2016;16(Suppl 6):s53–s9.
82. Rodríguez Murúa S, Farez MF, Quintana FJ. The immune response in multiple sclerosis. Annu Rev Pathol. 2022;17:121–39.
83. Efendi H. Clinically isolated syndromes: clinical characteristics, differential diagnosis, and management. Noro Psikiyatr Ars. 2015;52(Suppl 1):S1–s11.
84. Miljković D, Spasojević I. Multiple sclerosis: molecular mechanisms and therapeutic opportunities. Antioxid Redox Signal. 2013;19(18):2286–334.
85. Lavon I, Heli C, Brill L, Charbit H, Vaknin-Dembinsky A. Blood levels of co-inhibitory-receptors: a biomarker of disease prognosis in multiple sclerosis. Front Immunol. 2019;10:835.
86. Liu J, Zhang HX. CTLA-4 gene and the susceptibility of multiple sclerosis: an updated meta-analysis study including 12,916 cases and 15,455 controls. J Neurogenet. 2014;28(1–2):153–63.
87. Gyu Song G, Ho LY. CTLA-4 +49A/G and −318C/T polymorphisms and susceptibility to multiple sclerosis: a meta-analysis. Immunol Investig. 2013;42(5):409–22.
88. Wagner M, Sobczyński M, Karabon L, Bilińska M, Pokryszko-Dragan A, Pawlak-Adamska E, et al. Polymorphisms in CD28, CTLA-4, CD80 and CD86 genes may influence the risk of multiple sclerosis and its age of onset. J Neuroimmunol. 2015;288:79–86.
89. Karabon L, Kosmaczewska A, Bilinska M, Pawlak E, Ciszak L, Jedynak A, et al. The CTLA-4 gene polymorphisms are associated with CTLA-4 protein expression levels in multiple sclerosis patients and with susceptibility to disease. Immunology. 2009;128(1 Suppl):e787–96.
90. Mohammadzadeh A, Rad IA, Ahmadi-Salmasi B. CTLA-4, PD-1 and TIM-3 expression predominantly downregulated in MS patients. J Neuroimmunol. 2018;323:105–8.
91. Machcińska M, Kierasińska M, Michniowska M, Maruszewska-Cheruiyot M, Szewczak L, Rola R, et al. Reduced expression of PD-1 in circulating CD4+ and CD8+ Tregs is an early feature of RRMS. Int J Mol Sci. 2022;23(6).
92. Derakhshani A, Asadzadeh Z, Safarpour H, Leone P, Shadbad MA, Heydari A, et al. Regulation of CTLA-4 and PD-L1 expression in relapsing-remitting multiple sclerosis patients after treatment with fingolimod, IFNβ-1α, glatiramer acetate, and dimethyl fumarate drugs. J Personal Med. 2021;11(8).
93. Basile MS, Bramanti P, Mazzon E. The role of cytotoxic T-lymphocyte antigen 4 in the pathogenesis of multiple sclerosis. Genes. 2022;13(8).
94. Viglietta V, Bourcier K, Buckle GJ, Healy B, Weiner HL, Hafler DA, et al. CTLA4Ig treatment in patients with multiple sclerosis: an open-label, phase 1 clinical trial. Neurology. 2008;71(12):917–24.
95. Khoury SJ, Rochon J, Ding L, Byron M, Ryker K, Tosta P, et al. ACCLAIM: a randomized trial of abatacept (CTLA4-Ig) for relapsing-remitting multiple sclerosis. Mult Scler. 2017;23(5):686–95.
96. Saresella M, Piancone F, Marventano I, La Rosa F, Tortorella P, Caputo D, et al. A role for the TIM-3/GAL-9/BAT3 pathway in determining the clinical phenotype of multiple sclerosis. FASEB J. 2014;28(11):5000–9.
97. Lee HJ, Li CW, Hammerstad SS, Stefan M, Tomer Y. Immunogenetics of autoimmune thyroid diseases: a comprehensive review. J Autoimmun. 2015;64:82–90.
98. Lane LC, Wood CL, Cheetham T. Graves' disease: moving forwards. Arch Dis Child. 2023;108(4):276–81.
99. Danailova Y, Velikova T, Nikolaev G, Mitova Z, Shinkov A, Gagov H, et al. Nutritional management of thyroiditis of Hashimoto. Int J Mol Sci. 2022;23(9).

100. Chiorean AD, Vica ML, Bâlici Ș, Nicula GZ, Răcătăianu N, Bordea MA, et al. The C55A single nucleotide polymorphism in CTLA-4 gene, a new possible biomarker in thyroid autoimmune pathology such as Hashimoto's thyroiditis. Diagnostics. 2023;13(15):2517.
101. Huang F, He Q, Jiao X, Zhang H, Chang Q. Meta-analysis of CTLA-4 +49 gene polymorphism and susceptibility to Graves' disease. Crit Rev Eukaryot Gene Expr. 2020;30(5):377–90.
102. Shi M, Liu X, Song Q, Shi Y, Tai Q. Meta-analysis of the rs231775 locus polymorphism in the CTLA-4 gene and the susceptibility to Graves' disease in children. Open Life Sci. 2023;18(1):20220589.
103. Fouad NA, Saeed AM, Mahedy AW. Association of CTLA-4 +49 A/G and CT60 gene polymorphism with Graves' disease. Egypt J Immunol. 2017;24(2):63–70.
104. Kawabata M, Inoue N, Watanabe M, Kobayashi A, Hidaka Y, Miyauchi A, et al. PD-1 gene polymorphisms and thyroid expression of PD-1 ligands differ between Graves' and Hashimoto's diseases. Autoimmunity. 2021;54(7):450–9.
105. Pyzik A, Grywalska E, Matyjaszek-Matuszek B, Smoleń A, Pyzik D, Roliński J. Frequencies of PD-1- positive T CD3+CD4+, T CD3+CD8+ and B CD19+ lymphocytes in female patients with Graves' disease and healthy controls- preliminary study. Mol Cell Endocrinol. 2017;448:28–33.
106. Álvarez-Sierra D, Marín-Sánchez A, Ruiz-Blázquez P, de Jesús GC, Iglesias-Felip C, González Ó, et al. Analysis of the PD-1/PD-L1 axis in human autoimmune thyroid disease: insights into pathogenesis and clues to immunotherapy associated thyroid autoimmunity. J Autoimmun. 2019;103:102285.
107. Zhong Y, Lu TT, Liu XM, Liu BL, Hu Y, Liu S, et al. High levels of thyroid hormone impair regulatory T cell function via reduced PD-1 expression. J Clin Endocrinol Metab. 2021;106(9):2738–53.
108. Ortega-Rodríguez AC, Martínez-Hernández R, Monsiváis-Urenda A, Serrano-Somavilla A, Sánchez-Gutiérrez R, González-Amaro R, et al. Quantitative and functional analysis of PD-1+ NK cells in patients with autoimmune thyroid disease. J Clin Endocrinol Metab. 2020;105(11).
109. Han H, Fu X, Huang J, Zhang X, Yu J. PD-1/PD-L1 affects Graves progression through lymphocytes on the proliferation, apoptosis and inflammatory cytokine secretion of thyroid follicular epithelial cells. J Toxicol Sci. 2020;45(11):701–11.
110. Rendon A, Schäkel K. Psoriasis pathogenesis and treatment. Int J Mol Sci. 2019;20(6):1475.
111. Kamiya K, Kishimoto M, Sugai J, Komine M, Ohtsuki M. Risk factors for the development of psoriasis. Int J Mol Sci. 2019;20(18):4347.
112. Liu S, Xu J, Wu J. The role of co-signaling molecules in psoriasis and their implications for targeted treatment. Front Pharmacol. 2021;12:717042.
113. Liu P, He Y, Wang H, Kuang Y, Chen W, Li J, et al. The expression of mCTLA-4 in skin lesion inversely correlates with the severity of psoriasis. J Dermatol Sci. 2018;89(3):233–40.
114. Lee WS, Nam KH, Kim JH, Kim WJ, Kim JE, Shin EC, et al. Alleviating psoriatic skin inflammation through augmentation of Treg cells via CTLA-4 signaling peptide. Front Immunol. 2023;14:1233514.
115. Adamczyk M, Krasowska D. PD1/PD-L1 pathway in psoriasis and psoriatic arthritis: a review. Postepy Dermatol Alergol. 2021;38(6):925–30.
116. Bartosińska J, Zakrzewska E, Purkot J, Michalak-Stoma A, Kowal M, Krasowska D, et al. Decreased blood CD4+PD-1+ and CD8+PD-1+ T cells in psoriatic patients with and without arthritis. Postepy Dermatol Alergol. 2018;35(4):344–50.
117. Adamczyk M, Bartosińska J, Raczkiewicz D, Michalak-Stoma A, Krasowska D. The impact of biologic treatment on PD-1/PD-L1 pathway disturbances in psoriasis. J Clin Med. 2023;12(13).
118. Peled M, Strazza M, Azoulay-Alfaguter I, Silverman GJ, Scher JU, Mor A. Analysis of programmed death-1 in patients with psoriatic arthritis. Inflammation. 2015;38(4):1573–9.

119. Emre S, Süngü N, Hayran Y, Demirseren DD, Aktas A, Duman T. Investigation of the PD-1/PD-L1 expression in the lesional skins of patients with psoriasis. Dermatol Pract Concept. 2023;13(2).
120. Jung CJ, Yang HJ, Bang SH, Lee WJ, Won CH, Lee MW, et al. Clinicoprognostic and histopathological features of guttate and plaque psoriasis based on PD-1 expression. J Clin Med. 2021;10(21).
121. Maahs DM, West NA, Lawrence JM, Mayer-Davis EJ. Epidemiology of type 1 diabetes. Endocrinol Metab Clin N Am. 2010;39(3):481–97.
122. Powers AC. Type 1 diabetes mellitus: much progress, many opportunities. J Clin Invest. 2021;131(8).
123. Primavera M, Giannini C, Chiarelli F. Prediction and prevention of type 1 diabetes. Front Endocrinol. 2020;11:248.
124. Wang B, Du W, Jia Y, Zhang X, Ma G. Cytotoxic T-lymphocyte-associated protein 4 +49A/G polymorphisms contribute to the risk of type 1 diabetes in children: an updated systematic review and meta-analysis with trial sequential analysis. Oncotarget. 2017;8(6):10553–64.
125. Chen Z, Fei M, Fu D, Zhang L, Ma Y, Wang Y, et al. Association between cytotoxic T lymphocyte antigen-4 polymorphism and type 1 diabetes: a meta-analysis. Gene. 2013;516(2):263–70.
126. Si X, Zhang X, Luo Y, Tang W. Association between the CTLA-4 +49A/G polymorphism and type 1 diabetes: a meta-analysis. Genet Test Mol Biomarkers. 2012;16(11):1336–42.
127. Chen Y, Chen S, Gu Y, Feng Y, Shi Y, Fu Q, et al. CTLA-4 +49G/A, a functional T1D risk SNP, affects CTLA-4 level in Treg subsets and IA-2A positivity, but not beta-cell function. Sci Rep. 2018;8(1):10074.
128. Bruzzaniti S, Piemonte E, Bruzzese D, Lepore MT, Strollo R, Izzo L, et al. Progression of type 1 diabetes is associated with high levels of soluble PD-1 in islet autoantibody-positive children. Diabetologia. 2024;67(4):714–23.
129. Fujisawa R, Haseda F, Tsutsumi C, Hiromine Y, Noso S, Kawabata Y, et al. Low programmed cell death-1 (PD-1) expression in peripheral CD4(+) T cells in Japanese patients with autoimmune type 1 diabetes. Clin Exp Immunol. 2015;180(3):452–7.
130. Granados HM, Draghi A 2nd, Tsurutani N, Wright K, Fernandez ML, Sylvester FA, et al. Programmed cell death-1, PD-1, is dysregulated in T cells from children with new onset type 1 diabetes. PLoS One. 2017;12(9):e0183887.
131. Colli ML, Hill JLE, Marroquí L, Chaffey J, Dos Santos RS, Leete P, et al. PDL1 is expressed in the islets of people with type 1 diabetes and is up-regulated by interferons-α and-γ via IRF1 induction. EBioMedicine. 2018;36:367–75.
132. Liu C, Jiang J, Gao L, Hu X, Wang F, Shen Y, et al. A promoter region polymorphism in PDCD-1 gene is associated with risk of rheumatoid arthritis in the Han Chinese population of southeastern China. Int J Genomics. 2014;2014(1):247637.
133. Zou YuMing ZY, Zhang ZiTeng ZZ, Liu YanGang LY, Liu DengHui LD, Xu WeiDong XW. Are programmed cell death 1 gene polymorphisms correlated with susceptibility to rheumatoid arthritis?: a meta-analysis. 2017.
134. Zhou C, Gao S, Yuan X, Shu Z, Li S, Sun X, et al. Association between CTLA-4 gene polymorphism and risk of rheumatoid arthritis: a meta-analysis. Aging (Albany NY). 2021;13(15):19397.
135. Yu L, Shao M, Zhou T, Xie H, Wang F, Kong J, et al. Association of CTLA-4 (+ 49 A/G) polymorphism with susceptibility to autoimmune diseases: a meta-analysis with trial sequential analysis. Int Immunopharmacol. 2021;96:107617.
136. Razi B, Reykandeh SE, Alizadeh S, Amirzargar A, Saghazadeh A, Rezaei N. TIM family gene polymorphism and susceptibility to rheumatoid arthritis: systematic review and meta-analysis. PLoS One. 2019;14(2):e0211146.
137. Liu R, Wang X, Chen X, Wang S, Zhang H. TIM-3 rs1036199 polymorphism increases susceptibility to autoimmune diseases: evidence based on 4200 subjects. Biosci Rep. 2018;38(6):BSR20181235.

138. Oki M, Watanabe N, Owada T, Oya Y, Ikeda K, Saito Y, et al. A functional polymorphism in B and T lymphocyte attenuator is associated with susceptibility to rheumatoid arthritis. J Immunol Res. 2011;2011(1):305656.
139. Lin S-C, Kuo C-C, Chan C-H. Association of a BTLA gene polymorphism with the risk of rheumatoid arthritis. J Biomed Sci. 2006;13:853–60.
140. Gao J, Gai N, Wang L, Liu K, Liu X-H, Wei L-T, et al. Meta-analysis of programmed cell death 1 polymorphisms with systemic lupus erythematosus risk. Oncotarget. 2017;8(22):36885.
141. Xiao J-P, He W-T, Wang X-R, Wang J, Wang J, Pan H-F, et al. Association of PDCD1 gene polymorphisms with systemic lupus erythematosus and lupus nephritis: an up-date meta-analysis. Int J Clin Exp Med. 2016;9(11):20571–82.
142. Qi Y-y, Zhao X-y, Liu X-r, Wang Y-n, Zhai Y-l, Zhang X-x, et al. Lupus susceptibility region containing CTLA4 rs17268364 functionally reduces CTLA4 expression by binding EWSR1 and correlates IFN-α signature. Arthritis Res Ther. 2021;23:1–9.
143. Louthrenoo W, Kasitanon N, Wongthanee A, Kuwata S, Takeuchi F. CTLA-4 polymorphisms in Thai patients with rheumatoid arthritis, systemic lupus erythematosus, and systemic sclerosis. Int J Rheum Dis. 2021;24(11):1378–85.
144. Li W-X, Chen G-M, Yuan H, Yao Y-S, Li R-J, Pan H-F, et al. Polymorphisms of the TIM-1 and TIM-3 genes are not associated with systemic lupus erythematosus in a Chinese population. Mutagenesis. 2011;26(4):507–11.
145. Meng Q, Guo H, Hou S, Jiang Z, Kijlstra A, Yang P. Lack of an association of PD-1 and its ligand genes with Behcet's disease in a Chinese Han population. PLoS One. 2011;6(10):e25345.
146. Zhang Y, Xu W, Duan Z, Liu S, Pan H, Ye D. Lack of association between CTLA-4+ 49A/G and-318C/T polymorphisms and Behçet's disease risk: a meta-analysis. Clin Exp Rheumatol. 2012;30(3):S46.
147. Abbaspour-Aghdam S, Ahmadi M, Aslani S, Daneshmandpour Y, Mehdizadeh A, Valizadeh H, et al. Molecular analysis of CTLA4 gene in patients with Behçet's disease from an Iranian Northwest Azeri population. Gene Rep. 2020;19:100612.
148. Ataei M, Behfarjam F, Jadali Z. TIM-3 genetic variants and risk of Behçet disease in the Iranian population. An Bras Dermatol. 2019;94(4):429–33.
149. Cetin Y, Ilhan NF, Sen D, Karakas CS. The investigation of BTLA single-nucleotide polymorphisms in patients with Behcet disease in Elazıg province. Turk J Biochem. 2020;45(3):323–7.
150. Kroner A, Mehling M, Hemmer B, Rieckmann P, Toyka KV, Mäurer M, et al. A PD-1 polymorphism is associated with disease progression in multiple sclerosis. Ann Neurol. 2005;58(1):50–7.
151. Gyu Song G, Ho LY. CTLA-4+ 49 A/G and− 318 C/T polymorphisms and susceptibility to multiple sclerosis: a meta-analysis. Immunol Investig. 2013;42(5):409–22.
152. Yaghoobi E, Abedian S, Babani O, Maryam I. TIM-3 rs10515746 (A/C) and rs10053538 (C/A) gene polymorphisms and risk of multiple sclerosis. Iran J Public Health. 2016;45(5):644.
153. Al-Eitan L, Al Qudah M, Al Qawasmeh M. Association of multiple sclerosis phenotypes with single nucleotide polymorphisms of IL7R, LAG3, and CD40 genes in a Jordanian population: a genotype-phenotype study. Biomolecules. 2020;10(3):356.
154. Zanatta E, Ferrazzi B, Michelotto A, Cozzi F, Frigo AC, Alaibac M. PD-1 gene rs2227981 (PD-1.5) polymorphism analysis in patients with systemic sclerosis. Gene Rep. 2020;20:100776.
155. Gottenberg J-E, Loiseau P, Azarian M, Chen C, Cagnard N, Hachulla E, et al. CTLA-4+ 49A/G and CT60 gene polymorphisms in primary Sjögren syndrome. Arthritis Res Ther. 2007;9:1–3.
156. Chen S, Li Y, Deng C, Li J, Wen X, Wu Z, et al. The associations between PD-1, CTLA-4 gene polymorphisms and susceptibility to ankylosing spondylitis: a meta-analysis and systemic review. Rheumatol Int. 2016;36:33–44.

157. Mitchell AL, Cordell HJ, Soemedi R, Owen K, Skinningsrud B, Wolff AB, et al. Programmed death ligand 1 (PD-L1) gene variants contribute to autoimmune Addison's disease and Graves' disease susceptibility. J Clin Endocrinol Metabol. 2009;94(12):5139–45.
158. Borysewicz-Sańczyk H, Sawicka B, Wawrusiewicz-Kurylonek N, Głowińska-Olszewska B, Kadłubiska A, Gościk J, et al. Genetic association study of IL2RA, IFIH1, and CTLA-4 polymorphisms with autoimmune thyroid diseases and type 1 diabetes. Front Pediatr. 2020;8:481.
159. Ni J, Qiu L-J, Zhang M, Wen P-F, Ye X-R, Liang Y, et al. CTLA-4 CT60 (rs3087243) polymorphism and autoimmune thyroid diseases susceptibility: a comprehensive meta-analysis. Endocr Res. 2014;39(4):180–8.
160. Xu G, Zheng K, Lu X, Wang J, Chai Y, Wang J. Association between polymorphisms in the promoter region of T cell immunoglobulin and mucin domain-3 and myasthenia gravis-associated thymoma. Oncol Lett. 2015;9(3):1470–4.
161. Liang T, Wang XB, Cai PC, Tang ZM, Chen ZZ, Hu LH. Polymorphisms of the T-cell immunoglobulin and mucin domain molecule-3 are not associated with autoimmune Graves' disease in a Chinese Han Population. Clin Biochem. 2012;45(18):1624–8.
162. Hu Y, Xu K, Jiang L, Zhang L, Shi H, Cui D. Associations between three CTLA-4 polymorphisms and Hashimoto's thyroiditis risk: an updated meta-analysis with trial sequential analysis. Genet Test Mol Biomarkers. 2018;22(4):224–36.
163. Hua S, Fan B, Mao W, Xu R, Wang Y, Kuai L, et al. Association between PDCD1 gene polymorphisms and psoriasis susceptibility in the Chinese population. Int J Dermatol. 2021;60(11):1411–7.
164. Liang J, Zhang S, Luo Q, Li W, Tian X, Zhang F, et al. Lack of association between cytotoxic T-lymphocyte antigen-4+ 49A/G polymorphism and psoriasis and vitiligo: a meta-analysis of case–control studies. Gene. 2015;568(2):196–202.
165. Mohamed RA, Morgan DS, Hodeib M, Radwan A, Ali HF. The genetic influence of PD-1/PD-L1 axis single nucleotide polymorphisms on the incidence of type 1 diabetes mellitus in pediatric Egyptian patients. Egypt J Med Hum Genet. 2022;23(1):90.
166. Fathima N, Narne P, Ishaq M. Association and gene–gene interaction analyses for polymorphic variants in CTLA-4 and FOXP3 genes: role in susceptibility to autoimmune thyroid disease. Endocrine. 2019;64:591–604.
167. Brück P, Ramos-Lopez E, Bartsch W, Böhme A, Badenhoop K. TIM-3 polymorphisms in type 1 diabetes families. J Hum Genet. 2008;53(6):559–64.
168. Inuo M, Ihara K, Matsuo T, Kohno H, Hara T. Association study between B-and T-lymphocyte attenuator gene and type 1 diabetes mellitus or systemic lupus erythematosus in the Japanese population. Int J Immunogenet. 2009;36(1):65–8.

Chapter 8
Immune Checkpoints in Asthma

8.1 Introduction

Asthma is a heterogeneous disease affecting airways, which manifests various symptoms, including cough, chest tightness, shortness of breathing, wheezing, and variable airflow obstruction. Asthma prevalence has been increasing in recent decades. Various environmental and genetic factors affect the clinical phenotypes of the disease [1]. Allergic asthma is the most common form of asthma. It usually occurs in children with varying degrees of severity and can progress to severe asthma in adulthood. Sensitization to environmental allergens plays a key role in the onset of asthma in early life [2]. Historically, asthma has been considered a T helper 2 (Th2)-cell-mediated disease. Nevertheless, over time, it became clear that in addition to the Th2 response, more complex mechanisms are involved in the immunopathology of asthma. These findings led to a revision in the classification of asthma phenotype, which today is divided into two general categories: type 2-high asthma and type 2-low asthma. The role of immune checkpoints in the pathogenesis of autoimmune diseases and cancers has been well described. In addition to these clinical conditions, it has been found that immune checkpoints are important in the prevention or development of asthma. In this chapter, the evidence of the role of various immune checkpoints in the pathogenesis and outcome of asthma is discussed.

8.2 Immune Response in Asthma

Disruption of the epithelial barrier by various external environment elements, such as microbes, pollutants, tobacco smoke, allergens, and detergents, facilitates the penetration of substances into the tissue. Dendritic cells (DCs) recognize and

L. Tayebi, M. Abdolmaleki, *Immune System Regulation*,
https://doi.org/10.1007/978-981-95-8026-2_8

capture antigens by their receptors. DCs then migrate from the subepithelial layer to the draining lymph nodes and present allergens to $CD4^+$ T cells and differentiate them into Th2 cells (mainly driven by IL-4) [3]. The thymic stromal lymphopoietin (TSLP), IL-25, and IL-33 cytokines secreted by activated epithelial cells stimulate tissue type 2 innate lymphoid cells (ILC2s). Th2 cells and ILC2s, through secretion of IL-5, IL-9, and IL-13 cytokines, promote airway inflammation, including mucus production, activation of epithelium, mast cells, and eosinophils [3, 4]. Th2 switches the B cell response toward IgE production. IgE-dependent activation of mast cells leads to the release of several mediators (histamine, serotonin, lipid mediators, and proteases). In the delayed phase of the allergic response, the Th2 response is more extensive and is associated with eosinophil recruitment and the production of various cytokines [5].

8.2.1 *Mast Cell*

Mast cells are large granular cells resident in mucosal and epithelial tissues that are derived from the myeloid lineage. Classically, mast cells are divided into two phenotypes: connective tissue-type mast cells (CTMCs) and mucosal mast cells (MMCs). CTMCs produce tryptase, chymase and carboxypeptidase, cathepsin G, while MMCs contain only tryptase [6, 7]. Mast cells can recognize microbial particles and respond to pathogens. They also participate in wound healing and tissue repair. Masts are important cells in promoting allergic reactions and asthma. They express a high-affinity receptor for allergen-specific IgE (FcεRI). Antigen recognition by IgE-FcεRI stimulates mast cells [8, 9]. Activated mast cells release various substances. Some of them, such as proteases, proteoglycans, and neuropeptides, are stored in granules, and the other groups, including lipid mediators and cytokines, are de novo synthesized. Histamine is one of the most well-known mediators of mast cells, which exerts various effects, including increasing epithelial barrier permeability and inducing the production of various cytokines and chemokines. Prostaglandin and leukotriene are two main mediators derived from arachidonic acid that promote a set of inflammatory mechanisms, including bronchoconstriction and recruiting and stimulating immune cells, such as eosinophil and ILC2. Mast cells also secrete various cytokines, such as IL-1, IL-18, IL-6, IL-13, TNF-α, CXCL1, and IL-8, which are involved in the pathology of asthma [7–9].

8.2.2 *Eosinophil*

Eosinophils are a subset of granulocytes that are about 10–16 μm in diameter. Eosinophils in the bone marrow differentiate from the myeloid lineage under stimulation by IL3, GM-CSF, and IL-5. The presence of eosinophils in various organs, such as lymphatic and mucous tissues and skin, is involved in the formation of the immune response. Eosinophils are involved in both infectious and noninfectious situations. They are important cells in defense against helminth parasites. Eosinophils are also important players in allergic asthma [10, 11]. Two main types of granules are observed in eosinophils. Large specific granules contain mediators, such as major basic protein (MBP), eosinophil cationic protein (ECP), eosinophil peroxidase (EPO), and eosinophil-derived neurotoxin (EDN). Primary granules are smaller and contain Charcot-Leyden and hexagonal bipyramidal crystals [10]. Eosinophils express various cytokine and chemokine receptors on their surface, including IL-5, IL-4, IL-13, IL-33, and TSLP receptors. IL-5, produced by Th2 cells and mast cells, plays an important role in the stimulation of eosinophils. They also express CCR1 and CCR3. CCR1 is activated by chemoattractant cytokine ligand-3 (CCL-3) and CCL-5 (RANTES). CCR3 binds to monocyte chemoattractant protein-3 (MCP-3) and MCP-4. These chemokines are important for eosinophil recruitment to the airways during asthma. Eosinophils also express FcεR1, which leads to their activation by binding to IgE. Accumulation of eosinophils in airways during allergic inflammation can lead to tissue damage and fibrosis. These effects are mediated through the release of various factors, including EPO, MBP, TGF-β, IL4, and IL13 [10, 12, 13].

8.2.3 Innate Lymphoid Cells (ILCs)

ILCs belong to the innate immune system and lack antigen receptors of T and B cells. They mainly reside in mucosal tissues. In addition to antimicrobial defense, they also participate in tissue repair and remodeling. ILC1s play a role in eliminating bacteria and viruses. The expression of T-bet transcription factor and IFN-γ production are the characteristics of these cells. ILC2s are found in the skin, lung, gut, and adipose tissue and participate in the fight against parasites. Development and activation of these cells are dependent on IL-33, IL-25, and TSLP. After activation, they secrete large amounts of IL-5 and IL-13. Along with Th2 cells, ILC2s play a prominent role in asthma pathogenesis. ILC3s are mainly resident in the intestinal lamina propria and partially in the lung and liver. Like Th17 cells, RORγt is the main transcription factor of ILC3s. These cells activated after stimulation with IL-23 and IL-1β and secrete IL-17A, IL-22, and TNF-α [14, 15].

8.3 Phenotypes of Asthma

Due to the general respiratory symptoms, the classification of asthma subtypes is complicated. According to various criteria, including clinical, biological, physiological, pathological, treatment response state, and prognostic factors, different phenotypes of asthma have been described [16]. The first phenotypic classification of asthma was made in the 1940s, which consisted of two categories: extrinsic (allergic or related to atopy) and intrinsic (nonallergic or independent of atopy). Later, with the identification of Th cells, it has been revealed that the Th2 response plays a central role in atopic asthma [5]. Nevertheless, the Th2-inflammation hypothesis is not a perfect model to explain the mechanism of asthma. Th2 cells are important immune cells in asthma endotypes (a subtype of a disease, which is characterized by a distinct pathophysiological mechanism). However, poor efficacy of Th2-targeted treatments of asthma and the recurrence of symptoms in some patients indicate the presence of more complex underlying mechanisms [17]. Woodruff et al. suggested that the Th2 response in asthma can create two distinct phenotypes, including Th2-high and Th2-low asthma. The Th2-high phenotype is associated with high production of IL-13 and IL-5 and airway eosinophilia. IL-5 plays an essential role in the systemic eosinophilia of this asthma phenotype. In the Th2-low phenotype, other mechanisms, such as neutrophilic inflammation along with high levels of IL-17, are involved in the pathology of asthma [18]. Further studies revealed that in addition to the Th2 response, ILCs are also important players in the immunopathology of asthma. Therefore, T2-high and T2-low asthma (instead of Th2-high and Th2-low) are more accurate terms in asthma terminology [19].

8.3.1 T2-High Asthma

T2-high phenotype affects children and ranges from mild to severe disease. Th2 and ILC2 cells are responsible for the lung inflammatory response in the T2-high phenotype. Eosinophilia and secretion of cytokines IL-5, IL-4, IL-13, IL-9, and prostaglandin D2 (PGD2) are the characteristics of T2 inflammation. Due to the high frequency of eosinophils, T2-high asthma is also known as eosinophilic asthma. T2-high phenotype is divided into three main groups, including early-onset allergic asthma, late-onset eosinophilic asthma, and aspirin-exacerbated respiratory disease (AERD). The distinguishing features of these patients from T2-high nonatopic asthma are positive allergy skin tests and increased allergen-specific serum IgE [5, 20].

Early-onset asthma usually occurs in childhood and is characterized by allergen-specific IgE and atopy. Atopic march is determined by the symptoms of atopic dermatitis, allergic rhinitis, and asthma. Allergen-specific IgE levels are high in these patients and L-13, IL- 33, IL-4 and GATA3 genes are actively expressed [5, 14, 20]. Late-onset eosinophilic asthma occurs in adults and is usually more severe. It is defined by eosinophilia refractory to corticosteroid treatment. Late-onset asthma is less allergic, with an increased population of eosinophils in sputum, bronchus, and blood. During late-onset asthma, in the absence of atopy and IgE-dependent response, mucosal tissue-resident ILC2s contribute to asthma development. These cells cause epithelial cell proliferation and airway remodeling by secreting effector mediators (such as amphiregulin). IL-13, IL-5, eotaxin, and inducible nitric oxide synthase (iNOS) levels are increased in these patients. Severe late-onset asthma is defined by high eosinophilia, impaired lung function, and airflow obstruction [5, 14, 20].

8.3.2 T2-Low Asthma

The T2-low phenotype exhibits different characteristics from T2-high asthma, which include neutrophilic asthma (sputum neutrophilia, low eosinophil), mixed granulocytic asthma (sputum neutrophilia with high eosinophils), and paucigranulocytic asthma (neutrophil and eosinophil within normal range). Neutrophilic asthma is associated with Th1/Th17 cytokine (TNF-α, IL-22, L-17A, L-17F). Paucigranulocytic asthma is accompanied by airway smooth muscle hypertrophy. Based on various factors, T2-low asthma is divided into three groups: obesity associated asthma, smoking-associated asthma, and very late onset (over 50 years old) asthma. The T1 immune response (including Th1 and ILC1), which is associated with high production of IFN-γ, and the T3 immune response (driven by Th17 and ILC3), characterized by the production of IL-17 family and IL-22 cytokines, are the main immune responses that shape the T2- low phenotype [5, 14, 20, 21].

8.4 Role of Immune Checkpoints in Asthma Prevention or Development

8.4.1 CTLA-4

According to several meta-analyses, CTLA-4 +49 A/G polymorphism is related to susceptibility to asthma and is considered a risk factor in this disease [22–25]. It has been demonstrated that the expression of soluble CTLA-4 (sCTLA-4) is increased in asthmatic patients [26]. Based on a study, plasma levels of sCTLA-4 were significantly increased in both nonsteroid-treated and steroid-treated asthmatic patients. However, the expression of membrane CTLA-4 (mCTLA-4) on peripheral blood mononuclear cells (PBMCs) of the patients was comparable to that of control subjects [27]. Chan et al. showed that sCTLA-4 in asthma patients was negatively associated with forced expiratory volume in 1 s (FEV1)/forced vital capacity (FVC) [28]. Another study indicated that the plasma concentrations of sCTLA-4, sCD28, sCD80, and sCD86 were significantly increased during the primary acute attack in asthmatic children. As the acute phase of the disease subsided, the levels of these markers decreased [29]. It has also been reported that sCTLA-4 is elevated in both atopic and nonatopic asthma and is associated with disease severity [30]. sCTLA-4 can dampen the inhibitory signal of mCTLA-4/B7 axis by binding to B7 (CD86/CD80) molecules on antigen-presenting cells (APCs). On the other hand, sCTLA-4 may interfere with T cell activation by inhibiting the ligation of CD28 by B7.

Suppressing Th1 response and further activation of Th2 cells are possible functional mechanisms of sCTLA-4 in asthma [27, 28]. Based on these findings, sCTLA-4 levels are related to impaired lung function and the severity of asthma.

8.4.2 *PD-1*

The association of PD-1 polymorphisms with asthma has also been studied. For example, a study has shown that the PD-1.3 polymorphism of the PD-1 gene is related to IgE-mediated bronchial asthma and total serum IgE levels in the Russian population [31]. The association of the PD-1/PD-L1 pathway and asthma has been investigated in several mouse and human studies [32]. Neutrophilic asthma is one of the asthma phenotypes that occurs in adults as a severe disease. Helou et al. demonstrated that deletion of the PD-1 gene in a mouse model of acute neutrophilic asthma exacerbated airway hyperreactivity (AHR) and increased recruitment of inflammatory cells to the lung compared to wild-type (WT) mice in response to house dust mite challenge. The number of leukocytes, especially neutrophils and T cells, was increased in bronchoalveolar lavage (BAL). In addition, BAL of PD-1 knock-out (KO) mice contained higher amounts of inflammatory mediators, such as TNF-α, IL-17A, IFN-γ, and IL-6, as well as neutrophil-recruiting mediators, such as G-CSF, MCP-1, and CXCL-10. In general, deletion of PD-1 was associated with increased AHR. In addition, they showed that a PD-1 agonist is effective in reducing the recruitment of neutrophils, T cells, and alveolar macrophages to lung inflammation and, consequently, suppression of AHR. In PD-1-expressing mice treated with PD-1 agonist, a decrease in the levels of IFN-γ, IL-6, TNF-α, and IL-17 was observed in BAL. Therefore, targeting the PD-1 pathway may be one of the novel therapeutic approaches in modulating the immune response in asthma [33].

The correlation between PD-1/PD-L1 signaling and Treg/Th17 imbalance in asthmatic children has been investigated by Xi. They found that the Treg/Th17 ratio in the peripheral blood of mild persistent (MP) and moderate to severe persistent (MS) asthma groups was decreased compared to the mild intermittent (MI) group and healthy controls. Evaluation of PD-1/PD-L1 expression showed that the percentage of PD-1$^+$ Treg and PD-L1$^+$ Th17 cells was significantly higher in the MP and MS groups than in healthy controls and MI groups. Conversely, the percentage of PD-L1$^+$ cell Treg and PD-L1$^+$ Th17 was lower in the MP and MS groups. Furthermore, in vitro assessment of anti-PD-1 treatment effect on the differentiation of T cells showed that anti-PD-1 decreased Th17 differentiation and increased Treg differentiation. In addition, the administration of anti-PD-1 to the mouse model of asthma was associated with an elevated Treg/Th17 ratio [34].

As mentioned above, ILCs are important cells in asthmatic inflammation. ILC2s have similar functions to Th2 cells. These cells express some immune checkpoints on their surface, including CTLA-4, PD-1, CD200 receptor, TIGIT, and KLRG1 [35]. A research group evaluated the effect of the PD-1 pathway on the regulation of ILC2 response during airway inflammation. The results showed that the expression of PD-1 on pulmonary ILC2s was strongly increased in IL-33-challenged mice (in order to induce AHR). Activated ILC2s in PD-1-KO mice produced higher levels of IL-5, IL-13, and IL-9 compared to WT, indicating the modulatory effect of PD-1/PD-L1 axis in cytokine production of ILC2s. In addition, the lack of PD-1 decreased apoptosis and increased the proliferation of ILC2s. On the other hand, deletion of PD-1 altered metabolic activity and enhanced glycolytic metabolism in these cells. Interestingly, lung inflammation and AHR were ameliorated in IL-33-treated PD-1 KO mice compared to WT. Examining the effect of PD-1 agonist in human ILC2s culture revealed that PD-1 blockade dampened the production of IL-5 and IL-13. Moreover, the PD-1 agonist reduced ILC2-dependent AHR in humanized mice. In conclusion, these findings indicate the role of PD-1 in regulating the effector functions, survival, and proliferation of ILC2s in asthma [36].

8.4.3 TIM-3

TIM-3 is another inhibitory receptor that is involved in the regulation of immune response in asthma. A meta-analysis of 11 case-control studies revealed that the TIM-3574T>G polymorphism is associated with increased susceptibility to asthma and is considered a risk factor in this disease [37]. It has also been reported that +4259 T>G and −574 G>T polymorphisms are associated with asthma susceptibility in the Iranian population [38]. Nonetheless, the role of TIM-3 in allergic airway inflammation is controversial. Some studies have stated that TIM-3 is dispensable for the development of airway inflammation in mouse models [39, 40]. For example, by evaluating the effect of TIM-3 in the ovalbumin (OVA)-induced asthma mouse model, Boehne et al. indicated that TIM-3 KO mice and WT mice were comparable in various parameters, such as Th2 cytokine production and eosinophilic inflammation [41]. On the other hand, Kearley et al. showed that blockade of TIM-3 is effective in improving airway inflammation. Preliminary evaluations showed that the expression of TIM-3 on $CD4^+$ T cells of lung tissue was increased in the experimental model of allergen-induced airway inflammation. In the next step, they investigated the effect of anti-TIM-3 blocking antibodies after OVA challenge in mice injected with OVA-reactive Th2-polarized cells. The results showed that blocking TIM-3 reduced IL-5 and IL-13 levels in lung tissue homogenate and BAL, while IFN-γ was increased. Moreover, in the presence of anti-TIM-3, the levels of proinflammatory chemokines, including CCL-11 (eotaxin), CCL22, CCL2 (MCP-1), and CCL5 (RANTES), were decreased in the lung. In addition, lung tissue eosinophils were also reduced. They suggested that inhibition of TIM-3 signaling shifts the allergen-dependent T cell response toward a Th1 phenotype and may be beneficial in reducing allergen-induced airway inflammation [42]. Furthermore, increased expression of TIM-3 on $CD4^+$ T cells has been observed in allergic asthma patients. Inhibition of TIM-3 signaling by blocking antibodies increased the production of Th1 cytokines (IFN-γ and TNF-α) and decreased Th2 cytokines (IL-4,

IL-5, and IL-13) in PBMCs derived from the asthma patients, which indicates the relationship of TIM-3 with Th1/Th2 imbalance in asthma [43].

8.4.4 *CD200-CD200R*

The CD200-CD200R axis is one of the important regulators of immune homeostasis. CD200 is expressed on a wide range of immune cells and normal tissues. Upregulation of CD200 in hematologic malignancies is associated with tumor progression. CD200 receptor (CD200R) is highly expressed on tumor-infiltrating myeloid cells, including tumor-associated macrophages, myeloid-derived suppressor cells, and tumor-associated dendritic cells. CD200R lacks immunoreceptor tyrosine-based inhibitory motifs (ITIMs) in the cytoplasmic tail and exerts its inhibitory signal through the binding of adapter protein Dok2 to the NPxY motif [44–46].

CD200 is expressed on airway epithelium and submucosal cells. Moreover, CD200R is highly expressed on alveolar macrophages. The CD200-CD200R axis plays an important role in controlling the function of lung-resident macrophages and establishing airway homeostasis [47, 48]. CD200 is one of the genes that is downregulated in asthma and is associated with disease exacerbation [49]. Lauzon-Joset et al. showed that administration of recombinant CD200 (rCD200) to a rat model of allergic asthma abolished the AHR. In addition, IL-13 levels in BAL decreased, and IL-10 was upregulated. rCD200 reduced the recruitment of Th2 cells to the lungs, but not eosinophils [50]. The role of the CD200-CD200R axis in the regulation of the effector functions of ILC2s has been comprehensively studied by Shafiei-Jahani et al. They showed that in WT mice injected with IL-33, the expression of CD200R on pulmonary ILC2s was increased. Ex vivo culture of IL-33-activated pulmonary ILC2s cells in the presence of CD200-Fc chimeric protein led to a reduction of IL-5, IL-6, IL-9, IL-13, and GM-CSF production and elevated IL-10 levels. CD200-Fc also reduced the proliferation of ILC2s. Adding CD200-Fc to human peripheral blood ILC2s delivered similar results. In vivo investigation revealed that CD200-Fc abrogated IL-33-induced AHR in mice through inhibition of ILC2 function. CD200-Fc reduced mucous production and airway epithelium thickness. Similarly, in the humanized IL-33 mouse model, administration of CD200-Fc prevented AHR. These findings indicate that CD200R engagement can be a potential therapeutic strategy for ILC2-mediated asthma [51].

8.4.5 *VISTA*

V-domain Ig suppressor of T cell activation (VISTA) is a well-known immune regulatory receptor from the B7 family, which is expressed on various immune cells such as T cells, monocytes, macrophages, and DCs. PSGL-1 and VSIG-3 have been identified as VISTA ligands. VISTA, through its SH2-binding motif, can induce inhibitory signals in T cells and suppress their functions. VISTA is overexpressed in many cancers and is associated with poor prognosis [52, 53]. The regulatory role of VISTA in suppressing asthma has been demonstrated in murine models of airway inflammation. It has been reported that the deletion of the VISTA (PD-1H) gene or blocking the signaling of this inhibitory receptor augmented lung inflammation with the accumulation of eosinophils in the mouse model of asthma. In addition, IL-5, IL-13, IL-6, MCP-1, and TNF-α levels were elevated in BAL. On the other hand, the VISTA agonistic antibody suppressed pulmonary inflammation and ameliorated asthma [54]. Consistent with these findings, another study showed that administration of anti-VISTA blocking antibodies during allergen challenge caused eosinophilia in BAL and worsened the AHR. Moreover, Th2 cytokines (IL-5, IL-13) increased in BAL [55]. These results suggest the regulatory role of VISTA in controlling asthma.

8.4.6 BATLA

B and T lymphocyte attenuator (BTLA) belongs to the CD28 immunoglobulin superfamily, which inhibits cell function by binding to its ligand HVEM. BTLA is expressed on many immune cells, especially T and B cells. BTLA/HVEM axis plays an important role in suppressing the immune response in cancers [56]. The role of BTLA has been studied in lung diseases, such as infection (pneumonia), cancer (non-small cell lung cancer), and asthma [57]. BTLA, like PD-1, has a protective role in asthma. A study of an experimental model of acute allergic airway inflammation showed that BTLA and PD-1 were expressed on $CD4^+$ T cells present in BAL. Mice deficient for both BTLA and PD-1 had higher recruitment of inflammatory cells, including lymphocytes, eosinophils, and neutrophils, to the lungs. Importantly, BTLA and PD-1 were involved in reducing airway inflammation [58]. In line with this, it has been shown that IL-5 secretion and antigen-induced eosinophil recruitment to airways were increased in BTLA-KO mice [59].

8.4.7 TIGIT

T cell immunoglobulin and ITIM domain (TIGIT) is also considered one of the important immune checkpoints in cancer. The binding of TIGIT to its ligands CD155 and CD112 leads to the induction of inhibitory signals in T cells [60, 61]. Kourepini indicated that the in vitro polarization of naive T cells to Th2 was associated with the upregulation of TIGIT expression on Th2 cells. Meanwhile, $TIGIT^+$ Th2 cells produced higher amounts of IL-4 and IL-5. CD155 (TIGIT ligand) is highly expressed on DCs. It was found that inhibition of TIGIT-CD155 interaction by TIGIT and CD155 blocking antibodies suppressed the differentiation and cytokine production of Th2 cells co-cultured with DCs. They also showed that the percentage of TIGIT^{+} CD4^{+} T cells was increased in the draining mediastinal lymph nodes (MLNs) of mice with allergic airway inflammation. On the other hand, a large number of DCs expressing CD155 were observed in MLNs. Furthermore, TIGIT blocking antibodies decreased eosinophils and macrophages and dampened the production of IL-4, IL-13, and IL-5 in BAL and reduced airway inflammation in asthmatic mice [62].

8.4.8 LAG-3

Lymphocyte activation gene-3 (LAG-3) is an inhibitory molecule that is overexpressed on activated T cells and regulates their activity. LAG-3 can bind to MHC molecules on APCs and stop TCR signaling. In recent years, LAG-3 has been proposed as a promising target in cancer treatment. LAG-3 inhibition, along with PD-1 and CTLA-4 blockers, is effective in reinvigoration of the antitumor immune response [63]. It has been demonstrated that LAG-3 is an important immune checkpoint in regulating the suppressive activity of Treg cells. Double-negative Treg cells (DNT cells) belong to a subset of Tregs that lack FoxP3 expression but produce granzyme B and perforin. DNT cells constitute 1–3% of the T cell population. These cells can upregulate LAG-3 on their surface and play an important role in suppressing the functions of conventional T cells. Tian et al. showed that adoptive transfer of DNT cells to the OVA-induced allergic asthma mouse model ameliorated lung inflammation and mucus production. In addition, the infiltration of eosinophils and macrophages in the lung was decreased, and the population of CD11c^{+} MHC-II^{+} DCs in the mediastinal lymph node (mLN) was reduced. They found that the coculture of allergen-specific DNTs with DCs reduced the expression of costimulatory molecules CD40 and CD86 on DCs. LAG-3 participates in MHC-II antigen recognition by DNT. Importantly, deletion of the LAG-3 gene led to a reduction in the suppressive activity of OVA DNTs. Lag3$^{-/-}$ DNTs were unable to control inflammation and recruitment of inflammatory cells into the lung [64]. Other studies have also highlighted the role of LAG-3^{+} Treg cells in controlling the Th2 response and reducing allergic airway inflammation [65, 66].

8.5 Conclusion

The exploration of immune checkpoints in asthma presented in this chapter underscores the intricate balance between immune activation and regulation in the airways. The detailed examination of various checkpoint molecules reveals their crucial roles in modulating immune responses and their potential as therapeutic targets or biomarkers for asthma.

The chapter highlights the complexity of immune checkpoint interactions in asthma, with many molecules exhibiting context-dependent functions. For instance, while CTLA-4 and PD-1 generally play protective roles by suppressing excessive T cell responses, other checkpoints like TIGIT may contribute to disease pathogenesis by enhancing Th2 responses.

The emerging role of immune checkpoints in regulating ILC2 functions, particularly through the CD200-CD200R and PD-1 pathways, opens new avenues for therapeutic interventions. These findings suggest that targeting specific checkpoints could potentially modulate both adaptive and innate immune responses in asthma.

As research in this field progresses, integrating data from human studies and animal models will be crucial for developing a more nuanced understanding of immune checkpoint regulation in asthmatic conditions. This knowledge may pave the way for personalized treatment strategies, potentially allowing for fine-tuning of immune responses to alleviate asthma symptoms while minimizing side effects.

The future of asthma treatment may lie in harnessing the complex network of immune checkpoints to restore immune balance in the airways. However, this approach will require careful consideration of the potential risks, including the possibility of triggering autoimmune responses. Continued research into the tissue-specific and phenotype-specific roles of immune checkpoints will be essential for translating these findings into effective clinical applications.

In conclusion, while our understanding of immune checkpoints in asthma has grown significantly, many questions remain. The ongoing exploration of these pathways promises to yield new insights into the fundamental mechanisms of asthma pathogenesis and may lead to innovative approaches for managing this complex and heterogeneous disease.

Acknowledgments The authors gratefully acknowledge the valuable assistance provided by Maryam Sadr.

References

1. Papapostolou N, Makris M. Allergic asthma in the era of personalized medicine. J Personal Med. 2022;12(7):1162.
2. Akar-Ghibril N, Casale T, Custovic A, Phipatanakul W. Allergic endotypes and phenotypes of asthma. J Allergy Clin Immunol Pract. 2020;8(2):429–40.
3. Cevhertas L, Ogulur I, Maurer DJ, Burla D, Ding M, Jansen K, et al. Advances and recent developments in asthma in 2020. Allergy. 2020;75(12):3124–46.
4. Lambrecht BN, Hammad H, Fahy JV. The cytokines of asthma. Immunity. 2019;50(4):975–91.
5. Ricciardolo FLM, Guida G, Bertolini F, Di Stefano A, Carriero V. Phenotype overlap in the natural history of asthma. Eur Respir Rev. 2023;32(168)
6. Méndez-Enríquez E, Hallgren J. Mast cells and their progenitors in allergic asthma. Front Immunol. 2019;10:821.
7. Krystel-Whittemore M, Dileepan KN, Wood JG. Mast cell: a multi-functional master cell. Front Immunol. 2016;6
8. Banafea GH, Bakhashab S, Alshaibi HF, Natesan Pushparaj P, Rasool M. The role of human mast cells in allergy and asthma. Bioengineered. 2022;13(3):7049–64.
9. Baran J, Sobiepanek A, Mazurkiewicz-Pisarek A, Rogalska M, Gryciuk A, Kuryk L, et al. Mast cells as a target-a comprehensive review of recent therapeutic approaches. Cells. 2023;12(8)

10. McBrien CN, Menzies-Gow A. The biology of eosinophils and their role in asthma. Front Med. 2017;4:93.
11. O'Connell EM, Nutman TB. Eosinophilia in infectious diseases. Immunol Allergy Clin N Am. 2015;35(3):493–522.
12. Ramirez GA, Yacoub MR, Ripa M, Mannina D, Cariddi A, Saporiti N, et al. Eosinophils from physiology to disease: a comprehensive review. Biomed Res Int. 2018;2018:9095275.
13. Wechsler ME, Munitz A, Ackerman SJ, Drake MG, Jackson DJ, Wardlaw AJ, et al. Eosinophils in health and disease: a state-of-the-art review. Mayo Clin Proc. 2021;96(10):2694–707.
14. Huang C, Li F, Wang J, Tian Z. Innate-like lymphocytes and innate lymphoid cells in asthma. Clin Rev Allergy Immunol. 2020;59(3):359–70.
15. Matsuyama T, Machida K, Mizuno K, Matsuyama H, Dotake Y, Shinmura M, et al. The functional role of group 2 innate lymphoid cells in asthma. Biomolecules. 2023;13(6)
16. Agache I, Akdis C, Jutel M, Virchow JC. Untangling asthma phenotypes and endotypes. Allergy. 2012;67(7):835–46.
17. Anderson GP. Endotyping asthma: new insights into key pathogenic mechanisms in a complex, heterogeneous disease. Lancet (London, England). 2008;372(9643):1107–19.
18. Woodruff PG, Modrek B, Choy DF, Jia G, Abbas AR, Ellwanger A, et al. T-helper type 2-driven inflammation defines major subphenotypes of asthma. Am J Respir Crit Care Med. 2009;180(5):388–95.
19. Mjösberg JM, Trifari S, Crellin NK, Peters CP, van Drunen CM, Piet B, et al. Human IL-25- and IL-33-responsive type 2 innate lymphoid cells are defined by expression of CRTH2 and CD161. Nat Immunol. 2011;12(11):1055–62.
20. Kuruvilla ME, Lee FE, Lee GB. Understanding asthma phenotypes, endotypes, and mechanisms of disease. Clin Rev Allergy Immunol. 2019;56(2):219–33.
21. Robinson D, Humbert M, Buhl R, Cruz AA, Inoue H, Korom S, et al. Revisiting type 2-high and type 2-low airway inflammation in asthma: current knowledge and therapeutic implications. Clin Exp Allergy. 2017;47(2):161–75.
22. Zheng Y, Wang H, Luo L, Liao L, You L, Wang J, et al. A meta-analysis of the association between CTLA-4 genetic polymorphism and susceptibility of asthma. Medicine (Baltimore). 2018;97(28):e11380.
23. Nie W, Chen J, Xiu Q. Cytotoxic T-lymphocyte associated antigen 4 polymorphisms and asthma risk: a meta-analysis. PLoS One. 2012;7(7):e42062.
24. Yao YS, Wang LH, Chang WW, He LP, Li J, Jin YL, et al. Association between CTLA-4 exon-1 +49A/G polymorphism and asthma: an updated meta-analysis. Int J Clin Exp Med. 2015;8(3):3107–13.
25. Lee YH, Choi SJ, Ji JD, Song GG. The CTLA-4 +49 A/G and −318 C/T polymorphisms and susceptibility to asthma: a meta-analysis. Mol Biol Rep. 2012;39(8):8525–32.
26. Ip WK, Wong CK, Leung TF, Lam CW. Elevation of plasma soluble T cell costimulatory molecules CTLA-4, CD28 and CD80 in children with allergic asthma. Int Arch Allergy Immunol. 2005;137(1):45–52.
27. Wong CK, Lun SW, Ko FW, Ip WK, Hui DS, Lam CW. Increased expression of plasma and cell surface co-stimulatory molecules CTLA-4, CD28 and CD86 in adult patients with allergic asthma. Clin Exp Immunol. 2005;141(1):122–9.
28. Chan IH, Tang NL, Leung TF, Lam YY, Wong GW, Wong CK, et al. Association of plasma soluble CTLA-4 with lung function and gene polymorphism in Chinese asthmatic children. Int Arch Allergy Immunol. 2010;152(2):113–21.
29. Ip WK, Wong CK, Leung TF, Lam CW. Plasma concentrations of soluble CTLA-4, CD28, CD80 and CD86 costimulatory molecules reflect disease severity of acute asthma in children. Pediatr Pulmonol. 2006;41(7):674–82.
30. Shi HZ, Mo XY, Zhong XN. Soluble CTLA-4 in sera of patients with bronchial asthma. J Asthma. 2005;42(2):133–9.

31. Dmitrieva-Zdorova EV, Gabaeva MV, Seregin YA, Bodoev NV, Voronko OE. PDCD1 PD-1.3 polymorphism and allergic bronchial asthma in Russian and Buryat patients. J Asthma. 2017;54(1):46–52.
32. Kanannejad Z, Soleimanian S, Ghahramani Z, Sepahi N, Mohkam M, Alyasin S, et al. Immune checkpoint molecules in prevention and development of asthma. Front Immunol. 2023;14:1070779.
33. Helou DG, Quach C, Fung M, Painter JD, Hurrell BP, Eddie Loh YH, et al. Human PD-1 agonist treatment alleviates neutrophilic asthma by reprogramming T cells. J Allergy Clin Immunol. 2023;151(2):526–38.e8.
34. Xi X, Liu JM, Guo JY. Correlation of PD-1/PD-L1 signaling pathway with Treg/Th17 imbalance from asthmatic children. Int Arch Allergy Immunol. 2018;176(3–4):255–67.
35. Morita H, Saito H, Matsumoto K. Immune checkpoint molecules on ILC2s as potential therapeutic targets for allergic diseases. J Allergy Clin Immunol. 2022;149(1):60–2.
36. Helou DG, Shafiei-Jahani P, Lo R, Howard E, Hurrell BP, Galle-Treger L, et al. PD-1 pathway regulates ILC2 metabolism and PD-1 agonist treatment ameliorates airway hyperreactivity. Nat Commun. 2020;11(1):3998.
37. Wenping W, Jiaqi H, Yu M, Chuangli H, Shengfei Z. Association between gene polymorphisms of T cell immunoglobulin domain and mucin Domain-3 and risk of asthma: a systematic review and meta-analysis. Iran J Allergy Asthma Immunol. 2021;20(1)
38. Sadri M, Ganjalikhani-Hakemi M, Akbari P, Salehi R, Rastaghi S, Ghasemi R, et al. Association between +4259 T>G and −574 G>T polymorphisms of TIM-3 with asthma in an Iranian population. Iran J Allergy Asthma Immunol. 2017;16(4):321–8.
39. Barlow JL, Wong SH, Ballantyne SJ, Jolin HE, McKenzie AN. Tim1 and Tim3 are not essential for experimental allergic asthma. Clin Exp Allergy. 2011;41(7):1012–21.
40. Hiraishi Y, Nambu A, Shibui A, Nakanishi W, Yamaguchi S, Morita H, et al. TIM-3 is not essential for development of airway inflammation induced by house dust mite antigens. Allergol Int. 2016;65(4):459–65.
41. Boehne C, Behrendt AK, Meyer-Bahlburg A, Boettcher M, Drube S, Kamradt T, et al. Tim-3 is dispensable for allergic inflammation and respiratory tolerance in experimental asthma. PLoS One. 2021;16(4):e0249605.
42. Kearley J, McMillan SJ, Lloyd CM. Th2-driven, allergen-induced airway inflammation is reduced after treatment with anti-Tim-3 antibody in vivo. J Exp Med. 2007;204(6):1289–94.
43. Tang F, Wang F, An L, Wang X. Upregulation of Tim-3 on CD4(+) T cells is associated with Th1/Th2 imbalance in patients with allergic asthma. Int J Clin Exp Med. 2015;8(3):3809–16.
44. Ngwa C, Liu F. CD200-CD200R signaling and diseases: a potential therapeutic target? Int J Physiol Pathophysiol Pharmacol. 2019;11(6):297–309.
45. Nip C, Wang L, Liu C. CD200/CD200R: bidirectional role in cancer progression and immunotherapy. Biomedicine. 2023;11(12):3326.
46. Kotwica-Mojzych K, Jodłowska-Jędrych B, Mojzych M. CD200:CD200R interactions and their importance in immunoregulation. Int J Mol Sci. 2021;22(4)
47. Wissinger E, Goulding J, Hussell T. Immune homeostasis in the respiratory tract and its impact on heterologous infection. Semin Immunol. 2009;21(3):147–55.
48. Snelgrove RJ, Goulding J, Didierlaurent AM, Lyonga D, Vekaria S, Edwards L, et al. A critical function for CD200 in lung immune homeostasis and the severity of influenza infection. Nat Immunol. 2008;9(9):1074–83.
49. Aoki T, Matsumoto Y, Hirata K, Ochiai K, Okada M, Ichikawa K, et al. Expression profiling of genes related to asthma exacerbations. Clin Exp Allergy. 2009;39(2):213–21.
50. Lauzon-Joset JF, Langlois A, Lai LJ, Santerre K, Lee-Gosselin A, Bossé Y, et al. Lung CD200 receptor activation abrogates airway hyperresponsiveness in experimental asthma. Am J Respir Cell Mol Biol. 2015;53(2):276–84.
51. Shafiei-Jahani P, Helou DG, Hurrell BP, Howard E, Quach C, Painter JD, et al. CD200-CD200R immune checkpoint engagement regulates ILC2 effector function and ameliorates lung inflammation in asthma. Nat Commun. 2021;12(1):2526.

52. Huang X, Zhang X, Li E, Zhang G, Wang X, Tang T, et al. VISTA: an immune regulatory protein checking tumor and immune cells in cancer immunotherapy. J Hematol Oncol. 2020;13(1):83.
53. Martin AS, Molloy M, Ugolkov A, von Roemeling RW, Noelle RJ, Lewis LD, et al. VISTA expression and patient selection for immune-based anticancer therapy. Front Immunol. 2023;14:14.
54. Liu H, Li X, Hu L, Zhu M, He B, Luo L, et al. A crucial role of the PD-1H coinhibitory receptor in suppressing experimental asthma. Cell Mol Immunol. 2018;15(9):838–45.
55. Ohno T, Zhang C, Kondo Y, Kang S, Furusawa E, Tsuchiya K, et al. The immune checkpoint molecule VISTA regulates allergen-specific Th2-mediated immune responses. Int Immunol. 2018;30(1):3–11.
56. Sordo-Bahamonde C, Lorenzo-Herrero S, Granda-Díaz R, Martínez-Pérez A, Aguilar-García C, Rodrigo JP, et al. Beyond the anti-PD-1/PD-L1 era: promising role of the BTLA/HVEM axis as a future target for cancer immunotherapy. Mol Cancer. 2023;22(1):142.
57. Deng Z, Zheng Y, Cai P, Zheng Z. The role of B and T lymphocyte attenuator in respiratory system diseases. Front Immunol. 2021;12:635623.
58. Deppong C, Juehne TI, Hurchla M, Friend LD, Shah DD, Rose CM, et al. Cutting edge: B and T lymphocyte attenuator and programmed death receptor-1 inhibitory receptors are required for termination of acute allergic airway inflammation. J Immunol (Baltimore, Md: 1950). 2006;176(7):3909–13.
59. Tamachi T, Watanabe N, Oya Y, Kagami S, Hirose K, Saito Y, et al. B and T lymphocyte attenuator inhibits antigen-induced eosinophil recruitment into the airways. Int Arch Allergy Immunol. 2007;143(Suppl 1):50–5.
60. Harjunpää H, Guillerey C. TIGIT as an emerging immune checkpoint. Clin Exp Immunol. 2020;200(2):108–19.
61. Tang W, Chen J, Ji T, Cong X. TIGIT, a novel immune checkpoint therapy for melanoma. Cell Death Dis. 2023;14(7):466.
62. Kourepini E, Paschalidis N, Simoes DC, Aggelakopoulou M, Grogan JL, Panoutsakopoulou V. TIGIT enhances antigen-specific Th2 recall responses and allergic disease. J Immunol (Baltimore, Md: 1950). 2016;196(9):3570–80.
63. Ibrahim R, Saleh K, Chahine C, Khoury R, Khalife N, Cesne AL. LAG-3 inhibitors: novel immune checkpoint inhibitors changing the landscape of immunotherapy. Biomedicine. 2023;11(7):1878.
64. Tian D, Yang L, Wang S, Zhu Y, Shi W, Zhang C, et al. Double negative T cells mediate Lag3-dependent antigen-specific protection in allergic asthma. Nat Commun. 2019;10(1):4246.
65. Matsuda M, Doi K, Tsutsumi T, Fujii S, Kishima M, Nishimura K, et al. Regulation of allergic airway inflammation by adoptive transfer of CD4(+) T cells preferentially producing IL-10. Eur J Pharmacol. 2017;812:38–47.
66. Li X, Yang A, Huang H, Zhang X, Town J, Davis B, et al. Induction of type 2 T helper cell allergen tolerance by IL-10-differentiated regulatory dendritic cells. Am J Respir Cell Mol Biol. 2010;42(2):190–9.

Chapter 9
Immune Checkpoints and Pregnancy

9.1 Introduction

The immune relationship between mother and fetus has been the focus of immunologists for decades. From the immunological view, the embryo is the result of the mating of incompatible individuals in a population, and it can be compared with a semi-allograft transplant, which must be tolerated throughout pregnancy [1]. The semi-allogeneic graft embryo survival is known as an example of immune tolerance in the embryo by the mother. Several mechanisms have been proposed for the establishment of this tolerance, including the expression or lack of expression of histocompatibility antigens on fetal tissues, maternal immune tolerance to fetal antigens, and inhibiting the maternal anti-fetal immune responses. Fetal-placental tissue for nutrition needs a suitable environment in homeostatic conditions where the mother adapts her metabolism and immune system to the fetus [2]. During pregnancy, a large number of immune cells infiltrate the decidua, including natural killer (NK) cells, T cells, dendritic cells (DCs), and macrophages, which have a protective effect on the fetus. The absence of these immune cells negatively affects placental development and decidual formation. The immune system is precisely modulated during pregnancy; therefore, it is sensitive to the presence of microorganisms and eliminates infectious agents without harming the fetus [3]. Classically, it has been hypothesized that the T helper 2 (Th2) response is the dominant immune response during pregnancy, leading to the establishment of an anti-inflammatory state. However, it is now known that the immune response changes during pregnancy. In general, pregnancy can be divided into three stages. Initially, during embryo implantation and placentation, blastocytes invade the uterine epithelial barrier for implantation, which is accompanied by the presence of a strong Th1-dependent inflammatory response and the production of IL-6, IL-8, TNFα, IFN-γ, and IL-1 at this stage. The Th1 response also helps repair the uterine epithelium and clear the cellular debris. In the second phase of pregnancy, rapid fetal development occurs

L. Tayebi, M. Abdolmaleki, *Immune System Regulation*,
https://doi.org/10.1007/978-981-95-8026-2_9

and is immunologically associated with a Th2 response and the production of IL-4, IL-5, IL-10, and IL-13. Therefore, an anti-inflammatory state is established in this phase. In the final phase of pregnancy, the fetus has completed its development. Parturition, which is associated with the presence of immune cells in the myometrium and a proinflammatory environment, ends with the delivery and rejection of the placenta [3, 4].

There are a variety of different tolerance mechanisms during pregnancy. These mechanisms can act at a distance through hormones and molecules on the maternal immune system or locally on the level of the placenta. For example, progesterone is a hormone produced at high levels by the placenta and reduces maternal immune responses [5, 6]. Immune checkpoints are important molecules in the regulation of immune responses. The significance of these molecules in cancer is well-defined [7–9]. Immune checkpoints are also of particular importance in pregnancy. In general, innate and adaptive immune cells, including macrophages, NK, NKT-like, and T cells, express a range of inhibitory receptors on their surface during pregnancy, indicating their importance in regulating immune responses and maintaining tolerance towards the fetus [10]. Any disturbance in the tolerance of pregnancy can lead to recurrent pregnancy loss, miscarriage, and preeclampsia [11, 12]. Therefore, a successful pregnancy depends on efficient tolerance mechanisms, and the loss of such mechanisms can lead to abortion. This balance is influenced by internal (mother and fetus) and external (environmental) factors [5].

9.2 Components of the Maternal-Fetal Interface

The maternal-fetal interface consists of two main components, including the decidua and placenta. The placenta is derived from the trophectoderm of the blastocyst. Blastocyst is anchored to the decidua by invasive extravillous trophoblasts (EVTs) [1]. The placenta serves as a platform for fetal development. It is a combination of fetal and maternal tissue, and the fetus is connected to the placenta through the umbilical cord. The placenta is a highly vascularized organ with chorionic plate arteries, villi, and veins. Placental villi appear in the first week after fertilization and are completed in the third month [13]. Decidua is a platform of uterine tissue that exists only during pregnancy and is vital for a successful pregnancy. Decidua originates from the endometrium and consists of terminally differentiated endometrial stromal cells. Decidual cells are large, round cells with abundant glycogen and lipids, which differentiate from uterine stromal fibroblast-like cells in the endometrium [14]. Endometrial stromal cells (ESCs) undergo specific functional and morphological differentiation for the decidualization process. Decidualization is necessary for blastocyst implantation [15]. In humans, the placenta develops around the first week after conception. Polar trophoectoderm adheres to the endometrium, then proliferates and creates a trophoblast bilayer consisting of cytotrophoblasts (CTBs) and multinucleated syncytiotrophoblast (STB) cells. CTBs have great proliferative potential. CTB invasion to maternal decidua triggers embryonic development through vasculature remodeling and the interaction of endometrial decidual stromal cells with immune cells present in the decidua. Proliferation of CTBs and folding of the STB layer into the decidua cause the development of placental villi around 8 days post conception (dpc). Around 12 dpc, invasion of extra-embryonic mesenchyme into the villi forms the first villus mesenchymal cores. Villus structure consists of a trophoblastic bilayer (including mononuclear trophoblasts and an overlying multinucleated STB layer). STBs are in direct contact with maternal blood and are involved in absorbing nutrients and oxygen. CTBs at the tips of anchoring villi differentiate to extravillous trophoblast (EVT) by their rapid proliferation. The placenta mediates many important biological functions, including gas, nutrient, and waste exchange, and the production of hormones involved in fetal development. It also exerts its protective role by facilitating the transfer of maternal immunoglobulins to the fetus and preventing the passage of harmful compounds and microbes. The STB layer acts as a barrier to prevent the attachment and invasion of infectious agents. The high abundance of leukocytes, such as decidual NK (dNK) cells, creates an effective immunological defense at the maternal-fetal interface [16].

9.3 Immune Cells in Pregnancy

9.3.1 T Cells

T cells are the main cells of the immune system in pathogen recognition and elimination. T cells constitute approximately 10–20% of the immune cells present in the human decidua in the first trimester, of which 45–75% are $CD8^+$ T, and 30–45% are $CD4^+$ T cells [4, 17]. During pregnancy, these T-cells show tolerance to the fetus, so compared to their peripheral counterparts, $dCD8^+$ T cells cannot differentiate into effectors and have limited cytotoxicity function [18]. In addition to their importance in combating viral infections, decidual $CD8^+$ T cells are critical for establishing immune tolerance during pregnancy. These $CD8^+$ T cells produce less perforin and granzyme B and express various inhibitory receptors such as CTLA-4, PD-1, and TIM-3, suggesting the anti-inflammatory properties of these cells [4, 19]. In addition to $CD8^+$ T cells, $CD4^+$ Th cells are also essential in creating tolerance for a successful pregnancy. As previously mentioned, the proper ratio of Th1 and Th2 cells is closely related to a healthy pregnancy. Imbalance in T cell responses leads to miscarriage. Decidual dendritic cells can induce a Th2 response. Factors such as prostaglandin, progesterone, and estradiol also induce Th2 differentiation. IL-10 secreted by Th2 cells during normal pregnancy plays a role in placentation as well as in the regulation of inflammation and vascular function [4]. Furthermore, the Treg/Th17 balance is very important during pregnancy [20, 21]. A high frequency of Treg cells has been reported in both the peripheral blood and the decidua during pregnancy. Reduction of $CD25^+$ $FoxP3^+$ Tregs proportion leads to spontaneous abortion, preeclampsia, and spontaneous preterm birth [22, 23]. In addition to the increased number of Tregs at the maternal-fetal interface, they also increase in other peripheral tissues in pregnant women. Treg cells are involved in immune tolerance to the fetus by regulating inflammatory responses. Treg cells reduce cytokine production and the functions of $CD4^+$ T, $CD8^+$ T, and NK cells, thereby inhibiting the immune response to paternal antigens and inflammation [4, 14]. Th17, as a $CD4^+$ T subset, can exert a pro-inflammatory phenotype, and the elevated number of these cells is associated with spontaneous abortion and chorioamnionitis [24, 25]. In the first trimester of pregnancy, Th17 increases both in peripheral blood and decidua; also, Th17 cell numbers can prompt the migration and invasion of trophoblast. Therefore, coordination between the Th1/Th2/Th17/Treg paradigm demonstrates that T cell homeostasis is vital for a healthy pregnancy [25].

9.3.2 NK Cells

NK cells constitute approximately 60–70% of decidual lymphocytes in the first trimester of pregnancy, and most of them have the $CD16^-$ $CD56^{bright}$ phenotype. NK cells contribute to decidual angiogenesis and early embryonic development by secreting different factors such as vascular endothelial growth factor (VEGF), placental growth factor (PlGF), TGF-β, and IFN-γ [14]. dNK cells gradually increase with the beginning of implantation. They reach their maximum level by weeks 8–10 and make up 70% of decidual lymphocytes, then return to the normal level at term. The characteristics of dNK cells are the ability to produce growth factors, immune modulators, and low cytotoxicity [26]. In general, dNK cells can be divided into three categories: dNK1 ($CD39^+$ $KIR2DL^+$ $ITGB2^-$ $CD103^-$), dNK2 ($CD39^-$ $KIR2DL^+$ $ITGB2^+$ $CD103^-$), and dNK3 ($CD39^-$ $KIR2DL^-$ $ITGB2^+$) [27, 28]. The dNK cells play a vital role in some processes during pregnancy, such as embryo implantation, modulation of the immune system, differentiation of trophoblast and invasion, and remodeling of endothelial cells. Recent studies report that dNK cells provide osteoglycin and osteopontin for fetal development [29]. NK cells in peripheral blood are divided into two groups. The majority of peripheral NK (pNK) cells are $CD56^{dim}$ $CD16^+$, which constitute 90% of the population and produce cytotoxic cells. $CD56^+$ $CD16^-$ NK cells are less cytotoxic and can migrate to peripheral tissues [30]. Furthermore, pNK cells have a higher expression of TIM-3 and Galectin-1 and less IFN-γ secretion compared to non-pregnant women. NK cells present the largest fraction of lymphocytes in the endometrium in the early and late secretory phase of pregnancy. In contrast to pNK, the majority of the endometrium NK cells (eNK) are $CD56^+$ $CD16^-$, and the minority are cytotoxic with a $CD56^{dim}$ $CD16^+$ phenotype [31].

9.3.3 Macrophages

Monocytes have an immune role in immune homeostasis, inflammation, defense against infection, and tissue repair, and are the primary phagocytes and the most important antigen-presenting cells (APCs) in peripheral blood. In terms of cell surface markers, monocytes are found in three categories: classical ($CD14^{++}$ $CD16^{-}$), intermediate ($CD14^{+}$ $CD16^{+}$), and nonclassical ($CD14^{-}$ $CD16^{++}$) in circulation [32]. Myeloid cells constitute approximately 20 to 25% of the leukocytes present in the decidua [14]. Macrophages appear to be necessary for the support of pregnancy and embryogenesis. M1 macrophage has an immune system-activated phenotype and helps to contract the uterus during childbirth. M2 macrophage plays an anti-inflammatory and immunosuppressive role in protecting the fetus against environmental infections and rejection. Macrophages show dynamic changes during pregnancy [33]. Based on the expression of CD11c (complement receptor), decidua macrophages are divided into two groups: $CD11c^{hi}$ and $CD11c^{lo}$. In the first trimester, the majority of macrophages found in the decidua are $CD11c^{lo}$. These cells are involved in tissue growth and extracellular matrix formation. $CD11c^{hi}$ macrophages, which comprise a smaller population (about one-third) of decidua macrophages, express CD1a, CD1c, and CD1d and have antigen-presenting features. Macrophages have been shown to be involved in the inhibition of T cell activity and the control of inflammation during pregnancy by producing several factors, such as IL-10 and prostaglandin E2 [14]. Commonly, macrophages are produced from three main sources: early yolk sac macrophages, fetal liver monocytes, and bone marrow-derived monocytes. However, the origin of human decidual macrophages is unclear. According to studies, decidual macrophages can maintain themselves through self-renewal or replenishment from peripheral monocytes [34].

9.4 Role of Immune Checkpoints in Pregnancy

A successful pregnancy is the result of interaction and balance in the mother's immune system against the fetus as an allogeneic transplant with different genetic content. During pregnancy, the mother's immune system requires various changes to maintain this tolerance to the fetus stably. In this tolerance, the role of checkpoints is important. Inhibitory molecules signaling pathways play a critical role in the establishment of maternal-fetal tolerance. Many studies have explored the role of inhibitory receptors such as CTLA-4, PD-1, TIM-3, and TIGIT in the development of immune tolerance of the mother to the fetus [35–37]. Here, the expression pattern of inhibitory molecules on immune cells and their role in the modulation of immune responses during pregnancy are discussed.

9.4.1 PD-1

PD-1 is expressed on the surface of multiple immune cells, such as B, T, and NK cells. PD-L1 and PD-L2 are ligands of PD-1. PD-L1 is widely expressed in hematopoietic and non-hematopoietic cells, while PD-L2 is expressed by professional APCs. Phosphorylation of intracellular tyrosine sequences (ITIM and ITSM) provides inhibitory signals upon PD-1 binding; as a result, it modulates the immune system response [38]. PD-1 and PD-L1 are involved in maintaining maternal-fetal tolerance. Several studies have examined the expression of these molecules during pregnancy [39]. Immunofluorescence evaluation of endometrial and decidual tissues demonstrated that PD-1 expression on T cells increases in the first trimester and remains high throughout pregnancy [40]. It has been shown that PD-1 is overexpressed on decidual T cells in the first trimester of pregnancy compared to peripheral T cells. PD-1 expression on decidual $CD4^+$ T, $CD8^+$ T, and NKT-like cells was significantly increased in the first trimester of pregnant women compared to peripheral blood mononuclear cells (PBMCs) of these women and also PBMCs of non-pregnant women. PD-L1 was also overexpressed on decidual $CD4^+$ T, NKT-like, and $CD56^+$ NK cells compared to their counterparts in PBMCs of non-pregnant women [41]. Immunohistochemistry studies have shown that PD-L1 is consistently expressed by syncytiotrophoblasts and extravillous cytotrophoblasts [42, 43].

Regarding maternal-fetal immunity, it has been reported that the expression of PD-L1 on the surface of T cells and soluble PD-L1(sPD-L1) in the peripheral blood of pregnant people was significantly increased compared to non-pregnant people, which maintains immune tolerance [44]. Gu et al. showed that sPD-1 was significantly elevated in the peripheral blood of preeclamptic patients compared to normal pregnant women [45]. In line with this, another study has shown that sPD-L1 and galectin-9 elevate during normal pregnancies. In addition, these molecules are upregulated at the maternal-fetal interface [46]. Looking at the expression of PD-1 and PD-L1 in PBMCs of preeclamptic subjects, it has been demonstrated that PD-1 was upregulated on $CD4^+$ T, $CD8^+$ T, Treg, and NKT-like cells in third-trimester women with early-onset preeclampsia compared to the normal pregnant group. PD-L1 was also overexpressed on NKT-like cells of these patients. Interestingly, the cytotoxicity of $PD\text{-}1^+$ $CD8^+$ T cells was increased in early-onset preeclampsia [47]. However, another study has shown that PD-1 expression on decidual memory $CD8^+$ T cells is reduced in preeclampsia cases [48]. It has also been reported that PD-L1 expression is reduced in the decidua during early recurrent miscarriage. Downregulation of this ligand may affect the function of Treg cells at the maternal-fetal interface [49]. The importance of PD-1/PD-L1 interaction has been demonstrated by blocking PD-L1 with anti-PD-L1 monoclonal antibodies in a murine study, resulting in a five-fold increase in allogeneic spontaneous abortion rates in pregnant mice [50]. In addition, it has been proven that blocking PD-L1's effect depends on the presence of Treg cells. So, when the abortion-prone mice lacking Treg were injected with Treg cells from healthy pregnant mice, they experienced a normal pregnancy. Specifically, PD-1 signaling reduces the proliferation and function of effector T (Teff) cells, while enhancing the differentiation and suppressive capacity of Tregs [21, 38].

9.4.2 *CTLA-4*

CTLA-4 is expressed as an intracellular protein mainly in Treg cells. After activation, it is overexpressed on the surface of Teff and Treg cells. CTLA-4 deficiency significantly reduces Treg inhibitory capacity. CTLA-4 acts as a competitive receptor with T cell activation receptors, CD28, for binding to CD80/CD86 molecules. As an important suppression mechanism, CTLA-4 induces expression of indoleamine 2,3-dioxygenase (IDO) by APCs through CTLA-4-CD80/CD86 interaction, which suppresses the inflammatory response [51]. Wang et al. showed that the frequency of maternal decidual TIM-3$^+$ CTLA-4$^+$ CD8$^+$ T cells increases during pregnancy. They found that this cell population has a high potency for producing anti-inflammatory cytokines. A decrease in the number or dysfunction of these cells is associated with miscarriage. In addition, animal studies showed that CTLA-4 and TIM-3 blocking antibodies reduce the production of anti-inflammatory cytokines, such as TGF-β1 and IL-10, from decidual CD8$^+$ T cells and upregulate the production of TNF-α and IFN-γ, which leads to the susceptibility to miscarriage [52]. In line with this, they observed that CTLA-4 and TIM-3 expressions on dCD4$^+$ T cells help to maintain maternal-fetal tolerance. Inhibition of signaling of these inhibitory receptors was associated with increased production of inflammatory cytokines, such as TNF-α and IFN-γ, from the T cells and fatal loss, indicating the role of CTLA-4 and TIM-3 in the regulation of the CD4$^+$ T cell function [53]. Decidual CTLA-4$^+$ Tregs in early pregnancy cause immunosuppression in several ways: by increasing IDO through DCs, secretion of anti-inflammatory cytokines, and inhibiting the pro-inflammatory cytokines production. Therefore, CTLA-4 signaling plays an important role in establishing maternal-fetal tolerance in early pregnancy [38, 54]. The association between CTLA-4 gene polymorphisms and pregnancy outcome is summarized in Table 9.1.

9.4.3 *TIM-3*

TIM-3 was first detected on helper T cells and was also detected on other immune and nonimmune cells. TIM-3 has modulatory effects on the immune system by interacting with its ligands. For example, galectin-9 (Gal-9) has been identified as one of the TIM-3 ligands, which provides a strong regulatory effect on lymphocytes. TIM-3 inhibits the proliferation and function of NK and Teff cells [55]. TIM-3/Gal-9 axis is another important pathway in regulating immune responses during pregnancy. According to the study by Wu et al., serum sTIM-3 levels were increased in patients with unexplained recurrent spontaneous abortion compared to

Table 9.1 Relationships between immune checkpoint polymorphism and clinical outcome of pregnancy

Gene	SNP	Position	Population	Comment	Ref
PD-1	rs36084323	chr2:241859444	Japan	These SNPs were identified as risk factors for RPL	[74]
	rs3481962	+6371G > A at intron 2			
CTLA-4	rs3087243	chr2:203874196	Palestinian North India Iranian	1) −1661, −318, and −1722 variants revealed no significant association in the Palestinian population 2) GG of CTLA-4 + 49A/G showed a significant association with the recurrent miscarriage cases in Palestinian, North India, and Iranian populations	[75] [76] [77]
	rs4553808 (−1661)	chr2:203866282			
	rs5742909 (−318)	chr2:203867624			
	rs733618 (−1722)	chr2:203866221			
	rs231775 (+49)	chr2:203867991			
TIM-3	rs10053538	chr5:157110499	Han Chinese	These polymorphisms in the TIM-3 promoter may not be associated with unexplained recurrent spontaneous abortion in Han Chinese women	[78]
	rs10515746	chr5:157109557			

normal pregnant women. In addition, Th1 cells of these patients secreted higher levels of IFN-γ than the normal pregnant group. In contrast, IL-4 production from Th2 cells in normal pregnant women was higher than that of the spontaneous abortion group. They concluded that increased sTIM-3 could change the T cell response toward Th1, higher production of IFN-γ, and inhibition of the Th2 response [56]. Therefore, dysregulation of TIM-3/Gal-9 pathway is associated with disrupted immune tolerance to the fetus. Sun et al. found that TIM-3 is highly expressed in PBMCs and decidual cells during early pregnancy. NK cells were the main population expressing TIM-3. Approximately 90% of decidual NK cells were positive for TIM-3, which was much higher than their counterparts in the periphery. TIM-3 expression on pNK cells of recurrent spontaneous abortion cases was also lower than in normal pregnant women. On the other hand, TGF-β1 levels were decreased in these patients. They showed that TGF-β1 upregulates the TIM-3 expression on NK cells and the TIM-3/Gal-9 axis inhibits the cytotoxicity of these cells toward trophoblasts [57]. TIM-3 expression is reduced on T and NK cells in women with early-onset preeclampsia [58].

A study showed that TIM-3 is expressed by more than 60% of decidual NK cells. In addition, nearly 90% of NK cells in the peripheral blood of pregnant women were TIM-3 positive. In vitro studies revealed that decidual TIM-3$^+$ NK cells produced more IL-4 and less TNF-α than TIM-3$^-$ NK cells; thus, they are more effective in the induction of a Th2 response. In addition, these TIM-3$^+$ cells produced less perforin and had limited cytotoxicity, consistent with their role in immune tolerance to the fetus. On the other hand, approximately 75% of trophoblast cells were positive for Gal-9. Interestingly, the coculture of trophoblasts with pNK cells induced IL-4 production from these cells and reduced their cytotoxicity. Blocking TIM-3 antibodies disrupted the regulatory effects of trophoblasts on NK cells, indicating the importance of the TIM-3/Gal-9 signaling pathway in the interaction between these two cell types [59]. By examining the decidua of pregnant mice, Lu and colleagues showed that a large population of TIM-3^+ Treg cells was accumulated in the decidua, and approximately 90% of these TIM-3^+ Tregs also expressed PD-1. The TIM-3^+ Treg subset was the majority of the decidua Treg population in early pregnancy, whereas the percentage of Tregs in RPL was reduced, and TIM-3 was downregulated on $CD4^+$ T cells and Tregs. Despite the increased expression of Gal-9 in recurrent pregnancy loss patients, insufficient engagement of the TIM-3/Gal-9 axis may be one of the reasons for the impaired immune tolerance in these patients [60]. Wang et al. also showed that TIM-3^+ PD-1^+ $CD8^+$ T cells comprise approximately 15% of decidual T cells in early pregnancy. Following the coculture of $CD8^+$ T cells with trophoblasts, TIM-3 and PD-1 were upregulated on the surface of the T cells. These data suggest that trophoblasts at the maternal-fetal interface can promote the TIM-3^+ PD-1^+ $CD8^+$ T cells phenotype. TIM-3 and PD-1 blockade enhanced the cytotoxic capacity of decidual $CD8^+$ cells and reduced IL-4 and IL-10 production from these cells. Importantly, TIM-3 and PD-1 expressions on T cells were reduced in miscarriage. On the other hand, challenging pregnant CBA/J female mice with TIM-3 and/or PD-1 blocking antibodies made them more susceptible to fetal loss [61].

9.4.4 TIGIT

TIGIT is a protein receptor with a transmembrane glycoprotein structure, which is expressed by activated T cells, such as $CD4^+$T, $CD8^+$, and NK cells. TIGIT intermediate inhibitory signals to downregulate T cell activity. TIGIT has some ligands, including CD155 (Poliovirus Receptor (PVR or Necl-5) and CD112 (PVRL2 or nectin-2), that are expressed on APCs. The TIGIT/CD155 pathway significantly breaks up the ligation between CD155 and CD226, which usually causes Teff activation. It has been reported that TIGIT is expressed on peripheral blood and dNK and T cells during normal pregnancy. In addition, the expression of functional molecules, including granzyme B, CD107a, and IFN-γ, was lower in $TIGIT^+$ NK cells than in TIGIT-negative cells [62]. According to another study, the expression of TIGIT and CD155 in $CD4^+$ T cells of preeclamptic patients is reduced compared to normal pregnancy [63]. However, Li et al. did not observe a significant difference in the expression of CD226 and TIGIT on $CD4^+$ and $CD8^+$ T lymphocytes and Tregs of preeclamptic patients and normal pregnant women [64]. A study has reported that there is a subset of $CD4^+$ T cells with higher levels of TIGIT and low levels of FoxP3, HELIOS, PD-1, and CD25, in the first trimester of pregnancy in humans. This subset significantly inhibited the proliferation of $CD4^+$ T cells, but it did not affect the proliferation and production of $CD8^+$ T cytokines [65].

9.4.5 LAG-3

LAG-3 is a transmembrane protein encoded by the lag-3 gene. Because of the structural similarity of LAG-3 and CD4, it can bind to MHCII. The LAG-3/MHCII pathway negatively regulates the proliferation and activation of the T cells. Another major ligand of LAG-3 is fibrinogen-like protein 1 (FGL1), which creates an inhibitory signal. Therefore, LAG-3 presents another "exhaustion" marker for $CD8^+$ and $CD4^+$ T cells to respond to continuous antigen presentation. In addition, LAG-3 affects the Tregs' function. LAG-3-expressing Tregs produce higher levels of anti-inflammatory cytokines, such as IL-10 and TGF-β, which suppress immune responses. In early pregnancy, LAG-3^+ Treg cells were detected both in the decidua and periphery, which act as strong immunosuppressors in favor of mother-fetal tolerance in early pregnancy [66]. More studies are needed to clarify the role of LAG-3 in pregnancy.

9.5 Immune Checkpoints in Miscarriage

During a healthy pregnancy, the immune system should be able to defend against harmful pathogens and also accept semi-allogeneic embryos containing paternal antigens. Immune tolerance begins with implantation, continues throughout pregnancy, and ceases at birth. During this time, both innate and adaptive immune cells are crucial. For instance, NK cells, DCs, macrophages, and myeloid-derived suppressor cells are plentiful in the human decidua during implantation [67]. Miscarriages are increasing worldwide today, and if they occur more than twice, they are called recurrent spontaneous abortions (RSA). Some causes of abortion are known, such as chromosomal abnormalities, ovarian anatomical malformations, endocrine disorders, thrombophilic factors, and immune disorders, but almost 50% of the cases remain unknown [68]. Many studies report the relationship between recurrent spontaneous abortion in the mother and changes in the maternal immune system, but more studies are necessary to better understand the interaction between the mother's immune system and fetal cells. According to a study, the proportions of PD-1^+ Th1, PD-1^+ Th17, and PD-L1^+ Th17 cells were lower in the peripheral blood of women with recurrent pregnancy losses compared to the control group [69]. Furthermore, another study showed that decidual PD-L1 mRNA was decreased in recurrent early miscarriage cases compared to normal pregnant women [49]. Based on flow cytometry analysis, PD-1^+ Treg cells change in the peripheral blood and decidua in women with recurrent early miscarriages [49]. A study of women with RSA revealed that PD-1 and LAG-3 expression on $CD4^+$, cytotoxic $CD8^+$ T cells, and Treg cells derived from the peripheral blood of RSA patients was decreased. Impaired expression of TIM-3 and VISTA was also observed on $CD8^+$ T and NK cells. These results may confirm the effect of immune checkpoints in regulating pregnancy [70]. Decreased expression of TIM-3 on cytotoxic T cells has been reported in RSA patients [71]. Examination of dNK cells in miscarriage cases revealed that the proportion of TIM-3$^+$ NK cells in these patients was significantly lower than in normal pregnancies [59]. Zhang et al. compared the TIM-3/Gal-9 and PD-1/PL-1 expression in peripheral blood over 4 weeks of gestation after blastocyst transfer between women who had a normal pregnancy with live birth and those who miscarried. In women with normal pregnancy, the level of TIM-3$^+$ pNK cells was increased 1 month after blastocyst transfer; also, the concentration of serum PD-L1 was elevated. These changes may be associated with successful pregnancy outcomes [72]. Another study has explored the TIGIT, PD-1, ICOS, and BTLA expression on CD8$^+$ T cells in peripheral blood and decidual tissue of normal pregnant and unexplained RSA groups from 8 to 10 weeks of gestation. They found decreased levels of BTLA$^+$ CD8$^+$ T cells in the peripheral blood of the URSA group, but other immune checkpoints did not change. In decidual tissues, the differences were not significant. In decidual tissues, levels of PD-1$^+$ CD8$^+$, TIGIT$^+$ CD8$^+$, ICOS$^+$ CD8$^+$, and BTLA$^+$ CD8$^+$ T cells decreased slightly in the URSA group compared with the normal pregnant group [73].

9.6 Conclusion

The comprehensive examination of immune checkpoints in pregnancy presented in this chapter highlights several key conclusions. Firstly, the maternal-fetal interface represents a unique immunological environment, where tolerance must be carefully balanced with protective immunity. The intricate interplay of various immune cells, including T cells, NK cells, and macrophages, is essential for maintaining this balance.

Secondly, immune checkpoint molecules, particularly PD-1, CTLA-4, TIM-3, TIGIT, and LAG-3, play key roles in regulating maternal immune responses during pregnancy. These molecules are expressed on various immune cells and contribute to the establishment and maintenance of maternal-fetal tolerance. Their dysregulation has been associated with pregnancy complications, such as recurrent miscarriage and preeclampsia, and highlights their potential as biomarkers or therapeutic targets.

Thirdly, the dynamic nature of immune responses during pregnancy is evident, with different stages requiring distinct immune profiles. This temporal regulation is critical for successful implantation, fetal development, and parturition.

Lastly, the chapter emphasizes the complexity of pregnancy immunology and the need for further research. While significant progress has been made in understanding the role of immune checkpoints in pregnancy, many questions remain unanswered. Future studies should focus on elucidating the precise mechanisms by which these molecules contribute to maternal-fetal tolerance and exploring their potential in developing diagnostic tools or therapeutic interventions for pregnancy-related disorders.

In conclusion, the study of immune checkpoints in pregnancy not only advances our understanding of reproductive immunology but also opens new avenues for improving maternal and fetal health outcomes.

Acknowledgment The authors gratefully acknowledge the valuable assistance provided by Maryam Sadr.

References

1. Ander SE, Diamond MS, Coyne CB. Immune responses at the maternal-fetal interface. Sci Immunol. 2019;4(31):eaat6114.
2. Morelli SS, Mandal M, Goldsmith LT, Kashani BN, Ponzio NM. The maternal immune system during pregnancy and its influence on fetal development. Res Rep Biol. 2015:171–89.
3. Mor G, Cardenas I, Abrahams V, Guller S. Inflammation and pregnancy: the role of the immune system at the implantation site. Ann N Y Acad Sci. 2011;1221(1):80–7.
4. Colamatteo A, Fusco C, Micillo T, D'Hooghe T, de Candia P, Alviggi C, et al. Immunobiology of pregnancy: from basic science to translational medicine. Trends Mol Med. 2023;29(9):711–25.
5. Thellin O, Heinen E. Pregnancy and the immune system: between tolerance and rejection. Toxicology. 2003;185(3):179–84.
6. Siiteri PK, Stites DP. Immunologic and endocrine interrelationships in pregnancy. Biol Reprod. 1982;26(1):1–14.
7. Tang XY, Luo ZL, Xiong YL, Yang J, Shi AP, Zheng KF, et al. The proliferative role of immune checkpoints in tumors: double regulation. Cancers (Basel). 2022;14(21).
8. Borgeaud M, Sandoval J, Obeid M, Banna G, Michielin O, Addeo A, et al. Novel targets for immune-checkpoint inhibition in cancer. Cancer Treat Rev. 2023;120:102614.
9. Ziogas DC, Theocharopoulos C, Lialios PP, Foteinou D, Koumprentziotis IA, Xynos G, et al. Beyond CTLA-4 and PD-1 inhibition: novel immune checkpoint molecules for melanoma treatment. Cancers (Basel). 2023;15(10).
10. Li WX, Xu XH, Jin LP. Regulation of the innate immune cells during pregnancy: an immune checkpoint perspective. J Cell Mol Med. 2021;25(22):10362–75.
11. Deshmukh H, Way SS. Immunological basis for recurrent fetal loss and pregnancy complications. Annu Rev Pathol. 2019;14(1):185–210.
12. Yang F, Zheng Q, Jin L. Dynamic function and composition changes of immune cells during normal and pathological pregnancy at the maternal-fetal interface. Front Immunol. 2019;10:2317.
13. Lei J, Zhao M, Li L, Ji B, Xu T, Sun M, et al. Research progress of placental vascular pathophysiological changes in pregnancy-induced hypertension and gestational diabetes mellitus. Front Physiol. 2022;13:954636.
14. Mori M, Bogdan A, Balassa T, Csabai T, Szekeres-Bartho J. The decidua-the maternal bed embracing the embryo-maintains the pregnancy. Semin Immunopathol. 2016;38(6):635–49.
15. Murata H, Tanaka S, Okada H. Immune tolerance of the human decidua. J Clin Med. 2021;10(2).
16. Khorami-Sarvestani S, Vanaki N, Shojaeian S, Zarnani K, Stensballe A, Jeddi-Tehrani M, et al. Placenta: an old organ with new functions. Front Immunol. 2024;15:1385762.
17. Suryawanshi H, Morozov P, Straus A, Sahasrabudhe N, Max KE, Garzia A, et al. A single-cell survey of the human first-trimester placenta and decidua. Sci Adv. 2018;4(10):eaau4788.
18. Iwatani Y, Amino N, Tachi J, Kimura M, Ura I, Mori M, et al. Changes of lymphocyte subsets in normal pregnant and postpartum women: postpartum increase of NK/K (Leu 7) cells. Am J Reprod Immunol Microbiol. 1988;18(2):52–5.

19. Kinder JM, Turner LH, Stelzer IA, Miller-Handley H, Burg A, Shao T-Y, et al. CD8+ T cell functional exhaustion overrides pregnancy-induced fetal antigen alloimmunization. Cell Rep. 2020;31(12):107784.
20. Wienke J, Brouwers L, van der Burg LM, Mokry M, Scholman RC, Nikkels PG, et al. Human Tregs at the materno-fetal interface show site-specific adaptation reminiscent of tumor Tregs. JCI Insight. 2020;5(18).
21. Salvany-Celades M, van der Zwan A, Benner M, Setrajcic-Dragos V, Gomes HAB, Iyer V, et al. Three types of functional regulatory T cells control T cell responses at the human maternal-fetal interface. Cell Rep. 2019;27(9):2537–47. e5.
22. Care AS, Bourque SL, Morton JS, Hjartarson EP, Robertson SA, Davidge ST. Reduction in regulatory T cells in early pregnancy causes uterine artery dysfunction in mice. Hypertension. 2018;72(1):177–87.
23. Bai K, Li X, Zhong J, Ng EH, Yeung WS, Lee C-L, et al. Placenta-derived exosomes as a modulator in maternal immune tolerance during pregnancy. Front Immunol. 2021;12:671093.
24. Mjösberg J, Berg G, Jenmalm MC, Ernerudh J. FOXP3+ regulatory T cells and T helper 1, T helper 2, and T helper 17 cells in human early pregnancy decidua. Biol Reprod. 2010;82(4):698–705.
25. Saito S, Nakashima A, Shima T, Ito M. Th1/Th2/Th17 and regulatory T-cell paradigm in pregnancy. Am J Reprod Immunol. 2010;63(6):601–10.
26. Koopman LA, Kopcow HD, Rybalov B, Boyson JE, Orange JS, Schatz F, et al. Human decidual natural killer cells are a unique NK cell subset with immunomodulatory potential. J Exp Med. 2003;198(8):1201–12.
27. Vento-Tormo R, Efremova M, Botting RA, Turco MY, Vento-Tormo M, Meyer KB, et al. Single-cell reconstruction of the early maternal–fetal interface in humans. Nature. 2018;563(7731):347–53.
28. Keskin DB, Allan DS, Rybalov B, Andzelm MM, Stern JN, Kopcow HD, et al. TGFβ promotes conversion of CD16+ peripheral blood NK cells into CD16− NK cells with similarities to decidual NK cells. Proc Natl Acad Sci. 2007;104(9):3378–83.
29. Hanna J, Goldman-Wohl D, Hamani Y, Avraham I, Greenfield C, Natanson-Yaron S, et al. Decidual NK cells regulate key developmental processes at the human fetal-maternal interface. Nat Med. 2006;12(9):1065–74.
30. Li Y, Zhang J, Zhang D, Hong X, Tao Y, Wang S, et al. Tim-3 signaling in peripheral NK cells promotes maternal-fetal immune tolerance and alleviates pregnancy loss. Sci Signal. 2017;10(498):eaah4323.
31. Molvarec A, Blois SM, Stenczer B, Toldi G, Tirado-Gonzalez I, Ito M, et al. Peripheral blood galectin-1-expressing T and natural killer cells in normal pregnancy and preeclampsia. Clin Immunol. 2011;139(1):48–56.
32. Michlmayr D, Andrade P, Gonzalez K, Balmaseda A, Harris E. CD14+ CD16+ monocytes are the main target of Zika virus infection in peripheral blood mononuclear cells in a paediatric study in Nicaragua. Nat Microbiol. 2017;2(11):1462–70.
33. Jena MK, Nayak N, Chen K, Nayak NR. Role of macrophages in pregnancy and related complications. Arch Immunol Ther Exp. 2019;67:295–309.
34. Jiang X, Li L. Decidual macrophage: a reversible role in immunotolerance between mother and fetus during pregnancy. Arch Gynecol Obstet. 2024;309(5):1735–44.
35. Miko E, Meggyes M, Doba K, Barakonyi A, Szereday L. Immune checkpoint molecules in reproductive immunology. Front Immunol. 2019;10:846.
36. Chen Z, Huang J, Kwak-Kim J, Wang W. Immune checkpoint inhibitors and reproductive failures. J Reprod Immunol. 2023;156:103799.
37. Mohamed Khosroshahi L, Parhizkar F, Kachalaki S, Aghebati-Maleki A, Aghebati-Maleki L. Immune checkpoints and reproductive immunology: pioneers in the future therapy of infertility related disorders? Int Immunopharmacol. 2021;99:107935.
38. Zhang YH, Sun HX. Immune checkpoint molecules in pregnancy: focus on regulatory T cells. Eur J Immunol. 2020;50(2):160–9.

39. Mittelberger J, Seefried M, Franitza M, Garrido F, Ditsch N, Jeschke U, et al. The role of the immune checkpoint molecules PD-1/PD-L1 and TIM-3/Gal-9 in the pathogenesis of pre-eclampsia-a narrative review Medicina (Kaunas). 2022;58(2).
40. Taglauer ES, Trikhacheva AS, Slusser JG, Petroff MG. Expression and function of PDCD1 at the human maternal-fetal interface. Biol Reprod. 2008;79(3):562–9.
41. Meggyes M, Miko E, Szigeti B, Farkas N, Szereday L. The importance of the PD-1/PD-L1 pathway at the maternal-fetal interface. BMC Pregnancy Childbirth. 2019;19(1):74.
42. Petroff MG, Chen L, Phillips TA, Azzola D, Sedlmayr P, Hunt JS. B7 family molecules are favorably positioned at the human maternal-fetal interface. Biol Reprod. 2003;68(5):1496–504.
43. Veras E, Kurman RJ, Wang TL, Shih IM. PD-L1 expression in human placentas and gestational trophoblastic diseases. Int J Gynecol Pathol. 2017;36(2):146–53.
44. Okuyama M, Mezawa H, Kawai T, Urashima M. Elevated soluble PD-L1 in pregnant women's serum suppresses the immune reaction. Front Immunol. 2019;10:86.
45. Gu Y, Morgan J, Lewis DF, Cooper DB, McCathran CE, Wang Y. Maternal soluble PD-1 levels are significantly increased in women with preeclampsia. Am J Reprod Immunol. 2020;83(1):e13193.
46. Enninga EAL, Harrington SM, Creedon DJ, Ruano R, Markovic SN, Dong H, et al. Immune checkpoint molecules soluble program death ligand 1 and galectin-9 are increased in pregnancy. Am J Reprod Immunol. 2018;79(2).
47. Meggyes M, Miko E, Lajko A, Csiszar B, Sandor B, Matrai P, et al. Involvement of the PD-1/PD-L1 co-inhibitory pathway in the pathogenesis of the inflammatory stage of early-onset preeclampsia. Int J Mol Sci. 2019;20(3).
48. Morita K, Tsuda S, Kobayashi E, Hamana H, Tsuda K, Shima T, et al. Analysis of TCR repertoire and PD-1 expression in decidual and peripheral CD8(+) T cells reveals distinct immune mechanisms in miscarriage and preeclampsia. Front Immunol. 2020;11:1082.
49. Li G, Lu C, Gao J, Wang X, Wu H, Lee C, et al. Association between PD-1/PD-L1 and T regulate cells in early recurrent miscarriage. Int J Clin Exp Pathol. 2015;8(6):6512–8.
50. Tian M, Zhang Y, Liu Z, Sun G, Mor G, Liao A. The PD-1/PD-L1 inhibitory pathway is altered in pre-eclampsia and regulates T cell responses in pre-eclamptic rats. Sci Rep. 2016;6(1):27683.
51. Bucheit AD, Hardy JT, Szender JB, Oliva ICG. Conception and viable twin pregnancy in a patient with metastatic melanoma while treated with CTLA-4 and PD-1 checkpoint inhibition. Melanoma Res. 2020;30(4):423–5.
52. Wang S, Sun F, Li M, Qian J, Chen C, Wang M, et al. The appropriate frequency and function of decidual Tim-3(+)CTLA-4(+)CD8(+) T cells are important in maintaining normal pregnancy. Cell Death Dis. 2019;10(6):407.
53. Wang S, Chen C, Li M, Qian J, Sun F, Li Y, et al. Blockade of CTLA-4 and Tim-3 pathways induces fetal loss with altered cytokine profiles by decidual CD4(+)T cells. Cell Death Dis. 2019;10(1):15.
54. Jin LP, Fan DX, Zhang T, Guo PF, Li DJ. The costimulatory signal upregulation is associated with Th1 bias at the maternal–fetal interface in human miscarriage. Am J Reprod Immunol. 2011;66(4):270–8.
55. Meggyes M, Miko E, Polgar B, Bogar B, Farkas B, Illes Z, et al. Peripheral blood TIM-3 positive NK and CD8+ T cells throughout pregnancy: TIM-3/galectin-9 interaction and its possible role during pregnancy. PLoS One. 2014;9(3):e92371.
56. Wu M, Zhu Y, Zhao J, Ai H, Gong Q, Zhang J, et al. Soluble costimulatory molecule sTim3 regulates the differentiation of Th1 and Th2 in patients with unexplained recurrent spontaneous abortion. Int J Clin Exp Med. 2015;8(6):8812–9.
57. Sun J, Yang M, Ban Y, Gao W, Song B, Wang Y, et al. Tim-3 is upregulated in NK cells during early pregnancy and inhibits NK cytotoxicity toward trophoblast in Galectin-9 dependent pathway. PLoS One. 2016;11(1):e0147186.

58. Miko E, Meggyes M, Bogar B, Schmitz N, Barakonyi A, Varnagy A, et al. Involvement of Galectin-9/TIM-3 pathway in the systemic inflammatory response in early-onset preeclampsia. PLoS One. 2013;8(8):e71811.
59. Li YH, Zhou WH, Tao Y, Wang SC, Jiang YL, Zhang D, et al. The Galectin-9/Tim-3 pathway is involved in the regulation of NK cell function at the maternal-fetal interface in early pregnancy. Cell Mol Immunol. 2016;13(1):73–81.
60. Hu X, Zhu Q, Wang Y, Wang L, Li Z, Mor G, et al. Newly characterized decidual Tim-3+ Treg cells are abundant during early pregnancy and driven by IL-27 coordinately with Gal-9 from trophoblasts. Hum Reprod. 2020;35(11):2454–66.
61. Wang SC, Li YH, Piao HL, Hong XW, Zhang D, Xu YY, et al. PD-1 and Tim-3 pathways are associated with regulatory CD8+ T-cell function in decidua and maintenance of normal pregnancy. Cell Death Dis. 2015;6(5):e1738.
62. Wang Y, Li D, Yu T, Hu M, Xing J, Bai S, et al. Dynamics of TIGIT and PD-1 expression on NK cells during the course of normal pregnancy. Immunol Lett. 2021;230:42–8.
63. Kamrani A, Soltani-Zangbar MS, Shiri S, Yousefzadeh Y, Pourakbari R, Aghebati-Maleki L, et al. TIGIT and CD155 as immune-modulator receptor and ligand on CD4(+) T cells in preeclampsia patients. Immunol Investig. 2022;51(4):1023–38.
64. Li C, Liu H, Duan Z. Expression of the immune checkpoint molecules CD226 and TIGIT in preeclampsia patients. BMC Immunol. 2024;25(1):12.
65. Meggyes M, Nagy DU, Feik T, Boros A, Polgar B, Szereday L. Examination of the TIGIT-CD226-CD112-CD155 Immune Checkpoint Network during a healthy pregnancy. Int J Mol Sci. 2022;23(18):10776.
66. Dimova T, Nagaeva O, Stenqvist AC, Hedlund M, Kjellberg L, Strand M, et al. Maternal Foxp3 expressing CD4+ CD25+ and CD4+ CD25- regulatory T-cell populations are enriched in human early normal pregnancy decidua: a phenotypic study of paired decidual and peripheral blood samples. Am J Reprod Immunol. 2011;66(Suppl 1):44–56.
67. Weng J, Couture C, Girard S. Innate and adaptive immune systems in physiological and pathological pregnancy. Biology. 2023;12(3):402.
68. Kaur R, Gupta K. Endocrine dysfunction and recurrent spontaneous abortion: an overview. Int J Appl Basic Med Res. 2016;6(2):79–83.
69. Wang WJ, Salazar Garcia MD, Deutsch G, Sung N, Yang X, He Q, et al. PD-1 and PD-L1 expression on T-cell subsets in women with unexplained recurrent pregnancy losses. Am J Reprod Immunol. 2020;83(5):e13230.
70. Zych M, Kniotek M, Roszczyk A, Dąbrowski F, Jędra R, Zagożdżon R. Surface immune checkpoints as potential biomarkers in physiological pregnancy and recurrent pregnancy loss. Int J Mol Sci. 2024;25(17).
71. Zych M, Roszczyk A, Kniotek M, Dąbrowski F, Zagożdżon R. Differences in immune checkpoints expression (TIM-3 and PD-1) on T cells in women with recurrent miscarriages-preliminary studies. J Clin Med. 2021;10(18).
72. Zhang T, Zhao Y, Cheung WC, Gan YH, Huang L, Li M, et al. Serial changes in two immune checkpoint receptors and ligands, Tim-3/Gal-9 and PD-1/PD-L1 in peripheral blood prior to miscarriage: comparison with pregnancies resulting in a live birth. Am J Reprod Immunol. 2022;87(5):e13524.
73. Liang Q, Tong L, Xiang L, Shen S, Pan C, Liu C, et al. Distinct changes of in BTLA, ICOS, PD-1, and TIGIT expression on peripheral blood and decidual CD8+ T cells in women with unexplained recurrent spontaneous abortion. Biol Reprod. 2020;103(5):1012–7.
74. Hayashi Y, Nishiyama T, Nakatochi M, Suzuki S, Takahashi S, Sugiura-Ogasawara M. Association of genetic variants of PD 1 with recurrent pregnancy loss. Reprod Med Biol. 2018;17(2):195–202.
75. Helles EN, Ashour MJ, Sharif FA. CTLA-4 gene polymorphism in women with idiopathic recurrent pregnancy loss. Int J Genet Genom. 2016;4:31.
76. Nasiri M, Rasti Z. CTLA-4 and IL-6 gene polymorphisms: risk factors for recurrent pregnancy loss. Hum Immunol. 2016;77(12):1271–4.

77. Gupta R, Prakash S, Parveen F, Agrawal S. Association of CTLA-4 and TNF-α polymorphism with recurrent miscarriage among North Indian women. Cytokine. 2012;60(2):456–62.
78. Shen Y, Wang C, Hong D, Zeng B, Fang C, Yuan C, et al. The relationship between polymorphisms in the promoter region of Tim-3 and unexplained recurrent spontaneous abortion in Han Chinese women. Reprod Biol Endocrinol. 2013;11:1–7.

Chapter 10
Immune Checkpoints in Organ Transplantation: Mechanisms, Clinical Outcomes, and Therapeutic Challenges

10.1 Introduction

Organ transplantation is a promising treatment that has drastically improved the survival and quality of life of people with end-stage organ failure. Over the decades, knowledge in this field has been developed, and new techniques and methods have been invented. In the 1950s, immunological concepts of graft rejection were introduced, and immunosuppression methods, including radiation and chemical drugs, such as mercaptopurine and azathioprine, were employed to preserve the allograft. Gradually, other methods, such as human leukocyte antigen (HLA) typing, antibody screening, and organ preservation, were developed to improve graft survival. The first successful kidney transplant was performed in 1954 between identical twins. With the advancement of surgical methods, tissue selection protocols, and immunosuppression, 5-year survival for living-related donor kidney transplants (LRDKT) has reached 85%. The first liver transplant was performed in 1964, which failed, but by the late 1960s, some patients survived for up to a year. Presently, 5-year survival for liver transplantation is around 75% [1]. Cyclosporine A is a calcineurin inhibitor that suppresses lymphocyte proliferation. This agent was approved as an antirejection drug in 1983. Cyclosporine has been very effective in various organ transplants, including kidney, liver, pancreas, lung, heart, and bone marrow. Tacrolimus (FK506) is another calcineurin inhibitor that was approved for liver transplantation in 1994 and for kidney transplantation in 1997. Tacrolimus is more potent in suppressing the proliferation of T lymphocytes and has less toxicity. Sirolimus, or rapamycin, is another agent that was approved in 1999 for use in kidney transplant recipients. Sirolimus inhibits IL-2-induced proliferation of T cells and causes cell cycle arrest in the G1 phase. Mycophenolate mofetil (MMF) also inhibits the synthesis of purine nucleotides and disrupts DNA synthesis in lymphocytes. Glucocorticoids are general immunosuppressants that are usually used with other antirejection medicines [2]. Despite the efficacy of current anti-graft rejection therapies, they can cause

L. Tayebi, M. Abdolmaleki, *Immune System Regulation*,
https://doi.org/10.1007/978-981-95-8026-2_10

serious side effects, including susceptibility to infections, such as cytomegalovirus (CMV) or the development of malignancies. The other issues regarding the long-term use of calcineurin inhibitors are complications, like nephrotoxicity, cardiovascular disease, diabetes mellitus, hypertension, and dyslipidemia, which are associated with morbidity and mortality in patients. Novel immunomodulation strategies can reduce these side effects and toxicities. One of these methods is targeting co-stimulatory molecules that are involved in the activation of lymphocytes. CD28-B7, CD40-CD40L, and ICOS-ICOSL pathways are among these molecules. Belatacept is a fusion protein that inhibits the activation of T lymphocytes by disrupting the CD28-B7 interaction. The efficacy of this therapeutic agent in organ transplantation, especially kidney transplantation, has been proven in several studies [3, 4]. The outcome of transplantation substantially relies on immune tolerance in the allograft microenvironment, and immune checkpoints are key regulatory molecules in immune responses in this context. The function of the immune checkpoint in allograft transplantation has been explored in numerous researches. In the first part of this chapter, the expression of immune checkpoints, especially CTLA-4, PD-1, and TIM-3, in allograft transplants, including kidney, liver, and hematopoietic stem cell transplants, and the importance of these molecules in the clinical outcomes of transplants are discussed. In the following, the findings related to the use of belatacept in transplant recipients are reviewed. In the final section, the safety and efficacy of immune checkpoint inhibitors (ICIs) for the treatment of cancer in organ transplant patients are covered.

10.2 Immune Checkpoints in Kidney Allograft

T cell exhaustion is a well-known phenomenon in cancer. However, there is no comprehensive information about lymphocyte exhaustion in organ transplantation. The study conducted by Fribourg et al. has provided interesting findings in this regard. In this research, the immune checkpoint expression profile on peripheral blood T lymphocytes of kidney transplant patients was determined using time-of-flight mass cytometry (CyTOF). They found that the population of exhausted T cells (Tex) increased significantly at 6 months after transplantation. $CD4^+$ $PD\text{-}1^+$ $TIGIT^+$ $TIM\text{-}3^-$ $2B4^-$ cell subset had the highest frequency in the Tex population. Notably, the increase in the frequency of $CD4^+$ Tex and $CD8^+$ Tex was associated with the reduction of allograft fibrosis. In addition, the percentage of $CD4^+$ and $CD8^+$ Tex was related to estimated glomerular filtration rate (eGFR). Further investigations revealed that $PD\text{-}1^+$ $CD57^-$ $CD4^+$ T cells and $PD\text{-}1^+$ CD57- $CD8^+$ T cells produce less IL-2, IFN-γ, and TNF-α. The level of intracellular ATP production in these cells was low, which is consistent with the exhaustion state [5]. In line with these findings, a research group showed that the frequency of $CD4^+$ $PD1^+$ $CD57^-$ T cells and $CD8^+$ $PD1^+$ $CD57^-$ T cells subsets was significantly lower in acute rejection patients compared to the stable renal function group and healthy controls [6]. In summary, the findings demonstrate that T cell exhaustion development is related to the reduction of acute rejection rate and better clinical outcomes.

The expression of CTLA-4 in allograft transplantation and the relationship of its polymorphisms with the outcome of graft have been investigated in many studies (Table 10.1) [7–10]. A recent study reported that CTLA-4 mRNA expression in $CD8^+$ T cells was lower in more than half of graft recipients after transplantation compared to pretransplantation. In addition, soluble CTLA-4 (sCTLA-4) levels in the serum of about 60% of patients were reduced compared to before transplantation. The levels of sCTLA-4 in the serum of patients with rejection episodes were lower compared to those of stable patients. They suggested that decreased expression of CTLA-4 might be associated with clinical outcomes after transplantation [11]. According to a meta-analysis, the CTLA rs231775 polymorphism (+49A/G) is not considered a genetic risk in acute rejection after kidney transplantation [12], but Yang et al. reported that the GG genotype of CTLA4 +49A/G single-nucleotide polymorphism (SNP) was associated with acute rejection [10]. The rs5742909 (-318C/T) polymorphism in the CTLA4 gene was related to the risk of acute rejection in kidney transplant in African populations, although no correlation between this polymorphism and acute rejection of the transplant has been reported in overall populations [13]. Furthermore, it has been shown that the T-allele of rs5742909 had a protective effect in allograft recipients [7].

PD-1 is critical in maintaining allograft tolerance in kidney transplant patients. A study has shown that PD-1 expression was decreased in allograft rejection [14]. In another study, the relationship between PD-1 expression and renal function in kidney transplantation has been evaluated. This study showed that the percentage of

Table 10.1 Relationships between immune checkpoints polymorphisms and clinical outcome of kidney allograft

Gene	SNP	Position	Population	Comment	Ref
PD1.3	rs11568821	chr2:241851760	France	The A allele improved graft survival in kidney and lung transplant recipients receiving grafts from CMV-positive donors	[28, 29]
PD1.9	rs2227982	chr2:241851281	Iranian	Less significant frequency in the male acute rejection patients	
CTLA-4	rs3087243	chr2:203874196	Egyptian	AG genotype showed a significant impact on graft survival	[30]
	rs4553808 (−1661)	chr2:203866282	Iranian	−1661 showed less significant frequency in the male acute rejection patients	
	rs5742909 (−318)	chr2:203867624		−318 showed reduced acute kidney rejection	
	rs733618 (−1722)	chr2:203866221		−1722 showed a significant association with acute rejection in female patients	
	rs231775 (+49)	chr2:203867991	Korean	+49 has an association with acute rejection patients	[31]

$PD\text{-}1^+$ $CD4^+$ T cells was inversely related to the creatinine levels, and a higher frequency of $PD\text{-}1^+$ $CD4^+$ T cells was associated with lower levels of serum creatinine [15]. Furthermore, Wang et al. indicated upregulation of whole blood cells PD-1 mRNA levels in acute rejection, which can be considered as a predictive biomarker of graft rejection in kidney transplant patients [16]. A study of a mouse model of renal allografts has shown that most of the $CD8^+$ and $CD4^+$ T cells in the kidney had an increased expression of PD-1, especially in the first week after transplantation. In addition, the expression of PD-L1 was confirmed on tubular epithelial cells. Administration of PD-L1 blocking antibodies in these mice was associated with higher $PD\text{-}1^+$ T cell infiltration and increased tubular injury [17]. Gene deletion of PD-1 or PD-L1 in mice accelerated allograft rejection. Interestingly, inhibition of co-stimulation with CTLA-4Ig was not effective in preventing acute rejection. PD-1-deficient $CD4^+$ and $CD8^+$ T cells showed enhanced allo-activation, proliferation, and cytokine production compared to wild-type controls [18]. Based on this data, the PD-1/PD-L1 axis plays an essential role in the suppression of alloreactive T cells and inhibition of allograft rejection.

TIM-3 is also an important Immune checkpoint in the context of organ transplantation. Renesto et al. revealed that urinary TIM-3 mRNA expression was increased in kidney transplant recipients with confirmed acute rejection. They suggested that this marker can be useful in predicting acute rejection as a non-invasive method [19]. Moreover, Manfro et al., by evaluating TIM-3 in peripheral blood leukocytes or in urine cells of kidney transplant patients, found that the level of TIM-3 mRNA was significantly higher in patients with delayed graft function (DGF) or acute graft dysfunction (AGD). Therefore, this marker is helpful in the diagnosis of acute rejection [20]. Another study showed that urinary secretory TIM-3 (sTim-3) was significantly increased in kidney transplant patients experiencing acute rejection compared to those with stable renal function. In addition, urinary sTIM 3 levels in patients with steroid-resistant acute rejection (SRAR) were higher than those in patients with steroid-sensitive acute rejection (SSAR). Therefore, sTIM-3 is a potential indicator for evaluating kidney function and predicting kidney transplant rejection, as well as monitoring the response to anti-graft rejection therapy [21]. A cohort study evaluating the level of sTIM-3 and its soluble ligand galactosin-9 (sGal-9) in the serum of kidney transplant patients demonstrated that the level of sTIM-3 before transplantation (pre-TIM-3) in recipients with stable renal function was higher compared to the adverse outcome group. In addition, the level of sGal-9 after transplant (post-Gal-9) in the stable group was lower than that of people with adverse outcomes. They concluded that low pre-TIM-3 and high post-Gal-9 at the beginning of transplantation can be an indicator of the risk of rejection and worse outcome within 2 years after transplantation [22]. Another study has revealed that the expression of TIM-3 mRNA in the peripheral blood samples of kidney transplant patients who suffered acute allograft rejection was higher compared to the non-rejection group. The expression of TIM-3 after antirejection treatment was decreased [23].

Some studies have emphasized the importance of the BTLA/HVEM pathway in allografts. The expression of BTLA on peripheral blood $CD4^+$ T cells of kidney transplant patients with acute rejection was lower than that of the stable allograft group, while the expression of this molecule on $CD8^+$ T cells of acute rejection and stable group patients was increased [24]. Overexpression of BTLA has been reported in PBMCs of graft recipients after transplantation in both stable and acute rejection groups. BTLA expression levels gradually decreased in the stable group while remaining high in acute rejection, which has predictive value [25]. A study showed that the expression of BTLA and CD160 was increased on T cells of kidney transplant recipients with a sirolimus regimen. The expression of HVEM was decreased on $CD4^+$ T cells but was normal on $CD8^+$ T cells, while HVEM was upregulated on $CD4^+$ Tregs [26]. Zhang et al., by examining renal tissue biopsies, found that BTLA expression was higher in kidney transplant patients than in healthy controls. The expression of BTLA on peripheral blood T cells of kidney transplant recipients with acute rejection was significantly lower compared to the stable group. By establishing a kidney transplant model, they showed that rats transformed with adenovirus for BTLA ($BTLA^+$ group) experienced less kidney damage and allograft survival was better in this group. It was also found that the overexpression of BTLA limited the proliferation of T lymphocytes during mixed lymphocyte reaction (MLR) culture and reduced IL-2 and IFN-γ production in T cells [27].

10.3 Immune Checkpoints in Liver Allograft

Besides a kidney transplant, which is the most common allograft, the liver is also one of the most frequent transplants. The structure of the liver is due to the presence of immune cells, especially Kupffer cells or liver resident macrophages, NK, and T cells, which are specialized, and it is an important organ in clearing bloodstream infections. However, precise immunoregulatory mechanisms, such as the expression of immune checkpoints and their ligands, lower expression of MHC molecules, and production of anti-inflammatory cytokines, establish immune tolerance in the liver. The expression of PD-L1 on liver sinusoidal endothelial cells (LSECs) prevents the activation of T cells and induces tolerance in the tissue [32]. Several studies have investigated the role of immune checkpoints in liver transplantation (Table 10.2).

A retrospective study showed that the risk of acute transplant rejection was higher in liver transplant recipients with the +49A/+6230G haplotype of the CTLA-4 gene. On the other hand, recipients without this haplotype had a lower risk of acute rejection. An allele of +49A/G SNP is involved in full-length membrane-bound isoform of CTLA-4 (mCTLA4) production, while the presence of +6230G allele affects the expression of sCTLA-4 and reduces the production of this isoform. sCTLA-4 has a protective role against graft rejection through suppression of alloreactive T cell functions [33]. CT60 A/G polymorphism within the 3'-UTR of the CTLA-4 gene was associated with acute rejection after liver transplantation. Those without the CT60 G allele had a lower risk of rejection. This polymorphism is related to reduced levels of sCTLA-4 in the patients and an elevated risk of allograft rejection [34]. The expression of CTLA4 and PD-1 on $CD8^+$ and $CD4^+$ T cells of

Table 10.2 Relationships between immune checkpoint polymorphisms and clinical outcome of liver allograft

Gene	SNP	Position	Population	Comment	Ref
PD-1 PD-L1	rs4143815 rs41386349 rs11568821	chr9:5468257 chr2:241851697 chr2:241851760	Caucasian	Donor PD-L1 rs4143815 and recipient PD-1 rs11568821 were associated with acute rejection late after liver transplantation No association between rs11568821 and rs41386349 with acute rejection in the Caucasian population	[40, 41]
CTLA-4	rs231775 (+49) rs3087243 CT60	chr2:203867991 chr2:203874196	Iranian	Reported as a risk factor for liver transplantation, opposite to other study suggests that liver transplant recipients homozygous for the CLTA-4 +49 G allele have a reduced risk of acute rejection CT60 A/G does not influence acute rejection development in liver transplants	[41–44]
	rs733618 rs4553808	chr2:203866221 chr2:203866282	Caucasian	No significant difference in genotypic and allelic frequencies between liver transplantation recipients with and without acute rejection	

liver transplant recipients who experienced acute rejection was reduced. The expression of these molecules on T lymphocytes in the acute rejection group was significantly lower than in recipients with stable liver function [35]. FK506 is used as an immunosuppressant in liver transplantation. FK506-FK506 binding protein (FKBP) complex inhibits the intracellular signaling of T lymphocytes by inhibiting the dephosphorylation of calcineurin and prevents their proliferation. It has been demonstrated that FK506 increases the expression of CTLA-4 and PD-1 on T cells, especially $CD4^+$ T cells, which favors the survival of the liver allograft [36].

Most of the available information about the protective role of TIM-3 in liver transplantation comes from animal model studies. Kojima et al. assessed the interaction of TIM-3 and its ligand CEACAM1 in a mouse model of liver transplantation. They found that CEACAM1 knockout mice experienced more severe liver damage than wild-type (WT) mice. Moreover, the frequency of $TIM\text{-}3^+$ $CD4^+$ T cells in CEACAM1 knockout mice was lower compared to WT. In addition to conducting the inhibitory signal by TIM-3 in T lymphocytes, CEACAM1–TIM-3 interaction also augments TIM-3 expression and its stability on the cell surface. This study showed that in the absence of CEACAM1, the ability of TIM-3 to suppress liver damage was reduced, which indicates the importance of CEACAM1–TIM-3 crosstalk in regulating allo-reactive T cell responses [37]. Investigation of the mouse model of liver ischemia/reperfusion injury indicated that the TIM-3 blocking antibody caused inflammation development, increasing the infiltration of immune cells, including T cells, macrophages, and neutrophils, and liver damage. TIM-3 blockade led to increased production of IFN-γ from Th1 cells and subsequent activation of Kupffer cells and other innate immune cells [38]. In the murine model of orthotopic liver transplantation (OLT), disrupting TIM-3 signaling with a blocking antibody worsened hepatocellular injury. It also increased the infiltration of macrophages and neutrophils into the liver tissue. In the presence of a TIM-3 antagonist, the polarization of T cells toward the Th1/Th17 phenotype was enhanced. On the other hand, administration of stable-form Gal-9 (rGal-9) to mice increased TIM-3 levels and subsequently improved liver survival against IRI [39]. These data show that the TIM-3/Gal-9 signaling pathway plays an essential role in liver homeostasis.

10.4 Immune Checkpoints in Hematopoietic Stem Cell Transplantation

Allogenic hematopoietic stem cell transplantation (allo-HSCT) is an effective treatment for a range of hematological disorders, including malignancies, such as acute myeloid leukemia (AML), acute lymphoblastic leukemia (ALL), myeloid dysplastic syndromes (MDS), and myeloproliferativeneoplasms (MPN), or nonmalignant disorders, such as aplastic anemia and thalassemia. A major concern in this type of transplantation is graft versus host disease (GVHD), which leads to mortality and morbidity in transplant recipients. GVHD is an immune-dependent allogeneic response caused by the presentation of recipient antigens by recipient APCs to donor lymphocytes. GVHD occurs in 30–50% of allo-HSCT cases and mainly affects the skin, gastrointestinal tract, and liver. In leukemia patients, there is a form of GVHD called graft versus leukemia (GVL), in which donor lymphocytes are activated against the recipient's tumor antigens and destroy residual malignant cells, leading to induction of remission [45, 46].

Several studies have evaluated the relationship between immune checkpoints and clinical outcomes of allo-HSCT (Table 10.3). Garcia et al. presented the first reports on the association of CTLA-4 polymorphism with the clinical outcome of allo-HSCT from HLA-identical sibling donors. Their findings indicated that patients receiving transplants from donors with the CT60 AA genotype of the CTLA-4 gene had a higher incidence of acute GVHD than those with AG or GG genotypes. On the other hand, these patients had better clinical outcomes due to greater GVL reaction. They also found that the GG genotype of this polymorphism is associated with less production of sCTLA-4. sCTLA-4 can competitively inhibit the binding of membrane CTLA-4 (full-length isoform) expressed on the surface of T cells with B7 molecules (CD80/CD86) on APCs. The lack of sCTLA-4 can lead to more inactivation of T cells and a reduction in cellular immune response reduction and probably contributes to dampening the recognition of tumor antigens by T lymphocytes and increasing relapse rates [47]. According to a study, allo-HSCT with CTLA-4 -318 TT genotype donors was associated with an increased risk of disease relapse [48].

Table 10.3 Relationships between immune checkpoint polymorphisms and clinical outcome of allogeneic hematopoietic stem cell transplantation

Gene	SNP	Position	Comment	Ref.
PDCD-1	rs41386349 rs6705653	Intron 4	SNPs of Intron4 and exon5 are associated with post-HSCT GVHD All these SNPs are associated with post-HSCT CMV infection These exon 5 and promoter SNPs associated with post-HSCT disease relapse	[63]
	rs2227982	Exon 5		
	rs36084323 rs2227982	Promoter		
CTLA-4	rs62182595 rs5742909(−318) rs11571315 rs733618 rs11571316 rs573554201 rs4553808 rs16840252 rs945677329	Promoter	rs5742909 and rs231775 are associated with the risk of GVHD in patients with ALL and AML rs11571315, rs733618, and rs11571316 significantly contributed to the post-HSCT mortality in AML and ALL (−318) associated with GVHD post-HSCT	[63, 64]
	(+49) rs231775	Exon 1	Significant association was observed between recipients with +49A/GG allele and lower disease-free survival and overall survival compared to AA genotype A significantly reduced relapse rate in children who received a transplant from a donor with the CTLA-4 genotypes AG or GG in comparison with genotype AA rs231775 is associated with post-HSCT GVHD	[63, 65, 66]
	(CT60) rs3087243 rs231721 rs778932058 rs11571319	3′UTR	Significant association between the donor's CTLA-4 SNP of rs3087243 and transplant-related mortality in children undergoing allogeneic HSCT CT60 significantly contributed to the post-HSCT mortality in patients with AML and ALL	[63]
HAVCR2 (TIM -3)	rs10515746	chr5:157109557	CMV infection was more common in patients transplanted with TIM-3 rs10515746	[56]
BTLA	rs76844316 rs9288952	chr3:112469762 chr3:112466178	No strong association for a certain genotype at these SNPs in HSCT donors or recipients	[67]
LAG3	rs870849	chr12:6777854	No association between this SNP and HSCT donors or recipients	

Significant association of CTLA-4 polymorphisms, including CT60 (rs3087243), and polymorphic microsatellite marker with acute GVHD in thalassemia patients receiving allo-HSCT has been reported. In recipients with the CT60-AA genotype, the rate of acute GVHD (grade II-IV and grade III-IV) was higher [49]. In addition, Azarian et al., by examining 225 patients HSCT recipients from HLA-identical sibling donors, found that patients receiving allografts from donors with the CTLA-4 +49 GG genotype had a significantly higher risk of chronic GVHD compared to those with AG or those with the AA genotype [50]. A study of 164 patients after allo-HSCT showed that overall survival (OS) and relapse-free survival (RFS) were lower in donors with CTLA-4 rs4553808 (−1661 A/G) polymorphism. They suggested that the AG or GG genotype can be considered as an independent risk factor for OS and RFS [50]. A study evaluating CTLA 4 polymorphisms in 152 acute leukemia patients (including 83 ALL patients) after HLA haplotype-mismatched allo-HSCT revealed that ALL recipients with the +49 GG genotype had lower OS than GA and AA genotypes. They concluded that CTLA-4 +49 GG is an independent risk factor for OS in these patients [51].

It has been found that in myeloma and lymphoma patients following autologous stem cell transplantation (auto-SCT), PD-1 expression on T cells, NK cells, and monocytes was increased during early reconstitution, although the expression of this immune checkpoint on NK cells and monocytes gradually decreased and reached the normal level. PD-1$^+$ T cells of the patients showed an exhausted phenotype, and the increased frequency of these cells was associated with worse PFS. This study suggests that targeting PD-1 can help strengthen the conventional therapeutic regimen after auto-SCT [52]. Studying 105 allo-HSCT recipients, Simonetta et al. showed that the frequency of PD-1$^+$ CD4$^+$ T and PD-1$^+$ CD8$^+$ T cells was increased early after transplantation. PD-1 overexpression on CD8 T cells was transient and decreased progressively, but CD4 T cells had a stable PD-1 upregulation, which was evident up to 2 years after transplantation. Interestingly, PD-1$^+$ CD8$^+$ T cells had normal production of granzyme B and perforin, and their cytotoxic activity was not impaired [53]. Phenotypic and functional evaluation of peripheral blood T cells of AML patients receiving allo-HSCT showed that these cells had elevated expression levels of PD-1 and TIM-3. Additional phenotypic investigations demonstrated that these cells were antigen-experienced and mainly belonged to central memory (TCM) and effector memory (TEM) T cell subtypes. The production of IL-2, IFN-γ, and TNF-α in PD-1^{hi} TIM-3$^+$ T cells was reduced, which indicates the state of exhaustion in these cells. PD-1^{hi} TIM-3$^+$ T cell population showed a significant association with leukemia relapses posttransplantation. Interestingly, the increase in the frequency of this cell population occurred before the appearance of clinical symptoms of relapse. Therefore, they have predictive value and can be useful in the prediction of leukemia relapse [54]. Lee et al. investigated the phenotype of T cells in the bone marrow of multiple myeloma patients after auto-SCT. They found that the population of Treg cells increased in the bone marrow of these patients, while CD4 T cells decreased, and the ratio of CD4T:CD8T cells was lower than that of healthy donors. The main decrease in T lymphocytes was related to naïve subsets. Phenotypically, T cells were mainly differentiated and showed high levels of regulatory molecules and activation markers, including ICOS, PD-1, LAG-3, CTLA-4, granzyme B, and Ki-67. PD-1$^+$ T cells were mainly the TEM subset. The presence of PD-1^{hi} CD4$^+$ T cells was associated with early relapse and shorter PFS. In addition, patients with increased expression of LAG-3 on T cells (LAG-3^{hi} T cells), including LAG-3^{hi} CD4$^+$ T, LAG-3^{hi} CD8$^+$ T, and LAG-3^{hi} Treg cells, had a shorter PFS compared to LAG-3^{lo} group [55].

The association of TIM-3 polymorphism and allo-HSCT clinical outcomes has been investigated in some researches. Biały et al. found that transplant recipients with the CC and AC genotypes of the TIM-3 rs1036199 polymorphism (A > C) and the AA and CA genotypes of the rs10515746 polymorphism (C > A) had lower rates of acute GVHD. Recessive alleles of these polymorphisms were associated with a reduced risk of GVHD [56]. Evaluation of the expression of TIM-3 in peripheral blood hematopoietic stem cell transplantation (PBSCT) indicated that the increase in population of TIM-3$^+$ CD8$^+$ T cells in transplant recipients was related to severe acute GVHD and can be considered as a marker for acute GVHD in these patients [57]. In addition, a study of 42 allo-HSCT patients revealed that plasma levels of sTIM-3 were associated with acute GVHD. Patients with severe GVHD had markedly more sTIM-3 than those who developed mild GVHD [58]. Other studies have reported similar results [59]. It has been found that plasma levels of sTIM-3 were strongly related to no relapse mortality, and sTIM-3 has diagnostic value as a predictive biomarker of severe GVHD. It seems that sTIM-3 aggravates GVHD by blocking the interaction of membrane-bound TIM-3 with its ligand [60, 61]. The regulatory role of TIM-3 in the inhibition of GVHD has been shown in a mouse model of bone marrow transplantation. Veenstra et al. found that during GVHD, TIM-3 was overexpressed on donor T cells, and its ligand gal-9 was upregulated on nonhematopoietic cells. Blockade of TIM-3/Gal-9 interaction with TIM-3-Ig fusion protein worsened GVHD and lethality in recipient mice. Using TIM-3 KO donor T cells (TIM-3$^{-/-}$ T cells) showed similar results. Furthermore, in Gal-9 transgenic mice, the incidence of GVHD was reduced. In vitro and in vivo evaluations showed that blocking the TIM-3/Gal-9 pathway increases the proliferation and activation of donor T cells [62].

10.5 Role of Belatacept in Allograft Transplantation

Costimulatory pathways play a key role in the activation of adaptive immune responses during an alloimmune response. The CD28-CD80/86 pathway is critical for T cell activation. CD28Ig (Ig-fusion proteins) were designed to reduce T cell activation, although the binding affinity to CD80/86 was not strong. CTLA4Ig is another fusion protein that was produced to reduce CD28 signaling in T cells. CTLA4Ig consists of the extracellular domain of CTLA-4 and the constant fragment portion (Fc) of IgG1, which binds to CD80 and CD86 and disrupts the signaling of the CD28 pathway in T cells (Fig. 10.1). This factor is stronger in regulating T cell responses [68]. Despite the effectiveness of immunosuppressive drugs,

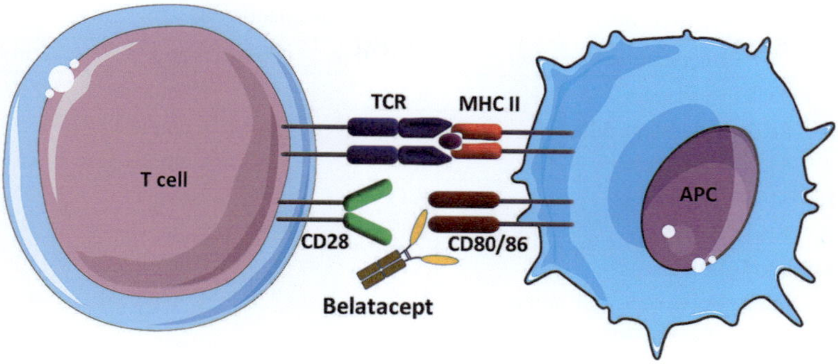

Fig. 10.1 Belatacept functions in the inhibition of T cell co-stimulatory signals. Recognition of the MHC-peptide complex on APC by the TCR provides the first activation signal for the T cell. The binding of CD28 to CD80/86 leads to the initiation of the second or co-stimulatory signal, resulting in T cell activation. Belatacept, a CTL4-4Ig fusion protein, similar to membrane-bound CTLA-4, competitively binds to CD80/86 and inhibits CD28-CD80/86 interaction. Created using elements from Servier Medical Art (https://smart.servier.com), licensed under CC BY 4.0 (https://creativecommons.org/licenses/by/4.0/)

mainly calcineurin inhibitors (including cyclosporin A and tacrolimus) in allograft survival and preventing acute rejection, these factors alone are not sufficient for long-term graft survival. In addition, long-term use of these drugs is associated with serious side effects such as nephrotoxicity, increased blood pressure, and posttransplant diabetes. Therefore, the strategy of blocking the co-stimulatory signal in T cells and reducing the allo-immune response has been considered [69]. The results of the clinical trials of belatacept, which is a high-affinity CTLA-4Ig, were promising in improving kidney transplant survival. Compared to cyclosporin A, belatacept showed acceptable effectiveness in maintaining immunosuppression and preventing graft rejection, and, of note, it had fewer toxicities. According to these promising results, belatacept was approved by the FDA in June 2011 as an additional treatment option for the prophylaxis of allograft rejection in kidney transplant recipients [70]. The clinical trials of belatacept in different organ transplantations are presented in Table 10.4.

The results of phase III trials, BENEFIT and BENEFIT-EXT, demonstrated that graft survival 1 year after kidney transplantation with belatacept was similar to that of cyclosporine-treated recipients. In addition, patients treated with belatacept had better renal function and less cardiac and metabolic toxicities, although posttransplant lymphoproliferative disorder was more common in these patients [71, 72]. Evaluation of the safety and efficacy of belatacept in renal transplantation over a 5-year period has shown that recipients with the belatacept regimen had stable renal function and a low rate of acute rejection. The rates of infections and neoplasms were similar to those treated with cyclosporine, but gastrointestinal disorders were higher in the belatacept group. Posttransplant lymphoproliferative disorder was not observed during treatment with belatacept. These results indicated the safety of belatacept during 5 years after allograft transplantation [73]. Zhang et al. investigated the effect of belatacept, along with the overexpression of another immune checkpoint, in a kidney transplant model with acute rejection. They found that

Table 10.4 Clinical trials involving belatacept in organ transplantation

Study ID	Intervention/treatment	Indication	Phase	Status	Enrollment
NCT02560558	Belatacept	KTx	4	Completed	166
NCT02078193	Belatacept, MMF	KTx	4	Completed	3
NCT00578448	Belatacept	KTx	2	Completed	14
NCT01953120	Belatacept	KTx	4	Completed	20
NCT01791491	Belatacept	KTx	2	Completed	16
NCT00569803	Belatacept	KTx	1	Completed	153
NCT01820572	Belatacept, tacrolimus, cyclosporine	KTx	3	Completed	446
NCT04786067	Belatacept	KTx	4	Recruiting	25
NCT04955366	Belatacept, abatacept	KTx	2	Recruiting	86
NCT04477629	Belatacept, tacrolimus, MMF, corticosteroid	HeartTx	2	Recruiting	12
NCT04180085	Belatacept, CNI	HeartTx	2	Recruiting	25
NCT02213068	Belatacept, tacrolimus, MMF	KTx	4	Completed	28
NCT00565773	Belatacept, sirolimus, alemtuzumab	KTx	2	Completed	40
NCT02738918	Belatacept	KTx	2	Completed	51
NCT02103855	Belatacept	PancreasTx	4	Completed	6
NCT02327403	Belatacept	KTx	2	Completed	15
NCT05345717	Belatacept	KTx	1/2	Recruiting	5
NCT01496417	Belatacept	KTx	–	Completed	20
NCT00402168	Belatacept, cyclosporine, tacrolimus	KTx	2	Completed	173
NCT04046549	Belatacept, VIB4920, ATG, methylprednisolone	KTx	2	Completed	25
NCT00114777	Cyclosporin, belatacept less intensive (LI), belatacept more intensive (MI)	KTx	3	Completed	595
NCT00455013	ATG, belatacept, sirolimus, tacrolimus, MMF	KTx	2	Completed	93
NCT01436305	Alemtuzumab, MMF basiliximab, tacrolimus, belatacept, methylprednisolone	KTx	2	Terminated	19
NCT00035555	Belatacept, cyclosporine, MMF corticosteroids	KTx	2	Completed	230
NCT02134288	Belatacept, everolimus	KTx	1	Terminated	8
NCT01729494	Alemtuzumab, ATG, belatacept, tacrolimus, MMF	KTx	4		316
NCT05017545	Carfilzomib, belatacept	KTx	1/2	Recruiting	15

(continued)

Table 10.4 (continued)

Study ID	Intervention/treatment	Indication	Phase	Status	Enrollment
NCT00346151	Belatacept, sirolimus ATG, methylprednisolone	KTx	2	Terminated	5
NCT00276250	Efalizumab, abatacept, belatacept	IsletTx	2	Completed	5
NCT00256750	Cyclosporine, belatacept less intensive (LI), belatacept more intensive (MI)	KTx	3	Completed	738
NCT04827979	Daratumumab, belatacept	KTx	1/2	Recruiting	15
NCT02137239	ATG, belatacept, MMF corticosteroids, everolimus, tacrolimus	KTx	2	Completed	58
NCT00555321	Tacrolimus, Basiliximab belatacept less intensive (LI), belatacept more intensive (MI), MMF	LiverTx	2	Terminated	260
NCT04177095	Belatacept, MMF, mTOR inhibitor, prednisone	KTx	4	Completed	17
NCT06055608	Sirolimus, belatacept, MMF, tacrolimus, ATG, tacrolimus	KTx	2	Recruiting	200
NCT03388008	Belatacept, tacrolimus, ATG, MMF, prednisone	LungTx	2	Completed	27
NCT01790594	Belatacept, methylprednisolone, ATG, tacrolimus, MMF	Pancreas and KTx	2	Terminated	46
NCT01856257	ATG, belatacept methylprednisolone, basiliximab, MMF, tacrolimus	KTx	2	Terminated	71
NCT06091995	Belatacept, tacrolimus	KTx	–	Active, not recruiting	300
NCT00501709	Belatacept, Raptiva	IsletTx	1/2	Completed	10
NCT03504241	Donor-derived mesenchymal stromal cells, alemtuzumab, belatacept sirolimus, MMF, prednisone	KTx	1	Active, not recruiting	8
NCT02152345	Belatacept, tacrolimus, MMF, ATG, methylprednisolone	KTx	4	Completed	57
NCT04066114	Lulizumab pegol, tocilizumab, belatacept, everolimus	KTx	1/2	Completed	10

(continued)

Table 10.4 (continued)

Study ID	Intervention/treatment	Indication	Phase	Status	Enrollment
NCT05562869	Belatacept	KTx	3	Recruiting	30
NCT00468403	Belatacept, basiliximab MMF, tacrolimus	IsletTx	2	Completed	10
NCT06336863	Belatacept	KTx	–	Enrolling by invitation	24
NCT06291103	Belatacep, tacrolimus	KTx	2/3	Not yet recruiting	290
NCT01921218	Belatacept, CNI, MMF, prednisone	KTx	3	Completed	13
NCT04877288	Belatacept, tacrolimus, cyclosporine, MMF, enteric-coated, mycophenolate sodium, corticosteroids	KTx	3	Recruiting	102
NCT05145296	Belatacept, daratumumab	KTx	–	Recruiting	12

MMF mycophenolate mofetil; *CNI* calcineurin inhibitor; *ATG* anti-thymocyte globulin; *KTx* kidney transplantation

administration of belatacept in BTLA overexpressing rats prolonged allograft survival. The levels of donor-specific antibodies (DSA) and the deposition of complement degradation products C4d decreased in the transplanted kidney. In the presence of belatacept plus overexpressed BTLA, the frequency of T cells was decreased. The production of inflammatory cytokines, including IFN-γ, was observed, while IL-4 and IL-10 were increased [74].

In addition to kidney transplantation, the effect of belatacept in allografts of other organs has also been investigated, although the available data are more limited compared to kidney transplantation. Klintmalm et al. evaluated the safety and efficacy of belatacept in liver transplantation in a phase II randomized study for the first time. They reported that the rate of acute rejection and graft loss was higher in the belatacept groups compared to the tacrolimus and MMF groups. In addition, more viral and fungal infections were observed in the belatacept groups, although they were not severe. Two of these patients experienced posttransplant lymphoproliferative disorder (PTLD). However, neurotoxic complications were low in the belatacept-treated groups [75]. Another study measuring the effectiveness of belatacept in hepatitis C-positive liver transplant patients who had perioperative kidney failure (3 patients) or posttransplant oliguria with low creatinine clearance (four patients) revealed that the combination of belatacept and mycophenolic acid is safe and effective in these patients [76].

Administration of CTLA-4Ig in the cardiac allograft mouse model led to interesting results. Chronic administration of the combination of CD40L blocking antibody and CTLA-4Ig improved allograft survival in mice. Similarly, in CD40L mice receiving CTLA-4Ig permanently, cellular rejection and DSA levels were significantly reduced, and this was associated with long graft survival. While short-term blockade of CD40L and CTLA-4Ig was not very effective [77], belatacept can be an effective alternative immunosuppressant in heart transplant patients who have kidney complications caused by calcineurin inhibitors. It has been found that belatacept improved kidney function in these patients [78]. There are a few case reports in which belatacept has been used as an immunosuppressant in heart transplant recipients [79–81].

Hui et al. reported a lung transplant recipient treated with belatacept. Three years after the transplant, he developed hemolytic uremic syndrome (HUS) caused by tacrolimus treatment. Conversion to a sirolimus regimen worsened the renal function, and belatacept was prescribed for immunosuppression. During this period, no evidence of acute cellular rejection was observed [82]. However, study of the efficacy and safety of belatacept in lung transplant patients showed that acute cellular rejection did not change before and after the administration of belatacept. Notably, GFR was increased in these patients. Also, there was no difference in the average rate of infections and average arterial pressure compared to calcineurin inhibitors [83]. A pilot randomized controlled trial was conducted to evaluate the effectiveness of belatacept in lung allograft recipients. The study was stopped due to the death of three participants treated with belatacept. Based on the results, there was no difference in acute cellular rejection, DSA development, and infection between the group treated with belatacept (in combination with tacrolimus and prednisone) and the control group (treated with tacrolimus, MMF, and prednisone) [84].

The use of belatacept to establish immunosuppression in islet allotransplantation in animal models has been promising. The combination of belatacept and sirolimus has been successful in preventing acute rejection of islet allo-transplantation in diabetic rhesus macaques. Belatacept, along with continuous administration of sirolimus, significantly improved allograft survival [85]. In addition, in islet transplanted-diabetic rhesus monkeys, administration of CTLA-4Ig strongly enhanced the efficacy of CD40-directed therapy. The combination of CTLA-4Ig and CD40 blocking antibody caused long-term allograft survival and prevented the development of DSA [86]. Posselt et al. showed that nonconventional immunosuppression regimens can be a good choice for allogeneic islet transplant survival. They found that belatacept or efalizumab (an antileukocyte functional antigen-1 antibody) was effective in inhibiting graft rejection. Belatacept had acceptable tolerability and safety in allograft recipient patients. All subjects treated with belatacept achieved insulin independence after single islet transplantation. No cases of PTLD or progressive multifocal leukoencephalopathy (PML) or serious infections were reported [87].

10.6 Immune Checkpoint Inhibitors in Transplantation

Immune checkpoint inhibitors (ICIs) are one of the most effective immunotherapies for malignancies, proven in cancer patients. So far, several ICIs have been approved by the FDA for the treatment of cancer, including anti-CTLA-4 blocking antibodies (ipilimumab, tremelimumab), anti-PD-1 (pembrolizumab, cemiplimab, nivolumab, dostarlimab), and anti-PD-L1 (atezolizumab, durvalumab, avelumab) (see Chap. 5). Due to the success of ICIs in the tumor therapy of non-transplanted patients, the use of these agents in transplanted patients with cancer was also considered. Immunosuppressants are mandatory to prevent graft damage and increase survival, but the development of cancer due to the harnessing of the immune system is an unwanted side effect that occurs in some recipients. Most cancers appear de novo after transplantation. In this category, cancers induced by viruses, such as EBV and human herpes virus, are particularly important. Some other cancers are caused by recurrence of malignancy in patients who were infected with cancer before transplantation. Unfortunately, activation of T cells following ICI therapy is not specifically against tumor cells, and the inactivation of PD-1 and CTLA-4 regulatory pathways can lead to allograft damage by activated lymphocytes [88].

Lipson et al. used ipilimumab for the first time to treat two kidney transplant patients with metastatic melanoma. Interestingly, it was safe and effective [89]. Since then, the use of ICIs in such patients has increased. A systematic review by Portuguese et al. analyzed 119 reported cases of solid organ transplant recipients who underwent ICI therapy for cancer treatment. The kidney and liver were the most transplanted organs, and the most common cancers were cutaneous melanoma, hepatocellular carcinoma, and cutaneous squamous cell carcinoma (cSCC), respectively. Most of the cases (90%) were treated with anti-PD-1. The objective response ratio (ORR) was 35.7% for melanoma and 18.5% for hepatocellular carcinoma (HCC). The highest ORR was related to cSCC (68.2%). The most common toxicity of ICI therapy was graft rejection. The median rejection time after administration of ICIs was about 3 weeks. Further, 41.2% of cases had graft rejection, and 23.5% ended in graft failure [90].

Immunosuppressive regimens have provided long-term survival for kidney transplant recipients, and a large percentage of patients experience survival of >10 years [91]. The risk of cancer increases during this long period of immunosuppression. Melanoma, renal cell carcinoma, urologic malignancies, cSCC, and non-small cell lung cancer (NSCLC) are common malignancies in kidney transplant recipients. Data related to ICI therapy in kidney transplant recipients with advanced cancer are mainly confined to case studies. Obviously, the risk of allograft rejection with immunotherapy was increased in many cases. However, the potency of ICIs in controlling tumor growth in these patients is a significant achievement [88, 92, 93]. A retrospective cohort study of 69 kidney transplant recipients was conducted to assess the effects of ICIs in the treatment of cancer in these patients. cSCC and melanoma were the most common cancers in this group. ICI therapy included pembrolizumab, nivolumab, or combination treatment with ipilimumab and nivolumab. The acute rejection rate was higher in patients treated with ICIs. Also, 42% percent of the ICI group developed acute rejection, of which 65.5% (19 patients) ended in graft failure. The ORR for cSCC and melanoma was evaluated as 40% and 36.4%, respectively. OS was increased in ICIs-treated cSCC patients compared to the non-ICI group [93].

HCC is the most common liver cancer and has a high morbidity and mortality rate. Surgical resection and liver transplantation are the main therapeutic strategies for the treatment of HCC patients. ICI therapy has shown promising results in the treatment of HCC. These immunotherapy agents improve OS and progression-free survival in patients [94–96]. However, the safety of administering ICIs to HCC patients who are candidates for liver transplantation needs to be clarified. Several studies have evaluated the outcome of ICI therapy in pretransplant HCC patients. A retrospective study evaluated the safety of administration of PD-1 inhibitors before liver transplantation in 16 HCC patients. Nine patients experienced acute rejection after liver transplantation (with a median time of 7 days after surgery); however, rejection resolved after immunosuppression regimen. The interval time between the last dose of ICI and liver transplantation was shorter in these patients [97]. Other studies have also reported the association of acute rejection with the administration of PD-1 inhibitors before liver transplantation. An important factor is the time between the last ICI treatment and the transplantation [98, 99].

ICI therapy after liver transplantation is also a feasible approach that has been noted in several studies. Based on these reports, melanoma, lung cancer, and HCC recurrence were the most common malignancies after liver transplantation, and the main ICI used was anti-PD-1 [100]. A study of 41 recipients diagnosed with cancer after liver transplantation evaluated the safety and efficacy of treatment with ICIs. According to this systematic review, HCC (22 cases), melanoma (10 cases), and SCC (5 cases) were the most frequent cancers. Twenty-five patients received nivolumab. Pembrolizumab, ipilimumab, and cemiplimab were used for other patients. Graft rejection occurred in 31.8% of patients, and six deaths due to rejection were reported. Examination of PD-L1 expression in tissue sections showed that allograft rejection and mortality were higher in PD-L1-positive patients. The overall response rate was about 25%, and ten patients responded to the treatment [101]. Similar studies have also indicated the role of PD-L1 as a biomarker in predicting the outcome of ICI therapy and liver graft rejection in these clinical conditions [102, 103].

Overall, despite the therapeutic advantages of ICIs in organ transplant recipients to control advanced cancers, the risk of graft rejection is a serious issue. Large-scale prospective cohort studies are necessary to better understand the function of these factors and to choose the best treatment protocol for the patients.

10.7 Conclusion

The exploration of immune checkpoints in organ transplantation presented in this chapter highlights the intricate balance between allograft tolerance and immune regulation. The detailed examination of CTLA-4, PD-1, and TIM-3 in various transplant settings reveals their crucial roles in modulating immune responses and their potential as biomarkers for predicting transplant outcomes.

The chapter features the complexity of immune checkpoint interactions in different organ transplants, with many molecules exhibiting context-dependent functions.

The association of checkpoint gene polymorphisms with transplant success rates provides valuable insights into the genetic basis of allograft tolerance and rejection.

While the success of belatacept in kidney transplantation has demonstrated the potential of targeting co-stimulatory pathways, its variable efficacy in other organ transplants emphasizes the need for organ-specific approaches. The challenges of using immune checkpoint inhibitors in transplant recipients with cancer further illustrate the delicate balance required in managing posttransplant immunosuppression.

As research in this field grows, integrating genomic, immunological, and clinical data will be important for developing more efficient approaches to transplant management. This knowledge may pave the way for personalized immunosuppression strategies, potentially allowing for fine-tuning of immune responses to maximize allograft survival while minimizing complications.

The future of transplantation medicine may lie in harnessing the complex network of immune checkpoints to promote long-term graft tolerance. However, this approach will require careful consideration of the potential risks, including increased susceptibility to infections and malignancies. Continued research into the tissue-specific and time-dependent roles of immune checkpoints will be essential for translating these findings into effective clinical applications.

In conclusion, while our understanding of immune checkpoints in transplantation has grown significantly, many questions remain. The ongoing exploration of these pathways promises to produce new insights into the fundamental mechanisms of allograft tolerance and may lead to innovative approaches for improving long-term transplant outcomes.

Acknowledgments The authors gratefully acknowledge the valuable assistance provided by Maryam Sadr.

References

1. Black CK, Termanini KM, Aguirre O, Hawksworth JS, Sosin M. Solid organ transplantation in the 21(st) century. Ann Transl Med. 2018;6(20):409.
2. Li Q, Lan P. Activation of immune signals during organ transplantation. Signal Transduct Target Ther. 2023;8(1):110.
3. Husain I, Luo X. Novel approaches to immunomodulation for solid organ transplantation. Annu Rev Med. 2024;75:369–80.
4. Perez CP, Patel N, Mardis CR, Meadows HB, Taber DJ, Pilch NA. Belatacept in solid organ transplant: review of current literature across transplant types. Transplantation. 2018;102(9):1440–52.
5. Fribourg M, Anderson L, Fischman C, Cantarelli C, Perin L, La Manna G, et al. T-cell exhaustion correlates with improved outcomes in kidney transplant recipients. Kidney Int. 2019;96(2):436–49.
6. Wang Y, Lin X, Wang C, Liu X, Wu X, Qiu Y, et al. Identification of PDCD1 as a potential biomarker in acute rejection after kidney transplantation via comprehensive bioinformatic analysis. Front Immunol. 2022;13:1076546.

7. Gorgi Y, Sfar I, Abdallah TB, Abderrahim E, Ayed SJ, Aouadi H, et al. Ctla-4 exon 1 (+49) and promoter (−318) gene polymorphisms in kidney transplantation. Transplant Proc. 2006;38(7):2303–5.
8. Duan Z, Zhang Y, Pan F, Zhang T, Zeng Z, Wang S, et al. Association between CTLA4 gene polymorphisms and acute rejection of kidney transplantation: a meta-analysis. J Nephrol. 2012;25(6):996–1002.
9. Misra MK, Kapoor R, Pandey SK, Sharma RK, Agrawal S. Association of CTLA-4 gene polymorphism with end-stage renal disease and renal allograft outcome. J Interferon Cytokine Res. 2014;34(3):148–61.
10. Yang C-H, Chen X-X, Chen L, Zheng D-H, Liu Q-S, Xie W-F. Association of cytotoxic T-lymphocyte antigen 4 +49A/G gene polymorphism with acute rejection risk in renal transplantation. Pediatr Transplant. 2017;21(4):e12916.
11. Çerçi Alkaç B, Soyöz M, Pehlivan M, Kılıçaslan Ayna T, Tatar E, Karahan Çöven H, et al. Assessment of CTLA-4 gene expression levels on $CD8^+$T cells in renal transplant patients and relation with serum sCTLA-4 levels. Biochem Genet. 2024;63:526.
12. Cargnin S, Galli U, Shin JI, Terrazzino S. CTLA-4 rs231775 and risk of acute renal graft rejection: an updated meta-analysis with trial sequential analysis. Sci Rep. 2020;10(1):12850.
13. Yang CH, Chen XX, Chen L, Zheng DH, Liu QS, Xie WF, et al. Relationship between cytotoxic T-lymphocyte antigen 4–318C/T (rs5742909) gene polymorphism and the risk of acute rejection in renal transplantation. Pediatr Transplant. 2017;21(7).
14. Carmona-Escamilla MA, Fonseca-Sánchez M, Chávez JP, Pizando LA, Soto V, Hernández-Mendoza SA, et al. Analyses of programmed cell death protein 1 in high immunologic-risk transplant patients. Transplant Proc. 2020;52(4):1132–5.
15. Mardomi A, KarajiBani M, Farnood F, Vahed SZ, Ardalan M. The frequency of peripheral PD-1(+) TCD4(+) cells is reversely associated with serum creatinine levels in recipients of kidney allografts. Transpl Immunol. 2023;81:101946.
16. Wang YW, Wang Z, Shi BY. Programmed death 1 mRNA in peripheral blood as biomarker of acute renal allograft rejection. Chin Med J. 2011;124(5):674–8.
17. Shim YJ, Khedraki R, Dhar J, Fan R, Dvorina N, Valujskikh A, et al. Early T cell infiltration is modulated by programed cell death-1 protein and its ligand (PD-1/PD-L1) interactions in murine kidney transplants. Kidney Int. 2020;98(4):897–905.
18. Wang L, Han R, Hancock WW. Programmed cell death 1 (PD-1) and its ligand PD-L1 are required for allograft tolerance. Eur J Immunol. 2007;37(10):2983–90.
19. Renesto PG, Ponciano VC, Cenedeze MA, Saraiva Câmara NO, Pacheco-Silva A. High expression of Tim-3 mRNA in urinary cells from kidney transplant recipients with acute rejection. Am J Transplant. 2007;7(6):1661–5.
20. Manfro RC, Aquino-Dias EC, Joelsons G, Nogare AL, Carpio VN, Gonçalves LF. Noninvasive Tim-3 messenger RNA evaluation in renal transplant recipients with graft dysfunction. Transplantation. 2008;86(12):1869–74.
21. Chen D, Peng W, Jiang H, Yang H, Wu J, Wang H, et al. Noninvasive detection of acute renal allograft rejection by measurement of soluble Tim-3 in urine. Mol Med Rep. 2017;16(1):915–21.
22. Yan L, Yang Y, Li YM, Fan JW, Wang XD, Bai YJ, et al. Soluble Tim-3/Gal-9 as predictors of adverse outcomes after kidney transplantation: a cohort study. Clin Biochem. 2022;102:19–25.
23. Joelsons G, Domenico T, Gonçalves LF, Manfro RC. Non-invasive messenger RNA transcriptional evaluation in human kidney allograft dysfunction. Braz J Med Biol Res. 2018;51(7):e6904.
24. Wang Z, Yang H, Liu X, Zhang J, Han Z, Tao J, et al. Role of B and T lymphocyte attenuator in renal transplant recipients with biopsy-proven acute rejection. Med Sci Monit. 2018;24:387–96.

25. Tian C, Liu YG, Yan JK, Liu SD, Zhao ST, Wang HW. B- and T-lymphocyte attenuator/herpes virus entry mediator as early indicators for acute rejection following kidney transplantation. Transplant Proc. 2013;45(1):157–62.
26. Bai Y, Shi Y, Li Y, Cai B, Zou Y, Wang L. Sirolimus-based regimen promotes inhibitory costimulatory signal of HVEM/BTLA/CD160/LIGHT pathway in allo-renal recipients. Transpl Immunol. 2013;28(1):38–47.
27. Zhang J, Zhang H, Wang Z, Yang H, Chen H, Cheng H, et al. BTLA suppress acute rejection via regulating TCR downstream signals and cytokines production in kidney transplantation and prolonged allografts survival. Sci Rep. 2019;9(1):12154.
28. Hoffmann TW, Halimi J-M, Büchler M, Velge-Roussel F, Goudeau A, Al-Najjar A, et al. Association between a polymorphism in the human programmed death-1 (PD-1) gene and cytomegalovirus infection after kidney transplantation. J Med Genet. 2010;47(1):54–8.
29. Forconi C, Gatault P, Miquelestorena-Standley E, Noble J, Al-Hajj S, Guillemain R, et al. Polymorphism in programmed cell death 1 gene is strongly associated with lung and kidney allograft survival in recipients from CMV-positive donors. J Heart Lung Transplant. 2017;36(3):315–24.
30. Ghoneim ME, Sheashaa H, Wafa E, Awadalla A, Ahmed AE, Sobh M, et al. Impact of CD 28, CD86, CTLA-4 and PD-1 genes polymorphisms on acute renal allograft rejection and graft survival among Egyptian recipients. Sci Rep. 2024;14(1):2047.
31. Kim H-J, Jeong K-H, Lee S-H, Moon J-Y, Lee T-w, Kang SW, et al. Polymorphisms of the CTLA4 gene and kidney transplant rejection in Korean patients. Transpl Immunol. 2010;24(1):40–4.
32. Kubes P, Jenne C. Immune responses in the liver. Annu Rev Immunol. 2018;36:247–77.
33. Tapirdamaz O, Pravica V, Metselaar HJ, Hansen B, Moons L, van Meurs JB, et al. Polymorphisms in the T cell regulatory gene cytotoxic T lymphocyte antigen 4 influence the rate of acute rejection after liver transplantation. Gut. 2006;55(6):863–8.
34. Muro M, Rojas G, Botella C, Miras M, Campillo JA, Minguela A, et al. CT60 A/G marker of the 3'-UTR of the CTLA4 gene and liver transplant. Transpl Immunol. 2008;18(3):246–9.
35. Liu Z, Yu X, Ren W, Zhang M, Wang H, Sun Y, et al. CD152 and PD-1 down-regulation on CD8 T cells is associated with human acute liver allograft rejection. Transplant Proc. 2014;46(10):3511–4.
36. Li J, Bai Y, Wang L, Wei H, Cai B, Yan L, et al. Regulatory effect of FK506 on CD152 and PD-1 in the liver allorecipients. Transplant Proc. 2008;40(5):1495–7.
37. Kojima H, Kadono K, Hirao H, Dery KJ, Torgerson T, Yao S, et al. T cell CEACAM1-TIM-3 crosstalk alleviates liver transplant injury in mice and humans. Gastroenterology. 2023;165(5):1233–48.e9.
38. Uchida Y, Ke B, Freitas MC, Yagita H, Akiba H, Busuttil RW, et al. T-cell immunoglobulin mucin-3 determines severity of liver ischemia/reperfusion injury in mice in a TLR4-dependent manner. Gastroenterology. 2010;139(6):2195–206.
39. Liu Y, Ji H, Zhang Y, Shen XD, Gao F, Nguyen TT, et al. Negative CD4^{+}TIM-3 signaling confers resistance against cold preservation damage in mouse liver transplantation. Am J Transplant. 2015;15(4):954–64.
40. Shi X-L, Mancham S, Hansen BE, de Knegt RJ, de Jonge J, van der Laan LJ, et al. Counter-regulation of rejection activity against human liver grafts by donor PD-L1 and recipient PD-1 interaction. J Hepatol. 2016;64(6):1274–82.
41. Thude H, Schipler AD, Treszl A, Peine S, Koch M, Sterneck M, et al. Lack of association between CTLA-4 and PDCD1 polymorphisms and acute rejection in German liver transplant recipients. Hum Immunol. 2013;74(8):1041–5.
42. Karimi MH, Motazedian M, Abedi F, Yaghobi R, Geramizadeh B, Nikeghbalian S. Association of genetic variation in co-stimulatory molecule genes with outcome of liver transplant in Iranian patients. Gene. 2012;504(1):127–32.

43. De Reuver P, Pravica V, Hop W, Boor P, Metselaar HJ, Hutchinson IV, et al. Recipient ctla-4+ 49 G/G genotype is associated with reduced incidence of acute rejection after liver transplantation. Am J Transplant. 2003;3(12):1587–94.
44. Azarpira N, Malekhosseini SA, Aghdaie MH, Daraie M. CTLA4 CT60 A/G gene polymorphism in liver transplant recipients. Exper Clin Transplant. 2010;8(3):210–3.
45. Rosik J, Szostak B, Machaj F, Pawlik A. The role of CTLA4 and its polymorphisms in solid organ and haematopoietic stem cell transplantation. Int J Mol Sci. 2021;22(6).
46. Köhler N, Ruess DA, Kesselring R, Zeiser R. The role of immune checkpoint molecules for relapse after allogeneic hematopoietic cell transplantation. Front Immunol. 2021;12:634435.
47. Pérez-García A, De la Cámara R, Román-Gómez J, Jiménez-Velasco A, Encuentra M, Nieto JB, et al. CTLA-4 polymorphisms and clinical outcome after allogeneic stem cell transplantation from HLA-identical sibling donors. Blood. 2007;110(1):461–7.
48. Wu J, Tang JL, Wu SJ, Lio HY, Yang YC. Functional polymorphism of CTLA-4 and ICOS genes in allogeneic hematopoietic stem cell transplantation. Clin Chim Acta. 2009;403(1–2):229–33.
49. Orrù S, Orrù N, Manolakos E, Littera R, Caocci G, Giorgiani G, et al. Recipient CTLA-4*CT60-AA genotype is a prognostic factor for acute graft-versus-host disease in hematopoietic stem cell transplantation for thalassemia. Hum Immunol. 2012;73(3):282–6.
50. Azarian M, Busson M, Lepage V, Charron D, Toubert A, Loiseau P, et al. Donor CTLA-4 +49 a/G*GG genotype is associated with chronic GVHD after HLA-identical haematopoietic stem-cell transplantations. Blood. 2007;110(13):4623–4.
51. Qin XY, Wang Y, Li GX, Qin YZ, Wang FR, Xu LP, et al. CTLA-4 polymorphisms and haplotype correlate with survival in ALL after allogeneic stem cell transplantation from related HLA-haplotype-mismatched donor. J Transl Med. 2016;14:100.
52. Richter S, Böttcher M, Stoll A, Zeremski V, Völkl S, Mackensen A, et al. Increased PD-1 expression on circulating T cells correlates with inferior outcome after autologous stem cell transplantation. Transplant Cell Ther. 2024;30(6):628.e1–9.
53. Simonetta F, Pradier A, Bosshard C, Masouridi-Levrat S, Dantin C, Koutsi A, et al. Dynamics of expression of programmed cell death Protein-1 (PD-1) on T cells after allogeneic hematopoietic stem cell transplantation. Front Immunol. 2019;10:1034.
54. Kong Y, Zhang J, Claxton DF, Ehmann WC, Rybka WB, Zhu L, et al. PD-1(hi)TIM-3(+) T cells associate with and predict leukemia relapse in AML patients post allogeneic stem cell transplantation. Blood Cancer J. 2015;5(7):e330.
55. Lee L, Alrasheed N, Khandelwal G, Fitzsimons E, Richards H, Wilson W, et al. Increased immune-regulatory receptor expression on effector T cells as early indicators of relapse following autologous stem cell transplantation for multiple myeloma. Front Immunol. 2021;12:618610.
56. Biały S, Siemaszko J, Sobczyk-Kruszelnicka M, Fidyk W, Solarska I, Nasiłowska-Adamska B, et al. Unravelling the potential of TIM-3 gene polymorphism in allogeneic hematopoietic stem cell transplantation - a preliminary study. Transpl Immunol. 2024;85:102084.
57. Pang N, Yu M, Xu J, Yuan H, Chen G, Wang D, et al. The level of Tim-3+CD8+ T cells can serve as a potential marker for evaluating the severity of acute graft-versus-host disease after haplo-PBSCT. Braz J Med Biol Res. 2023;56:e12997.
58. Nalini R, Roshandel E, Tavakoli Ardakani M, Kazemi MH, Ghaffari-Nazari H, Hajifathali A, et al. Soluble T cell immunoglobulin and mucin domain-3 (sTIM-3) predicts graft-versus-host disease (GVHD) in Iranian allogeneic hematopoietic stem cell transplantation. Int J Cancer Manag. 2022;15(4):e120888.
59. Hansen JA, Hanash SM, Tabellini L, Baik C, Lawler RL, Grogan BM, et al. A novel soluble form of Tim-3 associated with severe graft-versus-host disease. Biol Blood Marrow Transplant. 2013;19(9):1323–30.
60. McDonald GB, Tabellini L, Storer BE, Lawler RL, Martin PJ, Hansen JA. Plasma biomarkers of acute GVHD and nonrelapse mortality: predictive value of measurements before GVHD onset and treatment. Blood. 2015;126(1):113–20.

61. Abu Zaid M, Wu J, Wu C, Logan BR, Yu J, Cutler C, et al. Plasma biomarkers of risk for death in a multicenter phase 3 trial with uniform transplant characteristics post-allogeneic HCT. Blood. 2017;129(2):162–70.
62. Veenstra RG, Taylor PA, Zhou Q, Panoskaltsis-Mortari A, Hirashima M, Flynn R, et al. Contrasting acute graft-versus-host disease effects of Tim-3/galectin-9 pathway blockade dependent upon the presence of donor regulatory T cells. Blood. 2012;120(3):682–90.
63. Chen D-P, Chang S-W, Wang P-N, Lin W-T, Hsu F-P, Wang W-T, et al. The association between single-nucleotide polymorphisms of co-stimulatory genes within non-HLA region and the prognosis of leukemia patients with hematopoietic stem cell transplantation. Front Immunol. 2021;12:730507.
64. Gruhn B, Wittig S, Ernst T, Hammrich J. CTLA-4 polymorphisms: influence on transplant-related mortality and survival in children undergoing allogeneic hematopoietic stem cell transplantation. Blood. 2016;128(22):67.
65. Mossallam GI, Samra MA. CTLA-4 polymorphism and clinical outcome post allogeneic hematopoietic stem cell transplantation. Hum Immunol. 2013;74(12):1643–8.
66. Hammrich J, Wittig S, Ernst T, Gruhn B. CTLA-4 polymorphism rs231775: influence on relapse and survival after allogeneic hematopoietic stem cell transplantation in childhood. Eur J Haematol. 2019;102(3):251–5.
67. Takahashi H, Okayama N, Yamaguchi N, Nomura M, Miyahara Y, Mahbub M, et al. Analysis of relationships between immune checkpoint and methylase gene polymorphisms and outcomes after unrelated bone marrow transplantation. Cancer. 2021;13(11):2752.
68. Schroder PM, Fitch ZW, Schmitz R, Choi AY, Kwun J, Knechtle SJ. The past, present, and future of costimulation blockade in organ transplantation. Curr Opin Organ Transplant. 2019;24(4):391–401.
69. Iglesias M, Brennan DC, Larsen CP, Raimondi G. Targeting inflammation and immune activation to improve CTLA4-Ig-based modulation of transplant rejection. Front Immunol. 2022;13:926648.
70. Archdeacon P, Dixon C, Belen O, Albrecht R, Meyer J. Summary of the US FDA approval of belatacept. Am J Transplant. 2012;12(3):554–62.
71. Durrbach A, Pestana JM, Pearson T, Vincenti F, Garcia VD, Campistol J, et al. A phase III study of belatacept versus cyclosporine in kidney transplants from extended criteria donors (BENEFIT-EXT study). Am J Transplant. 2010;10(3):547–57.
72. Vincenti F, Charpentier B, Vanrenterghem Y, Rostaing L, Bresnahan B, Darji P, et al. A phase III study of belatacept-based immunosuppression regimens versus cyclosporine in renal transplant recipients (BENEFIT study). Am J Transplant. 2010;10(3):535–46.
73. Vincenti F, Blancho G, Durrbach A, Friend P, Grinyo J, Halloran PF, et al. Five-year safety and efficacy of belatacept in renal transplantation. J Am Soc Nephrol. 2010;21(9):1587–96.
74. Zhang H, Wang Z, Zhang J, Gui Z, Han Z, Tao J, et al. Combined immunotherapy with Belatacept and BTLA overexpression attenuates acute rejection following kidney transplantation. Front Immunol. 2021;12:618737.
75. Klintmalm GB, Feng S, Lake JR, Vargas HE, Wekerle T, Agnes S, et al. Belatacept-based immunosuppression in de novo liver transplant recipients: 1-year experience from a phase II randomized study. Am J Transplant. 2014;14(8):1817–27.
76. LaMattina JC, Jason MP, Hanish SI, Ottmann SE, Klassen DK, Potosky D, et al. Safety of belatacept bridging immunosuppression in hepatitis C-positive liver transplant recipients with renal dysfunction. Transplantation. 2014;97(2):133–7.
77. Unger LW, Muckenhuber M, Mahr B, Schwarz C, Pilat N, Granofszky N, et al. Chronic CD40L blockade is required for long-term cardiac allograft survival with a clinically relevant CTLA4-Ig dosing regimen. Front Immunol. 2022;13:1060576.
78. Launay M, Guitard J, Dorent R, Prevot Y, Prion F, Beaumont L, et al. Belatacept-based immunosuppression: a calcineurin inhibitor-sparing regimen in heart transplant recipients. Am J Transplant. 2020;20(2):553–63.

79. Enderby CY, Habib P, Patel PC, Yip DS, Orum S, Hosenpud JD. Belatacept maintenance in a heart transplant recipient. Transplantation. 2014;98(7):e74–5.
80. Kumar D, Yakubu I, Cooke RH, Halloran PF, Gupta G. Belatacept rescue for delayed kidney allograft function in a patient with previous combined heart-liver transplant. Am J Transplant. 2018;18(10):2613–4.
81. Schenk AD, Anderson DJ, Cole RT, Badell IR, Larsen CP. De novo belatacept in a kidney-after-heart transplant recipient. Transplant Direct. 2020;6(1):e515.
82. Hui C, Kern R, Wojciechowski D, Kukreja J, Golden JA, Hays SR, et al. Belatacept for maintenance immunosuppression in lung transplantation. J Investig Med High Impact Case Rep. 2014;2(3):2324709614546866.
83. Iasella CJ, Winstead RJ, Moore CA, Johnson BA, Feinberg AT, Morrell MR, et al. Maintenance belatacept-based immunosuppression in lung transplantation recipients who failed calcineurin inhibitors. Transplantation. 2018;102(1):171–7.
84. Huang HJ, Schechtman K, Askar M, Bernadt C, Mittler B, Dore P, et al. A pilot randomized controlled trial of de novo belatacept-based immunosuppression following anti-thymocyte globulin induction in lung transplantation. Am J Transplant. 2022;22(7):1884–92.
85. Lowe MC, Badell IR, Turner AP, Thompson PW, Leopardi FV, Strobert EA, et al. Belatacept and sirolimus prolong nonhuman primate islet allograft survival: adverse consequences of concomitant alefacept therapy. Am J Transplant. 2013;13(2):312–9.
86. Badell IR, Russell MC, Cardona K, Shaffer VO, Turner AP, Avila JG, et al. CTLA4Ig prevents alloantibody formation following nonhuman primate islet transplantation using the CD40-specific antibody 3A8. Am J Transpant. 2012;12(7):1918–23.
87. Posselt AM, Szot GL, Frassetto LA, Masharani U, Tavakol M, Amin R, et al. Islet transplantation in type 1 diabetic patients using calcineurin inhibitor-free immunosuppressive protocols based on T-cell adhesion or costimulation blockade. Transplantation. 2010;90(12):1595–601.
88. Kawashima S, Joachim K, Abdelrahim M, Abudayyeh A, Jhaveri KD, Murakami N. Immune checkpoint inhibitors for solid organ transplant recipients: clinical updates. Korean J Transplant. 2022;36(2):82–98.
89. Lipson EJ, Bodell MA, Kraus ES, Sharfman WH. Successful administration of ipilimumab to two kidney transplantation patients with metastatic melanoma. J Clin Oncol. 2014;32(19):e69–71.
90. Portuguese AJ, Tykodi SS, Blosser CD, Gooley TA, Thompson JA, Hall ET. Immune checkpoint inhibitor use in solid organ transplant recipients: a systematic review. J Natl Compr Cancer Netw. 2022;20(4):406–16.e11.
91. Hariharan S, Israni AK, Danovitch G. Long-term survival after kidney transplantation. N Engl J Med. 2021;385(8):729–43.
92. Lai HC, Lin JF, Hwang TIS, Liu YF, Yang AH, Wu CK. Programmed cell death 1 (PD-1) inhibitors in renal transplant patients with advanced cancer: a double-edged sword? Int J Mol Sci. 2019;20(9).
93. Murakami N, Mulvaney P, Danesh M, Abudayyeh A, Diab A, Abdel-Wahab N, et al. A multicenter study on safety and efficacy of immune checkpoint inhibitors in cancer patients with kidney transplant. Kidney Int. 2021;100(1):196–205.
94. Gao Q, Anwar IJ, Abraham N, Barbas AS. Liver transplantation for hepatocellular carcinoma after downstaging or bridging therapy with immune checkpoint inhibitors. Cancer. 2021;13(24).
95. Finn RS, Qin S, Ikeda M, Galle PR, Ducreux M, Kim TY, et al. Atezolizumab plus bevacizumab in unresectable hepatocellular carcinoma. N Engl J Med. 2020;382(20):1894–905.
96. Abou-Alfa GK, Lau G, Kudo M, Chan SL, Kelley RK, Furuse J, et al. Tremelimumab plus durvalumab in unresectable hepatocellular carcinoma. NEJM Evid. 2022;1(8):EVIDoa2100070.
97. Wang T, Chen Z, Liu Y, Jia Y, Ju W, Chen M, et al. Neoadjuvant programmed cell death 1 inhibitor before liver transplantation for HCC is not associated with increased graft loss. Liver Transplant. 2023;29(6):598–606.

98. Schnickel GT, Fabbri K, Hosseini M, Misel M, Berumen J, Parekh J, et al. Liver transplantation for hepatocellular carcinoma following checkpoint inhibitor therapy with nivolumab. Am J Transplant. 2022;22(6):1699–704.
99. Dave S, Yang K, Schnickel GT, Kono Y, Delebecque F, Arellano D, et al. The impact of treatment of hepatocellular carcinoma with immune checkpoint inhibitors on pre- and post-liver transplant outcomes. Transplantation. 2022;106(6):e308–e9.
100. Wassmer CH, El Hajji S, Papazarkadas X, Compagnon P, Tabrizian P, Lacotte S, et al. Immunotherapy and liver transplantation: a narrative review of basic and clinical data. Cancer. 2023;15(18).
101. Zhang P, Zhu G, Li L, Lai G, Wang Z, Sun C, et al. Immune checkpoint inhibitor therapy for malignant tumors in liver transplantation recipients: a systematic review of the literature. Transplant Rev (Orlando). 2022;36(4):100712.
102. Shi GM, Wang J, Huang XW, Huang XY, He YF, Ji Y, et al. Graft programmed death ligand 1 expression as a marker for transplant rejection following anti-programmed death 1 immunotherapy for recurrent liver tumors. Liver Transplant. 2021;27(3):444–9.
103. DeLeon TT, Salomao MA, Aqel BA, Sonbol MB, Yokoda RT, Ali AH, et al. Pilot evaluation of PD-1 inhibition in metastatic cancer patients with a history of liver transplantation: the Mayo Clinic experience. J Gastroint Oncol. 2018;9(6):1054–62.

Chapter 11
Immune Checkpoints and COVID-19: Insights Into Immunopathogenesis, Therapeutic Opportunities, and Vaccine Implications

11.1 Introduction

Coronavirus disease 19 (COVID-19) is an emerging disease caused by severe acute respiratory syndrome coronavirus 2 (SARS-CoV-2), which was first identified in December 2019 in China. The COVID-19 pandemic has spread rapidly across the world. The respiratory tract is primarily affected, and the disease can develop into severe lung infections or pneumonia [1]. During T cell activation, the immune system utilizes the different checkpoints to preserve co-inhibitory and co-stimulator signals. In chronic viral infections, persistent activation by photogenic antigens can lead to an exhaustion state in lymphocytes and antiviral immune response disruption. T cell exhaustion is recognized by the upregulation of inhibitory receptors and reduced proliferation capacity, cytokine production, or cytotoxicity of the lymphocytes. Recent findings show that the overexpression of immune checkpoints (ICs) also occurs in COVID-19 patients [2, 3]. Based on available data, there may be an association between disease severity and increased expression of ICs. In COVID-19, immune checkpoint expression, along with lymphopenia and inflammatory cytokines contribute to poor clinical outcomes. Overall, the upregulation of some immune checkpoints could potentially be used as a prognostic biomarker of the disease severity [4]. This chapter provides recent findings about the expression of ICs such as PD-1, CTLA-4, TIM-3, LAG-3, TIGIT, BTLA, and VISTA on immune cells in patients with SARS-CoV-2 infection. In the final sections, the safety and efficacy of immune checkpoint inhibitor (ICI) therapy in SARS-CoV-2-infected cancer patients, as well as the safety of COVID-19 vaccination in cancer patients undergoing ICI therapy, are discussed.

L. Tayebi, M. Abdolmaleki, *Immune System Regulation*,
https://doi.org/10.1007/978-981-95-8026-2_11

11.2 Emerging Coronaviruses

Before the COVID-19 pandemic, two other outbreaks caused by coronaviruses had occurred, including acute respiratory distress syndrome (SARS) and Middle East respiratory syndrome (MERS). Since these diseases have similarities in clinical features and pathogenesis, their genome structure, epidemiology, and pathogenesis are summarized here.

11.2.1 Genome Structure of SARS, MERS, and SARS-CoV-2

Coronaviruses (CoVs), as members of the *Nidovirales* order, consist of an envelope and a genome made of positive-sense RNA. The *Coronavirinae* subfamily comprises four genera named alpha, beta, gamma, and deltacoronaviruses [5]. SARS-CoV, MERS-CoV, and SARS-CoV-2 belong to *Betacoronaviruses* (β- CoVs). Coronaviruses contain a non-segmented, positive-sense RNA genome. The genome length ranges from 27.3 kb in human coronavirus 229E (HCoV-229E) to 31.3 kb for mouse hepatitis virus (MHV) [5, 6]. Coronaviruses genomes contain a 5′ cap structure and a 3′ poly-A tail. This genome directly translates to the replicase polyproteins participating in viral RNA synthesis. Two large open reading frames (ORF) have been identified for the replicase gene: ORF1a and ORF1b, lodged in the 5′ end, which account for two-thirds of the genome (~20 kb). ORF1a encodes polyprotein 1a (450–500 kDa), whereas ORF1a and ORF1b encode polyprotein1ab (750–800 kDa) together. These polyproteins are processed into nonstructural proteins (NSP) by viral encoded proteases and form a replication-transcription complex (RTC) located in a double-membrane vesicle [7]. The Rest of the genome contains other ORFs that encode structural and accessory proteins. Four major structural proteins are produced by these genes, including spike (S), membrane (M), envelope (E), and nucleocapsid (N) proteins, which are encoded within the 3′ end of the viral genome. The coronavirus virion has a spherical shape and is about 125 nm in diameter. Coronavirus contains spike projections on the surface that give it a solar corona look [5]. S proteins assemble as a homotrimer structure and form the viral surface spike, which is the main molecule for binding the virus to the host cell receptor. M protein is a small transmembrane molecule (~25–30 kDa); it is abundant in the virus and is involved in the formation of the virion shape. E protein (~8–12 kDa) is a highly variable molecule in coronaviruses and takes part in the assembly of the virus particle. It functions as an ion channel in SARS-CoV [5]. The N protein is highly phosphorylated with two RNA-binding domains and participates in nucleocapsid structure. The N protein helps to tether the genome to RTC. Hemagglutinin-esterase (HE) is another structural protein encoded by β-CoV. HE is a hemagglutinin that binds to sialic acid residues of cell surface glycoproteins. It seems that HE facilitates S protein-mediated cell entry of the virus [5, 8].

11.2.2 Epidemiology of SARS, MERS, and SARS-CoV-2

SARS, the first emerging disease in the twenty-first century, was a highly contagious respiratory infection. The outbreak began in Guangdong province in China in November 2002 [9]. By June 2003, around 5327 SARS cases and 345 deaths were recorded in China [10, 11]. The disease has spread in many countries, such as Vietnam, Thailand, Singapore, Taiwan, and others. The total number of SARS-positive cases and deaths was estimated at 8422 and 916, respectively. The mortality rate of SARS was about 10% [9, 10].

MERS is the other epidemic disease of the new century that started in 2012. It was initially discovered in Saudi Arabia in September 2012 [12]. The patient was a 60-year-old man who died due to disease complications. The causative agent has been identified as a type of coronavirus named MERS-CoV [13]. By April 2014, 282 patients died from MERS, and infected individuals reached 1364 cases in Saudi Arabia in 2016 [12, 14]. The disease spread to 27 countries, including Middle East countries, such as the United Arab Emirates, Jordan, Qatar, and other regions, like South Korea, etc. [12]. At the end of 2019, the total number of infected people was 2494 cases around the world, including 858 deaths. The mortality rate was very high and estimated at 37% [15, 16]. It seems that camels are the main reservoir of the virus in the Middle East, north and east of Africa; therefore, "dromedary camels" could transmit the disease to humans [16, 17].

The last emerging disease of β-CoV is COVID-19. It was discovered in Wuhan, China, in December 2019. The new coronavirus was named SARS-CoV-2. The disease became a public health emergency, and the World Health Organization (WHO) declared it a pandemic on March 11, 2020 [14, 18]. SARS-CoV-2 has infected hundreds of millions of people around the world. It has been shown that SARS-CoV-2 is 96.2% identical to a bat CoV RaTG13 [18, 19]. Direct contact is the main route of dissemination, and the virus is transmitted to another human via droplets released through coughing or sneezing, like SARS and MERS [20]. The severity of COVID-19 varies from asymptomatic and mild to acute and critical conditions that lead to acute respiratory distress syndrome (ARDS) and death. Elderly people and those with underlying diseases are more susceptible to COVID-19 infection.

11.2.3 Immunopathogenesis

Along with β-CoVs, other coronaviruses cause the common cold in humans, including 229E, HKU1, NL63, and OC43, although in some cases they lead to severe respiratory tract infections [21]. Various factors have been associated with the severity of SARS, MERS, and COVID-19, including lymphopenia, lymphocyte dysfunction, granulocyte and monocyte abnormalities, and increased production of inflammatory cytokines [22]. Innate immune cells like macrophages and dendritic cells (DCs) can detect pathogen-associated molecular patterns (PAMPs) of microbes through their specific receptors called pattern recognition receptors (PRRs). Retinoic acid-inducible gene I protein (RIG-I) and melanoma differentiation-associated protein 5 (MDA5) are two examples of PRRs that recognize double-stranded RNA (dsRNA) or uncapped viral mRNA. Sensing viral PAMPs can trigger intracellular signaling cascades followed by the secretion of type I interferons (IFNs) and pro-inflammatory cytokines [23]. Coronaviruses are equipped with escape mechanisms from the immune system, such as membrane-enclosed vesicles. These compartments are privileged sites for viral RNA replication, and they protect viral RNA from sensing by PRR expressed by innate immune cells [21]. The adaptive immune responses play a pivotal role in the elimination of infections. Decreased T and B cell counts and the dysfunction of these cells during coronavirus infection dampen virus-specific immune responses [22, 24]. SARS-CoV can prevent MDA5 recognition by capping its mRNAs [23]. SARS-CoV enters the epithelial cells, particularly ciliated epithelial cells and alveolar type II pneumocytes in the respiratory tract, through angiotensin-converting enzyme 2 (ACE2). S-protein is an important component that mediates the attachment and entry of the virus into the host cells. After the interaction of S-protein with ACE2, both the virus and the receptor are internalized; as a result, it may reduce surface ACE2 expression. ACE has pro-inflammatory properties and plays a protective role in acute lung injury [21, 23]. The internalization of ACE2 is one of the pathogenesis mechanisms of SARS-CoV [21]. RNA interference (RNAi) is an antiviral defense mechanism applied by eukaryotic cells. It has been demonstrated that SARS-CoV N protein can act as a suppressor of RNAi [25]. IFN-Is (IFN-α and IFN-β) are important cytokines against viral infections [26, 27]. Coronaviruses encode several genes that can function as IFN antagonists [21, 23]. ORF6 blocks the nuclear import of STAT1/STAT2/IRF9 and STAT1/STAT1 complexes that are involved in IFN- β and IFN-γ signaling pathways. In addition, ORF6 can prevent the expression of IFN-β. Furthermore, the overexpression of NSP3 encoded by the COV genome can inhibit IFN responses [21, 28].

MERS-CoV attaches to dipeptidyl peptidase-4 (DPP4) on the target cell through the S protein. DPP4 is expressed in several organs, such as epithelial cells of the lung, kidney, and liver. The virus can induce apoptosis in alveolar epithelial cells. It also induces apoptotic death of T cells through intrinsic and extrinsic pathways [29]. MERS-CoV-infected macrophages serve as virus reservoirs. Replication of the virus in monocyte-derived macrophages and immature DCs prevents these cells from effectively presenting pathogenic antigens to T cells [29, 30]. Papain-like protease (PLpro), belonging to the nonstructural proteins of MERS-CoV, reduces the production of IFNs and increases virus replication in the cells [29]. The 4a, 4b, and M proteins are inhibitors of IRF3 phosphorylation and suppress IFN-I production. Protein 4a also blocks the NF-κB pathway and nuclear localization of STAT1. NSP15 has endoribonuclease activity, which can inhibit dsRNA sensors in innate immune cells [31].

Some of the aforementioned mechanisms are common in SARS-CoV-2 infection. This virus enters epithelial cells through interaction with ACE2. Increased ACE2 expression in the pulmonary epithelium is a risk factor for disease severity [24]. Additionally, the virus can directly infect T cells and macrophages. Decreased numbers of $CD4^+$ T, $CD8^+$ T, B, and NK cells have been reported in patients with severe disease [32, 33]. Furthermore, T cell exhaustion and overexpression of immune checkpoint have been demonstrated during COVID-19 [22, 24, 34, 35]. SARS-CoV-2 can cause a delayed IFN response. In addition, through its structural and nonstructural OR accessory proteins, namely, N, NSP1-3, NSP 13-14, ORF3, ORF6, and ORF8, SARS-CoV-2 suppresses the secretion of IFN-I [36, 37]. NSP1 disrupts the innate immune responses against the virus by inhibiting RIG-1 [38]. Furthermore, RF8 affects antigen presentation to CD8 T cells by reducing the level of MHC-I on the cell surface and ultimately disrupts the CTL responses [39]. In some cases of COVID-19, excessive cytokine production (including IL2, IL-4, IL-6, IL-8, IL-1β, TNF-α, IFN-γ, etc.) occurs, which is known as cytokine storm, and leads to serious problems such as septic shock and multi-organ damage, including lung, kidney, liver, and spleen [22, 32]. Cytokine storm is the main cause of ARDS in COVID-19 patients [40].

11.3 COVID-19 & Immune Checkpoint

T cell exhaustion may be involved in poor clinical outcomes in patients with COVID-19 infection. According to similar conditions in other infectious diseases and cancer, upregulation of ICs can strongly lead to dysregulation of T cell responses. Several ICs, such as PD-1, TIM-3, CTLA-4, LAG-3, TIGIT, BTLA, VISTA are overexpressed in COVID-19 [3, 41, 42]. In addition, there may be a possible association between disease severity and the upregulation of IC receptors and ligands. Generally, the increased expression of some ICs can be considered as a prognostic biomarker for COVID-19 severity.

11.3.1 CTLA-4

CTLA-4 is an important IC that induces inhibitory signals in T cells and reduces their functions. CTLA-4 can compete with CD28 for binding to CD80/CD86 on antigen-presenting cells (APCs) and contributes to establishing immune tolerance [43–45]. CTLA-4/B7 pathway plays a crucial role in T cell exhaustion in severe COVID-19 [46]. Recent Studies have shown increased levels of CTLA-4 on the peripheral blood mononuclear cells (PBMCs) in critically ill COVID-19 patients. Overexpression of CTLA-4 correlates with $CD8^+$ T cell exhaustion and impaired virus-specific immune response in the patients [47, 48]. In addition to membrane form, elevated soluble CTLA-4 (sCTLA-4) in the serum of severe COVID-19 patients has been reported [49]. Moreover, it has been demonstrated that patients with CTLA-4 insufficiency had nonsevere COVID-19, lacked autoantibodies against type 1 IFNs, and tolerated mRNA vaccines with few adverse effects [50].

11.3.2 PD-1

PD-1 is mainly expressed on activated lymphocytes and has been considered a marker of T cell exhaustion [51]. PD-1/PD-L interactions manage several immune-related diseases, such as autoimmune diseases, viral infections, and cancers [52]. High levels of PD-1 expression are detected on T cells, NK cells, and B cells of severe COVID-19 patients [49, 53, 54]. Furthermore, other studies demonstrated up-regulated PD-1 and other ICs including CTLA-4, Tim-3, LAG-3, and VISTA on SARS-CoV-2–specific T cells in the advanced stage of COVID-19 [55].

Beserra et al. have demonstrated that the total count of lymphocytes and monocytes decreased in COVID-19 patients. The overexpression of PD-1 on $CD4^+$ T, $CD8^+$ T cells, and B cells was observed in these patients. Furthermore, sPD-L1 levels were higher in the patients compared to healthy individuals [56]. In addition, increased expression of PD-L1 on lymphocytes, monocytes, dendritic cells, and platelets has also been reported in COVID-19 [57]. A study has shown that the serum levels of sPD-L1, sTIM-3, and sGal-9 are elevated in COVID-19 patients, especially those requiring invasive mechanical ventilation. Post-COVID-19 follow-up of recovered patients showed that the expression of these molecules decreased 8 months after recovery. This study suggests that sPD-L1 and sTIM-3 in serum can be considered as markers related to the severity of the disease [58]. In line with this finding, the increase of sPD-L1 in COVID-19 is related to poor prognosis, and the increase of this molecule in the serum has been proposed as a prognostic marker in patients [59]. Blocking the PD-1/PD-L1 axis can potentially be effective for the treatment of the disease, but there is not enough clinical data to support this idea. Ex vivo studies have shown that blockade of PD-1 enhances the T cell function in COVID-19 patients and anti-PD-L1 improves the capacity of platelets to stimulate IFN-γ production [57].

11.3.3 TIM-3

TIM-3 is another important co-inhibitory receptor that is overexpressed on the surface of $CD4^+$ and $CD8^+$ T cells, NK cells, neutrophils, Tregs, and monocytes of patients with severe COVID-19 [47, 60–62]. Pathological examination of lung tissue sections has revealed a higher level of TIM-3 in the center of the pulmonary inflammatory storm in patients with COVID-19 [47]. Another research reported a higher level of TIM-3 and PD-1 in NK and T cells in men compared to female patients [63]. According to a case report, the levels of TIM-3^+ $CD4^+$ and TIM-3^+ $CD8^+$ T cells in the lung tissue of men were significantly higher than those in female patients [62]. A study group has shown that TIM-3 was overexpressed on NKT cells during SARS-CoV-2 infection. The expression of TIM-3 on these cells was directly related to the severity of the disease. Interestingly, the expression of apoptosis-related genes such as caspases was higher in TIM-3^+ NKT cells. In addition, the expression of other ICs, including PD-1, CTLA-4, and LAG-3, was observed in TIM-3$^+$ NKT. These cells had a higher expression of IFN-γ, IL-4, and IL-10 than the healthy control group [64]. A current study from massive-scale RNA sequencing confirmed higher levels of inhibitory receptors such as TIM-3, PD-1, and BTLA in lung tissues from men compared to women. In addition, there was a positive relationship between lung TIM-3$^+$ cells and age in men but not in women [47, 63]. Recent studies demonstrated that TIM-3 on CD4$^+$ T cells is upregulated in both moderate/severe COVID-19 patients hospitalized in the ICU. These studies can support the role of TIM-3 in T cell exhaustion during SARS-CoV-2 infection, and the TIM-3/Gal-9 axis could be a potential target in this clinical setting [62, 65, 66]. Some studies have reported increased circulating of sTIM-3 in patients with severe COVID-19. Increased sTIM-3 correlates with more severe stage disease [67].

11.3.4 LAG-3

LAG-3 expression is increased on activated T cells (CD4$^+$, CD8$^+$), B cells, and NK cells and is known as a marker for cell dysfunction [4, 47]. In COVID-19 patients, increased expression of LAG-3 on CD4$^+$ and CD8$^+$ T cells (including naïve, central memory, transitional memory, effector memory, and RA$^+$ effector memory T cells) has been reported [68]. Both LAG-3 and TIM-3 are upregulated on T cells in COVID-19 patients, and they have been detected on circulating CD4$^+$ and CD8$^+$ T cells in severe compared with mild and moderate COVID-19, so they can be identified as a marker for bad prognoses in these patients [55, 68]. Furthermore, it has been shown that the levels of sTIM-3 and sLAG-3 are significantly higher in severe COVID-19 patients than in the healthy control group [49]. Moreover, the higher TIM-3 expression on peripheral blood CD4$^+$ T cells was detected in severe COVID-19 patients than in moderate and severe diseases, which could be related to T cell exhaustion [69]. In addition, NK cells of COVID-19 patients appear to be exhausted based on the expression of LAG-3. Thus, the functional exhaustion of T cells and NK cells can play a critical role in serious illness and weak antiviral immune responses [70, 71].

11.3.5 TIGIT

TIGIT is another inhibitory molecule, which is expressed on immune cells such as T cells and NK cells. It has been demonstrated that TIGIT is significantly upregulated on peripheral blood T cells in patients with acute COVID-19 compared with healthy controls [47, 55]. In contrast, studies have also observed no significant differences in TIGIT expression in COVID-19 patients, but it was considerably lower than that of the control group and normal TIGIT expression on cytotoxic T cells (CTLs) [4, 68]. Overall, the function of TIGIT is more debatable, and it suggests that the overexpression of TIGIT, CTLA-4, and TIM-3 was not related to exhaustion and disorder of T cells [55, 69]. Follicular helper T cells (Tfh) play a vital role in enhancing the response of B cells. These cells are involved in the germinal center reactions of the lymph node by providing co-stimulation for the expansion of B cells and the production of high-affinity antibodies. It has been found that the increase of circulating Tfh expressing TIGIT (TIGIT$^+$ cTfh) is associated with the decrease of S1 (a subunit of the virus spike protein) IgG titer in SARS-CoV-2 infection. Further, in vitro studies have shown that TIGIT$^+$ cTfh derived from COVID-19 patients have a lower capacity to activate B cells compared to TIGIT$^-$ cTfh cells. The gene expression profile of the TIGIT$^+$ cTfh cells showed lower expressions of CD40L, IL-21, and IL-17 compared to the TIGIT-negative population, which weakens their ability to help B cells in co-culture [72]. TIGIT$^+$ Tregs are considered to have strong suppressive properties and are able to inhibit the immune system response in infections. It has been shown that TIGIT$^+$ FOXP3$^+$ Tregs increase in COVID-19, and the increase in the number of this cell population is related to lung dysfunction, worse outcomes, and more severe disease [73].

11.3.6 BTLA

BTLA is an inhibitor expressed on B, T, and NK cells. The function and structure of BTLA are similar to those of CTLA-4 and PD-1 to inhibit lymphocyte effector functions during immune response. Overexpression of BTLA has been observed on transitional memory T cells and effector memory T cells in COVID-19 and malaria patients compared to controls [68]. Schultheiß et al. indicated that the expression of BTLA increased on circulating CD4$^+$ and CD8$^+$ T cells of COVID-19 patients [74]. In another study, increased levels of sBTLA were observed in patients with severe COVID-19 [49]. It has also been demonstrated that the expression of BTLA is related to the SARS-CoV-2 viral levels and severity of COVID-19 [42].

11.3.7 VISTA

VISTA is an IC that plays an initial and central role in controlling myeloid migration and the regulation of APCs' activity. VISTA is known as a primary target for controlling the earliest phases of innate inflammation [70]. It has been shown that VISTA was up-regulated in CD4$^+$ and CD8$^+$ T cells in mild and moderate COVID-19 patients. VSIG3 (known as IgSF11) acts as a major ligand of VISTA, showing specific binding and inhibitory function [70, 71]. In addition, according to another study, there are significantly increased VISTA molecules in the SARS-CoV-2-specific T cells (CD154$^+$ CD4$^+$, CD137$^+$ CD8$^+$ T cells) stimulated by antigens [55, 70]. Overall, VISTA on T cells, myeloid cells, and monocytes has a significant potential role in driving cytokine storms after viral infection [47, 70].

11.3.8 NKG2A

CD94/NK group 2 member A (NKG2A) is listed in novel IC proteins that are overexpressed on CTLs and NK cells in the early phase of SARS-CoV-2 infection. Overexpression of NKG2A decreases NK cell activity and increases $CD8^+$ T cell exhaustion [47]. $CD8^+$ T cells and NK cells are key immune cells in antiviral immune responses. Remarkably, these cell populations displayed functional exhaustion in severe COVID-19 cases as compared with mild disease patients and healthy controls. Interestingly, it is reported that the number of NK and $CD8^+$ T cells returned after therapy [75, 76].

11.4 Cancer ICI Therapy and COVID-19

Limited information is available on the interaction of COVID-19 infection and ICI therapy in cancer patients. Cancer development is correlated with the dysfunction of immune cells and the increase of immunosuppressive factors in favor of tumor expansion. The COVID-19 outcomes are worse in the presence of some underlying diseases, especially cancer. Moreover, conventional cancer treatments, such as chemotherapy and radiotherapy, make the patient more vulnerable to infections. ICIs can restore the function of immune cells and strengthen the antitumor immune response. ICI therapy plays a pivotal role in tumor growth inhibition by restoring T cell function and increasing the production of important cytokines, such as IFN-γ. $CD8^+$ T cells are very important in eliminating virus-infected cells. In viral infections, including SARS-CoV-2, the function of T lymphocytes decreases during the exhaustion process. Therefore, ICIs are potentially able to reactivate these cells, which leads to improvement of the antiviral immune response [77, 78]. However, in severe infections where T cells are completely exhausted, the efficacy of ICIs is diminished. Despite the beneficial effects, ICIs cause immune-related adverse events (irAEs) in some patients (see Chap. 6). ICI-induced pulmonary irAEs are reported in some cancer patients, especially in non-small cell lung cancer (NSCLC), which sometimes is life-threatening [79]. Pneumonitis caused by COVID-19 is not clearly distinguishable from ICI-related pulmonary complications in terms of clinical and laboratory signs, and they have many similarities. Cytokine release syndrome (CRS) is another adverse event that rarely happens in cancer patients treated with ICIs. CRS is an inflammatory condition with extensive secretion of inflammatory cytokines, especially IL-6 and IFN-γ. The clinical symptoms range from fever, myalgia, and malaise to lung failure and severe organ toxicity. In addition, CRS can occur as a result of infections like SARS-CoV-2. CRS in COVID-19 patients is relatively common, and it leads to lung tissue damage. CRS can become more expanded and appear as a cytokine storm, which can promote ARDS. Therefore, considering these similarities, it is not easy to distinguish whether lung damage is a direct result of ICI immunotherapy or SARS-CoV-2 infection. It is difficult to determine the effect of ICIs on COVID-19 outcomes in cancer patients undergoing ICI therapy [80–82].

Early reports suggested that ICIs might worsen the infection of COVID-19 and can act as a risk factor for COVID-19 and exacerbate the disease. However, several studies challenged this hypothesis. It has been shown that cancer treatment with ICIs does not increase the rate of COVID-19 [83]. The results of a meta-analysis indicated that ICIs had no negative effect on the severity and mortality of COVID-19, and in this regard, there was no difference with the control group [81]. In a cohort study, Tan et al. showed no difference in the severity and mortality of COVID-19 in cancer patients who were receiving ICIs compared to the control group [84]. Luo et al. reported that PD-1 inhibitor is not associated with increased severity of COVID-19 in lung cancer patients receiving this immunotherapy [85]. Moreover, a meta-analysis has shown that the ICIs do not affect the severity, hospitalization, or mortality of COVID-19 in cancer patients [86]. A systematic review by assessing 15,497 COVID-19 patients, including 3220 cancer patients receiving ICI from 25 studies, revealed that there was no significant difference in hospital admission and mortality rate between ICI patients compared to non-ICI patients [87]. Based on a propensity-matched analysis of the On Covid registry by Mostaghim et al., previous ICI therapy of cancer patients does not exacerbate COVID-19 outcomes [88]. Interestingly, according to some studies, ICIs in cancer patients can strengthen humoral and cellular immunity against COVID-19 infection [60, 89]. Overall, cancer ICI therapy (anti-PD-1/CTLA-4) does not interfere with the immune response to COVID-19 and is not considered a risk factor. It does not have negative effects on the clinical outcome of COVID-19, and the administration of ICIs in these patients can be continued. Several clinical trials have been designed on the efficacy of ICIs, including nivolumab, ipilimumab, and pembrolizumab in COVID-19 patients (Table 11.1); however, the results have not yet been published.

Table 11.1 Clinical trials evaluating ICIs in COVID-19

NCT number	Interventions	Status	Phase	Study design
NCT04343144	Nivolumab	Unknown	2	Evaluating the efficacy of nivolumab in COVID-19
NCT04413838	Nivolumab	Unknown	2	Evaluating the efficacy of nivolumab in obese individuals with COVID-19
NCT04356508	Nivolumab	Unknown	2	Study of nivolumab in COVID-19 patients
NCT05597800	Nivolumab, ipilimumab, and chemotherapy	Not yet recruiting	2	Evaluating the ICIs and chemotherapy combination in advanced NSCLC patients with HIV, HBV, HCV, and COVID-19
NCT04335305	Pembrolizumab, tocilizumab	Terminated	2	Evaluating the efficacy and safety of tocilizumab/pembrolizumab combination in COVID-19 pneumonia

11.5 Covid-19 Vaccination and Cancer ICI Therapy

Cancer patients are more susceptible to SARS-CoV-2 infection. They are prone to severe disease and morbidity due to COVID-19. Furthermore, during hospitalization, the risk of being exposed to the virus increases the COVID-19 incidence in these patients. Therefore, it seems that cancer patients are among the high-priority populations for COVID-19 vaccination. However, due to the weakened immune system in some cancer patients (immunocompromised patients), the humoral immune response to the vaccine may not be as expected [90–92]. Cumulative data show that COVID-19 vaccination in cancer patients undergoing cancer therapy, including chemotherapy (such as alkylating agents, TK inhibitors, and mTOR inhibitors) and radiotherapy, is associated with lower seropositivity or decreased antibody titers compared to healthy individuals. However, vaccination in these patients has acceptable safety and efficacy and can enhance the immune response against COVID-19. Therefore, COVID-19 vaccines are beneficial for cancer patients. In most patients, side effects related to the vaccines are similar to normal non-cancer people [92].

A serious concern in cancer patients undergoing ICI therapy is whether the COVID-19 vaccines are safe and effective in these patients. This issue has been evaluated in the clinical setting. Studies showed that ICI therapy does not have a significant effect on the seroconversion rate of cancer patients who receive the COVID-19 vaccine, although antibody titers may have decreased [92]. For example, a systematic review and meta-analysis analyzing 19 studies, including 2477 cancer patients receiving ICI, showed that COVID-19 vaccination is effective and safe in these patients. After two doses of the COVID-19 vaccine, there was no significant difference in seroconversion rates between ICI-receiving patients compared to non-ICI patients and non-cancer patients [93]. Mei et al. indicated that treating cancer patients with anti-PD-1 does not affect the efficacy of COVID-19 vaccination [94]. On the other hand, according to a prospective study, COVID-19 vaccination enhanced the effectiveness of ICI immunotherapy with anti-PD-1 in NSCLC patients. COVID-19 vaccination was associated with progression-free survival (PFS) and better overall survival (OS) in stage III-IV NSCLC patients with ICI treatment [95].

The adverse events of the COVID-19 vaccine in ICI-receiving patients are similar to those in non-cancer populations, which manifest as a range of local or systemic side effects, including pain at the site of injection, headache, muscle pain, fatigue, local rash, fever, and flu-like symptoms [92]. COVID-19 vaccination has been reported to be safe in lung cancer patients undergoing ICI therapy [96]. A retrospective study showed that COVID-19 vaccination is not related to an increase in the rate of severe irAEs in patients undergoing ICI therapy [97]. In melanoma patients receiving ICI, the response to COVID-19 vaccination was similar to that of healthy individuals [98]. In 130 patients with advanced skin cancer treated with ICI who received the COVID-19 vaccine, side effects were generally mild pain at the injection site and fatigue. Grade 3 irAEs, including colitis, hepatitis, myositis, and myocarditis, occurred in eight patients. Remarkably, no cases of CRS (> grade 2) were observed. This study indicated that the rate of irAEs did not increase after receiving the vaccine and that the COVID-19 vaccination was safe in these patients [99]. Taken together, COVID-19 vaccination is effective in ICI-treated cancer patients, and it is well tolerated in these patients.

11.6 Conclusion

The exploration of immune checkpoint expression in COVID-19 presented in this chapter highlights the intricate balance between immune activation and regulation in SARS-CoV-2 infection. The detailed examination of various checkpoint molecules reveals their crucial roles in modulating immune responses and their potential as prognostic markers for disease severity.

The chapter features the complexity of immune checkpoint interactions in COVID-19, with many molecules exhibiting context-dependent functions. The association of checkpoint expression with T cell exhaustion provides valuable insights into the mechanisms of severe disease and potential therapeutic approaches.

While the success of immune checkpoint inhibitors in cancer therapy has raised concerns about their use in COVID-19 patients, the evidence suggests that ICI therapy does not significantly worsen COVID-19 outcomes in cancer patients. This finding opens up possibilities for maintaining cancer treatments during the pandemic.

The safety and efficacy of COVID-19 vaccination in patients undergoing ICI therapy is a key finding, supporting the importance of vaccination in this vulnerable population. However, the potential for reduced antibody responses in some cancer patients emphasizes the need for personalized approaches.

Integrating immunological, clinical, and epidemiological data will be crucial for developing more efficient approaches to COVID-19 management. This knowledge may be useful for targeted therapies that modulate immune checkpoint expression to improve outcomes in severe cases.

The ongoing exploration of immune checkpoints in COVID-19 may suggest new insights into the fundamental mechanisms of antiviral immunity and may lead to innovative approaches for managing possible future pandemics. However, many questions remain, and continued research is essential to fully understand the role of immune checkpoints in COVID-19 pathogenesis and recovery.

Acknowledgments The authors gratefully acknowledge the valuable assistance provided by Maryam Sadr.

References

1. Maniruzzaman M, Islam MM, Ali MH, Mukerjee N, Maitra S, Kamal MA, et al. COVID-19 diagnostic methods in developing countries. Environ Sci Pollut Res Int. 2022;29(34):51384–97.

2. Mohammed RN, Tamjidifar R, Rahman HS, Adili A, Ghoreishizadeh S, Saeedi H, et al. A comprehensive review about immune responses and exhaustion during coronavirus disease (COVID-19). Cell Commun Signal. 2022;20(1):79.
3. Alahdal M, Elkord E. Exhaustion and over-activation of immune cells in COVID-19: challenges and therapeutic opportunities. Clin Immunol (Orlando, Fla). 2022;245:109177.
4. Al-Mterin MA, Alsalman A, Elkord E. Inhibitory immune checkpoint receptors and ligands as prognostic biomarkers in COVID-19 patients. Front Immunol. 2022;13:870283.
5. Fehr AR, Perlman S. Coronaviruses: an overview of their replication and pathogenesis. In: Coronaviruses. Springer; 2015. p. 1–23.
6. Ashour HM, Elkhatib WF, Rahman M, Elshabrawy HA. Insights into the recent 2019 novel coronavirus (SARS-CoV-2) in light of past human coronavirus outbreaks. Pathogens. 2020;9(3):186.
7. Ziebuhr J. The coronavirus replicase. In: Coronavirus replication and reverse genetics. Springer; 2005. p. 57–94.
8. Chen Y, Liu Q, Guo D. Emerging coronaviruses: genome structure, replication, and pathogenesis. J Med Virol. 2020;92(4):418–23.
9. Chan-Yeung M, Xu RH. SARS: epidemiology. Respirology. 2003;8:S9–S14.
10. Zhong N-S, Wong GW. Epidemiology of severe acute respiratory syndrome (SARS): adults and children. Paediatr Respir Rev. 2004;5(4):270–4.
11. Meo S, Alhowikan A, Al-Khlaiwi T, Meo I, Halepoto D, Iqbal M, et al. Novel coronavirus 2019-nCoV: prevalence, biological and clinical characteristics comparison with SARS-CoV and MERS-CoV. Eur Rev Med Pharmacol Sci. 2020;24(4):2012–9.
12. Ahmadinejad F, Honardoost M-A, Amiri M, Jami M-S. Genetics and epidemiology of Middle East Respiratory Syndrome-Coronavirus (MERS-CoV). Int J Epidemiol Res. 2015;2(4):204–8.
13. Chafekar A, Fielding BC. MERS-CoV: understanding the latest human coronavirus threat. Viruses. 2018;10(2):93.
14. Al-Omari A, Rabaan AA, Salih S, Al-Tawfiq JA, Memish ZA. MERS coronavirus outbreak: implications for emerging viral infections. Diagn Microbiol Infect Dis. 2019;93(3):265–85.
15. Tacke F, Alvarez D, Kaplan TJ, Jakubzick C, Spanbroek R, Llodra J, et al. Monocyte subsets differentially employ CCR2, CCR5, and CX3CR1 to accumulate within atherosclerotic plaques. J Clin Invest. 2007;117(1):185–94.
16. Nassar M, Bakhrebah M, Meo S, Alsuabeyl M, Zaher W. Middle East Respiratory Syndrome Coronavirus (MERS-CoV) infection: epidemiology, pathogenesis and clinical characteristics. Eur Rev Med Pharmacol Sci. 2018;22(15):4956–61.
17. Du L, Yang Y, Zhou Y, Lu L, Li F, Jiang S. MERS-CoV spike protein: a key target for antivirals. Expert Opin Ther Targets. 2017;21(2):131–43.
18. Guo Y-R, Cao Q-D, Hong Z-S, Tan Y-Y, Chen S-D, Jin H-J, et al. The origin, transmission and clinical therapies on coronavirus disease 2019 (COVID-19) outbreak–an update on the status. Mil Med Res. 2020;7(1):1–10.
19. Bulut C, Kato Y. Epidemiology of COVID-19. Turk J Med Sci. 2020;50(SI-1):563–70.
20. Lauer SA, Grantz KH, Bi Q, Jones FK, Zheng Q, Meredith HR, et al. The incubation period of coronavirus disease 2019 (COVID-19) from publicly reported confirmed cases: estimation and application. Ann Intern Med. 2020;172(9):577–82.
21. Frieman M, Baric R. Mechanisms of severe acute respiratory syndrome pathogenesis and innate immunomodulation. Microbiol Mol Biol Rev. 2008;72(4):672–85.
22. Yang L, Liu S, Liu J, Zhang Z, Wan X, Huang B, et al. COVID-19: immunopathogenesis and Immunotherapeutics. Signal Transduct Target Ther. 2020;5(1):1–8.
23. De Wit E, Van Doremalen N, Falzarano D, Munster VJ. SARS and MERS: recent insights into emerging coronaviruses. Nat Rev Microbiol. 2016;14(8):523.
24. Chatterjee SK, Saha S, Munoz MNM. Molecular pathogenesis, immunopathogenesis and novel therapeutic strategy against COVID-19. Front Mol Biosci. 2020;7:196.
25. Cui L, Wang H, Ji Y, Yang J, Xu S, Huang X, et al. The nucleocapsid protein of coronaviruses acts as a viral suppressor of RNA silencing in mammalian cells. J Virol. 2015;89(17):9029–43.

26. Fensterl V, Sen GC. Interferons and viral infections. Biofactors. 2009;35(1):14–20.
27. Teijaro JR. Type I interferons in viral control and immune regulation. Curr Opin Virol. 2016;16:31–40.
28. Dandekar AA, Perlman S. Immunopathogenesis of coronavirus infections: implications for SARS. Nat Rev Immunol. 2005;5(12):917–27.
29. Skariyachan S, Challapilli SB, Packirisamy S, Kumargowda ST, Sridhar VS. Recent aspects on the pathogenesis mechanism, animal models and novel therapeutic interventions for Middle East respiratory syndrome coronavirus infections. Front Microbiol. 2019;10:569.
30. Choudhry H, Bakhrebah MA, Abdulaal WH, Zamzami MA, Baothman OA, Hassan MA, et al. Middle East respiratory syndrome: pathogenesis and therapeutic developments. Future Virol. 2019;14(4):237–46.
31. Banerjee A, Baid K, Mossman K. Molecular pathogenesis of Middle East Respiratory Syndrome (MERS) coronavirus. Curr Clin Microbiol Rep. 2019;6(3):139–47.
32. Cao X. COVID-19: immunopathology and its implications for therapy. Nat Rev Immunol. 2020;20(5):269–70.
33. Bo X, C-y FAN, A-l WANG, Y-l ZOU, Y-h YU, Cong H, et al. Suppressed T cell-mediated immunity in patients with COVID-19: a clinical retrospective study in Wuhan, China. J Infect. 2020;81(1):e51–60.
34. Diao B, Wang C, Tan Y, Chen X, Liu Y, Ning L, et al. Reduction and functional exhaustion of T cells in patients with coronavirus disease 2019 (COVID-19). Front Immunol. 2020;11:827.
35. De Biasi S, Meschiari M, Gibellini L, Bellinazzi C, Borella R, Fidanza L, et al. Marked T cell activation, senescence, exhaustion and skewing towards TH17 in patients with COVID-19 pneumonia. Nat Commun. 2020;11(1):1–17.
36. Lei X, Dong X, Ma R, Wang W, Xiao X, Tian Z, et al. Activation and evasion of type I interferon responses by SARS-CoV-2. Nat Commun. 2020;11(1):1–12.
37. Bouayad A. Innate immune evasion by SARS-CoV-2: comparison with SARS-CoV. Rev Med Virol. 2020;30(6):1–9. https://doi.org/10.1002/rmv.2135.
38. Thoms M, Buschauer R, Ameismeier M, Koepke L, Denk T, Hirschenberger M, et al. Structural basis for translational shutdown and immune evasion by the Nsp1 protein of SARS-CoV-2. bioRxiv. 2020.
39. Zhang Y, Zhang J, Chen Y, Luo B, Yuan Y, Huang F, et al. The ORF8 protein of SARS-CoV-2 mediates immune evasion through potently downregulating MHC-I. bioRxiv. 2020.
40. Ye Q, Wang B, Mao J. The pathogenesis and treatment of theCytokine Storm'in COVID-19. J Infect. 2020;80(6):607–13.
41. Barnova M, Bobcakova A, Urdova V, Kosturiak R, Kapustova L, Dobrota D, et al. Inhibitory immune checkpoint molecules and exhaustion of T cells in COVID-19. Physiol Res. 2021;70(Suppl 2):S227.
42. Saheb Sharif-Askari N, Saheb Sharif-Askari F, Mdkhana B, Al Heialy S, Alsafar HS, Hamoudi R, et al. Enhanced expression of immune checkpoint receptors during SARS-CoV-2 viral infection. Mol Ther Methods Clin Dev. 2021;20:109–21.
43. Aghbash PS, Eslami N, Shamekh A, Entezari-Maleki T, Baghi HB. SARS-CoV-2 infection: the role of PD-1/PD-L1 and CTLA-4 axis. Life Sci. 2021;270:119124.
44. Fife BT, Bluestone JA. Control of peripheral T-cell tolerance and autoimmunity via the CTLA-4 and PD-1 pathways. Immunol Rev. 2008;224(1):166–82.
45. Rowshanravan B, Halliday N, Sansom DM. CTLA-4: a moving target in immunotherapy. Blood. 2018;131(1):58–67.
46. Mortaz E, Jamaati H, Dezfuli NK, Sheikhzade H, Hashemian SM, Roofchayee ND, et al. Changes in PD-1-and CTLA-4-bearing blood lymphocytes in ICU COVID-19 patients treated with Favipiravir/Kaletra or Dexamethasone/Remdesivir: a pilot study. Iran J Allergy Asthma Immunol. 2023;22(1):99–109.
47. Tan J, Li Y. Immune checkpoint alterations and their blockade in COVID-19 patients. Blood Sci. 2022;4(4):192–8.

48. Zahran AM, Nafady-Hego H, Rashad A, El-Badawy O, Nasif KA, Mostafa AT, et al. Increased percentage of apoptotic and CTLA-4 (CD152) expressing cells in CD4+/CD8+ cells in COVID-19 patients. Medicine. 2022;101(38):e30650.
49. Kong Y, Wang Y, Wu X, Han J, Li G, Hua M, et al. Storm of soluble immune checkpoints associated with disease severity of COVID-19. Signal Transduct Target Ther. 2020;5(1):192.
50. Ochoa S, Abers MS, Rosen LB, Rump A, Howe K, Lieberman JA, et al. Management and outcome of COVID-19 in CTLA-4 insufficiency. Blood Adv. 2023;7(19):5743–51.
51. Sharma P, Allison JP. The future of immune checkpoint therapy. Science. 2015;348(6230):56–61.
52. Chamoto K, Al-Habsi M, Honjo T. Role of PD-1 in immunity and diseases. In: Emerging concepts targeting immune checkpoints in cancer and autoimmunity. Springer; 2017. p. 75–97.
53. Bergantini L, d'Alessandro M, Cameli P, Cavallaro D, Gangi S, Cekorja B, et al. NK and T cell immunological signatures in hospitalized patients with COVID-19. Cells. 2021;10(11):3182.
54. Wildner NH, Ahmadi P, Schulte S, Brauneck F, Kohsar M, Lütgehetmann M, et al. B cell analysis in SARS-CoV-2 versus malaria: increased frequencies of plasmablasts and atypical memory B cells in COVID-19. J Leukoc Biol. 2021;109(1):77–90.
55. Shahbaz S, Xu L, Sligl W, Osman M, Bozorgmehr N, Mashhouri S, et al. The quality of SARS-CoV-2–specific T cell functions differs in patients with mild/moderate versus severe disease, and T cells expressing coinhibitory receptors are highly activated. J Immunol. 2021;207(4):1099–111.
56. Beserra DR, Alberca RW, Branco A, de Mendonça OL, de Souza Andrade MM, Gozzi-Silva SC, et al. Upregulation of PD-1 expression and high sPD-L1 levels associated with COVID-19 severity. J Immunol Res. 2022;2022:9764002.
57. Bonam SR, Hu H, Bayry J. Role of the PD-1 and PD-L1 axis in COVID-19. Future Microbiol. 2022;17:985–8.
58. Chavez-Galan L, Ruiz A, Martinez-Espinosa K, Aguilar-Duran H, Torres M, Falfan-Valencia R, et al. Circulating levels of PD-L1, TIM-3 and MMP-7 are promising biomarkers to differentiate COVID-19 patients that require invasive mechanical ventilation. Biomolecules. 2022;12(3):445.
59. Sabbatino F, Conti V, Franci G, Sellitto C, Manzo V, Pagliano P, et al. PD-L1 dysregulation in COVID-19 patients. Front Immunol. 2021;12:695242.
60. Yatim N, Boussier J, Tetu P, Smith N, Bruel T, Charbit B, et al. Immune checkpoint inhibitors increase T cell immunity during SARS-CoV-2 infection. Sci Adv. 2021;7(34):eabg4081.
61. Rezaei M, Tan J, Zeng C, Li Y, Ganjalikhani-Hakemi M. TIM-3 in leukemia; immune response and beyond. Front Oncol. 2021;11:753677.
62. Martín-Quirós A, Maroun-Eid C, Avendaño-Ortiz J, Lozano-Rodríguez R, Valentín Quiroga J, Terrón V, et al. Potential role of the Galectin-9/TIM-3 axis in the disparate progression of SARS-CoV-2 in a married couple: a case report. Biomed Hub. 2021;6(1):48–58.
63. Wu H, He P, Ren Y, Xiao S, Wang W, Liu Z, et al. Postmortem high-dimensional immune profiling of severe COVID-19 patients reveals distinct patterns of immunosuppression and immunoactivation. Nat Commun. 2022;13(1):269.
64. Yang J, Chang T, Tang L, Deng H, Chen D, Luo J, et al. Increased expression of Tim-3 is associated with depletion of NKT cells in SARS-CoV-2 infection. Front Immunol. 2022;13:796682.
65. Modabber Z, Shahbazi M, Akbari R, Bagherzadeh M, Firouzjahi A, Mohammadnia-Afrouzi M. TIM-3 as a potential exhaustion marker in CD4+ T cells of COVID-19 patients. Immun Inflamm Dis. 2021;9(4):1707–15.
66. Golden-Mason L, Palmer BE, Kassam N, Townshend-Bulson L, Livingston S, McMahon BJ, et al. Negative immune regulator Tim-3 is overexpressed on T cells in hepatitis C virus infection and its blockade rescues dysfunctional CD4+ and CD8+ T cells. J Virol. 2009;83(18):9122–30.
67. Ueland T, Heggelund L, Lind A, Holten AR, Tonby K, Michelsen AE, et al. Elevated plasma sTIM-3 levels in patients with severe COVID-19. J Allergy Clin Immunol. 2021;147(1):92–8.
68. Herrmann M, Schulte S, Wildner NH, Wittner M, Brehm TT, Ramharter M, et al. Analysis of co-inhibitory receptor expression in COVID-19 infection compared to acute plasmodium

falciparum malaria: lAG-3 and TIM-3 correlate with t cell activation and course of disease. Front Immunol. 2020;11:1870.
69. Hsieh W-C, Lai E-Y, Liu Y-T, Wang Y-F, Tzeng Y-S, Cui L, et al. NK cell receptor and ligand composition influences the clearance of SARS-CoV-2. J Clin Invest. 2021;131(21):e146408.
70. ElTanbouly MA, Zhao Y, Schaafsma E, Burns CM, Mabaera R, Cheng C, et al. VISTA: a target to manage the innate cytokine storm. Front Immunol. 2021;11:595950.
71. Wang J, Wu G, Manick B, Hernandez V, Renelt M, Erickson C, et al. VSIG-3 as a ligand of VISTA inhibits human T-cell function. Immunology. 2019;156(1):74–85.
72. Edner NM, Houghton LP, Ntavli E, Rees-Spear C, Petersone L, Wang C, et al. TIGIT(+)Tfh show poor B-helper function and negatively correlate with SARS-CoV-2 antibody titre. Front Immunol. 2024;15:1395684.
73. de Lima MHF, Machado CC, Nascimento DC, Silva CMS, Toller-Kawahisa JE, Rodrigues TS, et al. The TIGIT(+) T regulatory cells subset associates with nosocomial infection and fatal outcome in COVID-19 patients under mechanical ventilation. Sci Rep. 2023;13(1):13599.
74. Schultheiß C, Paschold L, Simnica D, Mohme M, Willscher E, von Wenserski L, et al. Next-generation sequencing of T and B cell receptor repertoires from COVID-19 patients showed signatures associated with severity of disease. Immunity. 2020;53(2):442–55.e4.
75. Antonioli L, Fornai M, Pellegrini C, Blandizzi C. NKG2A and COVID-19: another brick in the wall. Cell Mol Immunol. 2020;17(6):672–4.
76. Zheng M, Gao Y, Wang G, Song G, Liu S, Sun D, et al. Functional exhaustion of antiviral lymphocytes in COVID-19 patients. Cell Mol Immunol. 2020;17(5):533–5.
77. Luo B, Li J, Hou X, Yang Q, Zhou Y, Ye J, et al. Indications for and contraindications of immune checkpoint inhibitors in cancer patients with COVID-19 vaccination. Future Oncol. 2021;17(26):3477–84.
78. Vivarelli S, Falzone L, Grillo CM, Scandurra G, Torino F, Libra M. Cancer management during COVID-19 pandemic: is immune checkpoint inhibitors-based immunotherapy harmful or beneficial? Cancer. 2020;12(8):2237.
79. Guo X, Chen S, Wang X, Liu X. Immune-related pulmonary toxicities of checkpoint inhibitors in non-small cell lung cancer: diagnosis, mechanism, and treatment strategies. Front Immunol. 2023;14:1138483.
80. Yang Y, Xu G. SARS-CoV-2 infection and COVID-19 vaccination in cancer patients undergoing immune checkpoint inhibitors. Cell Death Dis. 2023;14(6):390.
81. Switzer B, Haanen J, Lorigan PC, Puzanov I, Turajlic S. Clinical and immunologic implications of COVID-19 in patients with melanoma and renal cell carcinoma receiving immune checkpoint inhibitors. J Immunother Cancer. 2021;9(7):e002835.
82. Bersanelli M. Controversies about COVID-19 and anticancer treatment with immune checkpoint inhibitors. Immunotherapy. 2020;12(5):269–73.
83. Klebanov N, Pahalyants V, Murphy WS, Theodosakis N, Zubiri L, Klevens RM, et al. Risk of COVID-19 in patients with cancer receiving immune checkpoint inhibitors. Oncologist. 2021;26(5):e898–901.
84. Tan R, Yun C, Seetasith A, Sheinson D, Walls R, Ngwa I, et al. Impact of immune checkpoint inhibitors on COVID-19 severity in patients with cancer. Oncologist. 2022;27(3):236–43.
85. Luo J, Rizvi H, Egger JV, Preeshagul IR, Wolchok JD, Hellmann MD. Impact of PD-1 blockade on severity of COVID-19 in patients with lung cancers. Cancer Discov. 2020;10(8):1121–8.
86. Minkove SJ, Sun J, Li Y, Cui X, Cooper D, Eichacker PQ, et al. Comprehensive adjusted outcome data are needed to assess the impact of immune checkpoint inhibitors in cancer patients with COVID-19: results of a systematic review and meta-analysis. Rev Med Virol. 2022;32(5):e2352.
87. Ruiz JI, Lopez-Olivo MA, Geng Y, Suarez-Almazor ME. COVID-19 outcomes in patients with cancer receiving immune checkpoint inhibitors: a systematic review. J Immunother Precis Oncol. 2023;6(2):103–10.
88. Mostaghim A, Minkove S, Aguilar-Company J, Ruiz-Camps I, Eremiev-Eremiev S, Dettorre GM, et al. Previous immune checkpoint inhibitor therapy is associated with decreased

COVID-19-related hospitalizations and complications in patients with cancer: results of a propensity-matched analysis of the OnCovid registry. Int J Infect Dis. 2024;139:13–20.
89. Mellinghoff SC, Vanshylla K, Dahlke C, Addo MM, Cornely OA, Klein F, et al. Case report: clinical management of a patient with metastatic non-small cell lung cancer newly receiving immune checkpoint inhibition during symptomatic COVID-19. Front Immunol. 2021;12:798276.
90. Wu JT, La J, Branch-Elliman W, Huhmann LB, Han SS, Parmigiani G, et al. Association of COVID-19 vaccination with SARS-CoV-2 infection in patients with cancer: a US Nationwide Veterans Affairs Study. JAMA Oncol. 2022;8(2):281–6.
91. Barrière J, Re D, Peyrade F, Carles M. Current perspectives for SARS-CoV-2 vaccination efficacy improvement in patients with active treatment against cancer. Eur J Cancer (Oxford, England: 1990). 2021;154:66–72.
92. Almasri M, Bshesh K, Khan W, Mushannen M, Salameh MA, Shafiq A, et al. Cancer patients and the COVID-19 vaccines: considerations and challenges. Cancer. 2022;14(22):5630.
93. Ruiz JI, Lopez-Olivo MA, Geng Y, Suarez-Almazor ME. COVID-19 vaccination in patients with cancer receiving immune checkpoint inhibitors: a systematic review and meta-analysis. J Immunother Cancer. 2023;11(2):e006246.
94. Mei Q, Hu G, Yang Y, Liu B, Yin J, Li M, et al. Impact of COVID-19 vaccination on the use of PD-1 inhibitor in treating patients with cancer: a real-world study. J Immunother Cancer. 2022;10(3):e004157.
95. Qian Y, Zhu Z, Mo YY, Zhang Z. COVID-19 vaccination is associated with enhanced efficacy of anti-PD-(L)1 immunotherapy in advanced NSCLC patients: a real-world study. Infect Agent Cancer. 2023;18(1):50.
96. Harada D, Tamura T, Ninomiya K, Kubo T, Kuyama S, Tachibana S, et al. Safety of anti-SARS-CoV-2 messenger RNA vaccine in lung cancer patients undergoing anticancer chemotherapy: a multicenter, prospective, observational, patient-reported outcome study. Thorac Cancer. 2023;14(3):231–6.
97. Gilbert D, Hu J, Medina T, Kessler ER, Lam ET. Safety of COVID-19 vaccines in subjects with solid tumor cancers receiving immune checkpoint inhibitors. Hum Vaccin Immunother. 2023;19(1):2207438.
98. Niewolik J, Mikuteit M, Cossmann A, Vahldiek K, Gutzmer R, Müller F, et al. Immunogenicity of COVID-19 vaccination in melanoma patients under immune checkpoint blockade. Oncology. 2022;100(7):392–8.
99. Strobel SB, Machiraju D, Kälber KA, Hassel JC. Immune-related adverse events of COVID-19 vaccination in skin cancer patients receiving immune-checkpoint inhibitor treatment. Cancer Immunol Immunother. 2022;71(8):2051–6.

MIX
Papier aus verantwortungsvollen Quellen
Paper from responsible sources
FSC® C105338
FSC
www.fsc.org

If you have any concerns about our products,
you can contact us on
ProductSafety@springernature.com

In case Publisher is established outside the EU,
the EU authorized representative is:
Springer Nature Customer Service Center GmbH
Europaplatz 3, 69115 Heidelberg, Germany

Printed by Libri Plureos GmbH
in Hamburg, Germany